THOMAS STEPHEN GARVIN EAKINS

IRISH MASTERS OF MEDICINE

Irish Masters
of
MEDICINE

DAVIS COAKLEY

The publication of this book has been supported by Upjohn Ireland

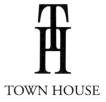

TOWN HOUSE

Published in 1992 by
Town House
42 Morehampton Road
Donnybrook
Dublin 4

British Library Cataloguing in Publication Data available

ISBN: 0-948524-41-3

Cover: *Portrait of Almroth Wright by Sir Gerald Kelly, RA. (Courtesy of St Mary's Hospital, London)*

Managing editor: Treasa Coady
Text editor: Elaine Campion
Designer: Bill Murphy
Colour origination: The Kulor Centre
Printed by Butler and Tanner Ltd, Frome and London

To the memory of Paul Wagstaff (1944–1989)

This book has been written to mark the quatercentenary of the foundation of Trinity College Dublin and the tercentenary of the granting of the William and Mary Charter to the Royal College of Physicians of Ireland.

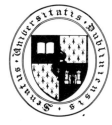

Trinity College Dublin

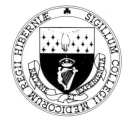

Royal College of Physicians of Ireland

CONTENTS

List of colour plates

List of black and white illustrations

ACKNOWLEDGEMENTS

While researching this book I received assistance from many friends and I also had the pleasure of making new friendships. Professor Kevin Breathnach of University College Dublin and Professor James Malone of St James's Hospital, Dublin, both read the typescript and I am very grateful to them for their constructive criticism. Dr Denis Burkitt and Professor Jeremy Swan were most helpful, and I also obtained enthusiastic assistance from the relatives of a number of doctors whose biographies appear in the following pages. I would in particular like to thank Lady Isabel Butterfield, Professor Dirmid Collis, Dr Robert Collis Jun., Ms Mary Donovan, Dr Michael Hayes, Mrs Nora Hayes, Dr Dorothy McGeeney, Dr Kevin McGeeney, Dr Barbara Phillips, Mr John Stevenson, Dr Joly Stevenson, Dr Barbara Stokes, and Mr John Wilson-Wright. It is a pleasure to thank Sir Peter Froggatt for his encouragement and help, and for agreeing so willingly to write the preface to the Irish edition. Professor Alan Browne was helpful in many ways, particularly with the obstetrical content. Dr Kevin McGeeney first drew my attention to Arthur Leared and Dr R G Thompson brought the achievements of Charles MacMunn to my notice. Both were very generous with their assistance. Professor James Watson of Cold Spring Harbor, New York, wrote to me about Bill Hayes, and he also kindly gave me permission to quote from his book *The Double Helix*. Dr Brian West and Professor Trevor West allowed me access to the diary of Edward Hallaran Bennett, which gave me a new perspective on nineteenth-century Irish medicine.

I am most grateful to the following who either supplied me with information or helped me in other ways: Dr Seamus Cahalane, Dr Anne Caird, Professor John Cairns, Revd James Coombes, Dr Robert Cox, Sir John Crofton, Dr James Deeny, Dr William Fennell, Professor John Fraher, Dr Patrick Freyne, Professor Eithne Gaffney, Dr J Gleeson, Professor Stuart Glover, Mr Kieran Hickey, Professor David Hopwood, Professor Ian Howie, Professor Conor Keane, Dr Ron Kirkham, Mr Victor Lane, Dr Clayton Love, Professor J B Lyons, Professor David McConnell, Mr TED McDermott, Mrs Joan McGeachin, Dr Edward Martin, Professor Norman Moore, Professor Patrick Moore, Dr Seán O'Briain, Professor Eoin O'Brien, Mr Gerald O'Neill, Dr Liam O'Sé, Mr Patrick Plunkett, Professor John Scott, Mr Raymond Refausse, Dr Michael Rowan, Dr Kim Ryder, Professor K A Stacey, Professor Eamon Sweeney, Mr Salter Stirling, Dr Mervyn Taylor, Dr Bernard Walsh, Dr Michael Walshe, Professor Conor Ward and Professor Frank Winder.

I would like to thank Professor Ian Temperley, dean of the Faculty of Health Sciences, Trinity College Dublin; Professor Stephen Doyle, president of the

Royal College of Physicians of Ireland; Professor Donald Weir, chairman of the Faculty of Health Sciences' Quatercentenary Committee, and Professor Peter Gatenby, chairman of Trinity College Dublin Medical Alumni Association, for their interest in the project. I would also like to thank Ms Jean O'Hanlon, secretary of the Quatercentenary Committee, for her assistance. Dr Frederick Falkiner, another member of this committee, helped me in a number of ways and he also organised support from Trinity Trust, for which I am grateful. I was particularly encouraged by the support and interest of Professor John Feely, registrar of the Royal College of Physicians of Ireland, and of Professor Brian Keogh, treasurer of the college.

I relied heavily on the assistance of Ms Mary O'Doherty, librarian in the Royal College of Surgeons in Ireland, and Mr Robert Mills, librarian in the Royal College of Physicians of Ireland. They were both very patient and courteous in dealing with my requests, and Mary O'Doherty went to great lengths to trace obscure references for me. I also wish to thank Ms Áine Keegan, Old Reading Room, Trinity College; Geoffrey Davenport, librarian, Royal College of Physicians, London; and Ian Milne, librarian, Royal College of Physicians, Edinburgh.

I am very grateful to Denis Murphy, general manager of Upjohn Ireland, and Rory O'Connor, US senior product manager for Upjohn USA, for supporting this book with substantial sponsorship. Upjohn has supported many academic and research developments in Ireland over the years and it is particularly appropriate that the company should be associated with this celebration of Irish medical achievement.

Most of the photographs in this book were taken by David Smyth and I wish to thank him for his patience and co-operation. It was a pleasure to work again with Treasa Coady and Elaine Campion of Town House. My secretary, Gay O'Kennedy, contributed to the preparation of the book in many ways and I had to spend long hours writing and researching in order to keep up with her!

Finally I would like to thank my wife Mary. Without her support and understanding it would not have been possible for me to undertake this project amidst all my other commitments. Her advice and help at all stages were invaluable and her interest in the book made the task a pleasure.

PREFACE

Ireland's great literary tradition is highly acclaimed, but it is only doctors for the most part who know of her equally proud medical one. Rooted through the centuries, it reached its finest flowering during the nineteenth century when Dublin became a medical Mecca and Ireland could boast an unusually comprehensive system of medical care, which was the envy of wealthier countries. Few areas of medical science have failed to benefit from an often eponymously commemorated Irish pioneer, whether home-based or from the extensive Irish diaspora.

Professor Coakley's purpose is 'to highlight those achievements of Irish doctors which have enhanced the knowledge and practice of medicine on an international level', and he effects this through perceptive and highly informative vignettes of forty-two well-chosen subjects from the last three hundred years. Many were called but not all could be chosen: some luminaries are smuggled in as subsidiary characters, but others had to be omitted, evidencing the wealth of talent available and the *embarras du choix* facing the author. The result is a whole which is more coherent than an aggregate of its constituent biographical sketches, and is a convincing proof of the author's growing authority. It is a fitting and timely tribute to Irish medicine in a year in which we celebrate the quatercentenary of the foundation of Trinity College and the tercentenary of the granting of the William and Mary Charter to the Royal College of Physicians of Ireland.

The prosecutor Kirillovich in Dostoevsky's *The Brothers Karamazov*, speaks of his compatriots as being 'immoderate...an astonishing blend of good and evil; we love enlightenment...and at the same time we riot in taverns...we are broad natures...able to accommodate every possible contradiction...we are broad like Mother Russia herself; we find room for everything, we reconcile ourselves to everything'. Ireland also has her contradictions, but she has a breadth of talent in her children, appropriate to the 'broad acres' occupied by the extended Irish diaspora. It is one of the many achievements of Professor Coakley that he considers his subjects against this wider international scene in which many were to practise and all to medically enrich – a refreshing draught against the xenophobia of many previous perspectives and a draught his subjects would have welcomed.

Peter Froggatt
Pro-Chancellor
University of Dublin

INTRODUCTION

The foundation stone of Trinity College was laid in 1592 by an apothecary named Thomas Smith, who was lord mayor of Dublin at the time. The new university displayed little interest in medicine during its early years. It was stated at the commencements in 1616 that only one medical degree had been conferred in the first twenty-three years of the existence of the college. William Bedell, who became provost in 1627, suggested that the college should become involved in medical teaching, but he resigned two years later and his plans were not developed. In 1654 John Stearne, fellow and registrar of Trinity College, was encouraged to establish a Fraternity of Physicians. The building which the university gave him for this purpose was known as Trinity Hall. It had originally been constructed as a bridewell and was situated just outside the college walls. The fraternity developed into the College of Physicians and it was incorporated by Royal Charter in 1667. John Stearne was the first president of the College of Physicians and he was also appointed as the first regius professor of physic in Trinity. The college maintained a close association with the university and medical lectures were given in Trinity Hall.

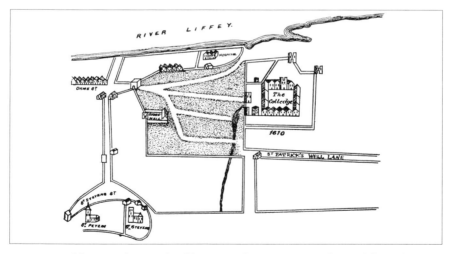

0.1   *Detail from Speed's map of Dublin (1610) showing Trinity College and the Bridewell. The latter was built by Dublin Corporation in 1604 as 'a place of punishment for offenders, and for putting idle persons to work'. It was given to Trinity College in 1617. After serving as student accommodation for some years, it was leased to John Stearne in 1654 for his Fraternity of Physicians.*

Parallel with these developments in medical education, efforts were also being made to encourage the study of the natural sciences in Ireland. A group of intellectuals, including several doctors such as Patrick Dun, Allen Mullen, William Petty and Thomas Molyneux, were members of the Dublin Philosophical Society which was established in 1683. The society encouraged original research and its members were delighted when they saw Dublin gain recognition in international scientific circles, largely through their efforts. At the end of the first year of the society's existence we find the philosopher William Molyneux writing to his brother Thomas, who was at that time on the Continent:

> Thus, Tom, you see that learning begins to peep out amongst us. The tidings, that our name is in the journals of Amsterdam, was very pleasing to me, and really, without vanity, I think our city and nation may be herein something beholding to us, for I believe the name Dublin has hardly ever before been printed or heard amongst foreigners on a learned account.[1]

Unfortunately the enthusiasm for original work did not survive beyond the lives of the founder members and the society did not meet after 1708.

Strains developed in the relationship between the university and the College of Physicians and the latter sought a new charter which would make it an independent institution. This charter was procured in 1692 from King William of Orange and Queen Mary by Sir Patrick Dun, and according to its provisions the provost and senior fellows of Trinity College lost all rights of involvement in the selection of the president of the College of Physicians. Sir Patrick Dun was elected the first president of the college under the new charter. Negotiations between the university and the College of Physicians resulted in an agreement in 1701 which regulated the granting of degrees in medicine. A medical school was built in Trinity which stood on the site now occupied by the Berkeley Library and it was formally opened by the provost on 10 August 1711. Sir Patrick Dun was almost certainly the main driving force behind these developments in medical education. In a will which he signed two months after the opening of the new medical school he left money to support 'one or two Professors of Physick' in the College of Physicians, whose appointment would be made jointly by the College

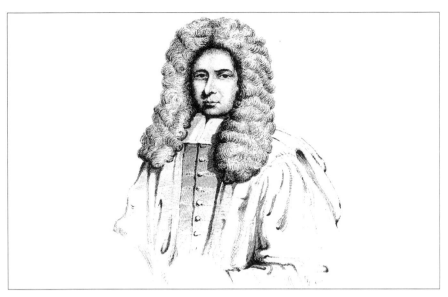

0.2   Sir Patrick Dun, one of the most dynamic and far-seeing presidents of the Royal College of Physicians of Ireland. (Courtesy of RCPI)

of Physicians and Trinity College. He died in 1713 and his bequest was used to support professorial chairs and to build Sir Patrick Dun's Hospital as a teaching hospital. The professors of the 'School of Physic' were under the control of both Trinity College and the College of Physicians. Lectures on anatomy, chemistry and botany were delivered in the Anatomy House of Trinity College, and lectures on medicine, pharmacology, physiology and obstetrics were given at Sir Patrick Dun's Hospital. The fellows of the College of Physicians also held their meetings at Dun's Hospital. It is highly appropriate that the funds which have accrued from the recent sale of Sir Patrick Dun's Hospital are being used both to build a new medical school for Trinity College at St James's Hospital and to develop postgraduate medical education at the Royal College of Physicians of Ireland.

Although eighteenth-century Dublin is now remembered for its elegance and fashion, many of its citizens lived in misery and squalor. The poor were housed in overcrowded slums and there were virtually no hospital facilities for the sick at the beginning of the century. As the century progressed several altruistic individuals, many of them doctors, established voluntary hospitals to meet the needs of the sick poor. The Charitable Infirmary, the first voluntary hospital in Ireland and Great

Britain, opened its doors in 1728. It was followed by others such as Dr
Steevens' Hospital in 1733, Mercer's Hospital in 1741, the Rotunda
Hospital in 1745 and the Meath Hospital in 1753. Despite the
opportunities for the study of disease which these hospitals presented,
Dublin contributed little to the growth of medical knowledge during
this period. The Medico-Philosophical Society was founded in 1756 to
remedy this unsatisfactory situation by encouraging original
observation. George Cleghorn, professor of anatomy in Trinity College,
highlighted the importance of developing medical knowledge when he
spoke to his colleagues in the new society:

> True it is that the Practice of Physick in Dublin has long been in the
> hands of Men eminent for Learning and Abilities, some of whom have
> given the strongest Proofs of their Zeal for the good of the Public, and
> the Advancement of their Profession by a diligent Application to
> Experimental Philosophy and by appropriating the whole of their
> Fortune for the Establishment of Hospitals and Schools of Physick; but
> sorry am I to observe that the laudable endeavours of these Patriots have
> not yet produced all the Good consequences that might be expected
> from them, and still it is alleged that Ireland contributes to promote
> medical Knowledge less than her Neighbours.... Hence it is, that the
> Fame of our most celebrated Practitioners have seldom reached beyond
> the limits of our own Coast, and not withstanding our Hospitals have
> been crowded with Patients for 30 years yet this fertile Field of
> observation hath been so ill cultivated that none of its Fruits have
> appeared to the World.[2]

Several members of this society, such as Cleghorn, Clossy and Rutty,
made significant contributions to medicine. Samuel Clossy emigrated to
the United States where he made an historical contribution to the
development of medical education. He was the first of a long line of
Irish doctors who would pursue careers in the United States and make
notable contributions to the development of medical science.

The death of George Cleghorn led to a period of decline in the
Trinity medical school, and its dominant position in Irish medical
education was further threatened in 1784 when the Royal College of
Surgeons in Ireland was established. Soon the College of Surgeons began
to organise its own teaching in both surgery and medicine, and in the
early years of the nineteenth century it attracted many able men such as

Abraham Colles and John Cheyne onto its staff. The British government needed a large supply of military surgeons at this time to service its fleet during the Napoleonic wars. This demand led to the establishment of a plethora of private medical schools in Dublin. The dwindling fortunes of the medical school at Trinity were saved by the appointment of the dynamic James Macartney as professor of anatomy and surgery in 1813. Student numbers increased again and Macartney built a new medical school. Part of this school still exists today and is incorporated into the current medical school building.

Cheyne, Colles and Macartney laid the groundwork for what was to become known as the Irish school of medicine. During this period Dublin produced giants of international medicine, such as Robert Graves, William Stokes and Dominic Corrigan. Others such as Arthur Jacob, Robert Adams, John Houston, Robert Smith and William Wilde also made significant contributions to medicine at this time. Their achievements are all the more remarkable when one considers that they were accomplished during a period of great national deprivation and suffering which culminated in the Great Famine.

The establishment of medical schools in the new Queen's Colleges of Belfast, Cork and Galway in the middle of the last century brought about the demise of many of the private medical institutions. In 1854 Newman established a medical school as part of his Catholic University. This medical school was based in Cecilia Street and it was incorporated into University College Dublin in 1908. The medical schools in Dublin, Belfast, Cork and Galway shared the high standards of the older schools in Trinity College and the College of Surgeons. They produced medical graduates who were well trained by the method of bedside clinical teaching that had been championed by Graves and Stokes. Many of these graduates, whether by choice or necessity, set out to build their careers abroad. This pattern has continued into our own times and Irish graduates have been involved in the provision of health care in many countries throughout the world, in developed regions and in the Third World. Many of these Irish doctors have made fundamental contributions to the development of medical science and practice.

The purpose of this book is to highlight those achievements of Irish doctors which have enhanced the knowledge and practice of medicine on an international level. The work of most of the doctors whose biographies appear in this book has been included in international anthologies, such as R H Major's *Classic Descriptions of Disease* or Garrison and Morton's *A Medical Bibliography*. The latter provides a chronological bibliography of the most important contributions to world literature on medicine and related sciences. I consulted widely when drawing up the list of doctors whose biographies appear in this book, but the final selection was my own. I have included biographies of two Scotsmen, George Cleghorn and John Cheyne, because they both spent their professional lives in Dublin and played a key role in the development of Irish medicine. In making the selection I have cast my net widely; biographies of specialists in medicine, surgery, obstetrics, paediatrics, pathology, radiology, anaesthesia and the basic medical sciences are included. Some of the original work described was carried out in Ireland, but the contributions of the Irish medical diaspora mentioned earlier are represented by research undertaken in different parts of the world, in places as far afield as Africa, North America, England, India and continental Europe. I have included biographies of three living men who worked abroad — Denis Burkitt, William Hayes and Jeremy Swan, but I have not included a biography of any doctor currently living in Ireland as the choice would have been invidious.

One of my aims in writing this book is to document the significant medical advances made by Irish doctors, often against great difficulties. Many of them forfeited personal wealth in order to carry out research on the major health issues of their day, and one of them, Adrian Stokes, lost his life in pursuit of his goals. I hope that the work of these great men will emphasise the importance of creating and supporting an ethos of research within our medical schools and hospitals and that the biographies may inspire medical students and young Irish doctors to face the challenges posed by the major health issues of our own time.

ALLEN MULLEN
c 1653–1690

1 *One of Ireland's first medical scientists*

Allen Mullen, in collaboration with other distinguished members of the Dublin Philosophical Society, such as Thomas Molyneux and William Petty, brought medicine in Dublin to the attention of a European audience for the first time. Born around the year 1653, he was a son of Patrick Mullen of Ballicoulter in the north of Ireland. He entered Trinity College at the age of eighteen and graduated BA in the summer of 1676. Two years later he became a Bachelor of Physic. He was awarded the degree of MD in 1684 and he also became a fellow of the Royal College of Physicians.

Mullen built up a large and lucrative practice among the gentry and was the most distinguished of Trinity's early medical graduates. His success in practice was almost certainly related to his fame for curing gout, for which he used a vegetable which may have been colchicum infused in brandy! He was presented with an unusual opportunity to display his skills in anatomy when an elephant was burnt accidentally whilst on exhibition in Essex Street in 1681. In a communication to Sir William Petty of the Royal Society of London in 1682, Mullen described the difficulties under which he performed the dissection. A crowd had assembled at the scene and everyone was intent on obtaining a piece of the unfortunate elephant:

To prevent his being taken away by the multitude, the manager, Mr Wilkins, procured a file of musqueteers to guard him, till he should build a shed where he might securely disjoint him, in order to the making of a skeleton: this he got finished at seven o'clock at night, and about eight I heard of his design. Being desirous to inform myself in the structure of the elephant, I made search for him, and having found him, I proffered my service to him; of which when he accepted, I endeavoured to persuade him to discharge some butchers which he had in readiness to order the elephant after their way, and to leave the whole management of the matter to me, and to such as I thought fit to employ, designing a general dissection, and that the icons of each part should be taken in order by some painters, with whom upon this occasion I could prevail: but my endeavours proved fruitless, because that, about ten a'clock that night, when we went to the shed, to find what condition the elephant was in, he emitted very noisom steams.[1]

As the elephant was very near the Council Chambers, it was likely that the lord mayor would order the immediate removal of the animal and punish the manager for causing a public disorder. Mullen therefore decided to make use of the butchers as assistants and to proceed with the dissection overnight by candlelight. He communicated his findings to the Royal Society, through Dr William Petty, and it is one of the earliest extant anatomical accounts of the elephant. His second contribution to the Royal Society was communicated in a letter to Robert Boyle; it contained a detailed account of the tunics of the eye and other ocular structures. In 1682 both papers were published in London in a book entitled *An Anatomical Account of the Elephant Accidentally Burnt in Dublin....Together With a Relation of new Anatomical Observations in the Eyes of Animals.*

FRIENDSHIP WITH ROBERT BOYLE

Mullen decided to visit London, probably to oversee the publication of his book and also to meet the scientific leaders of the time. He bore a letter of introduction to the Irish physicist, Robert Boyle, from Narcissus Marsh, the provost of Trinity College Dublin, who wrote:

Sir, the bearer hereof is one Mr Mullan, Batchelor in Physic of this

College, who has been successful in several things that he has undertaken, especially in anatomy, wherein he has good skill; and had an opportunity the last Summer to exercise it on an occasion that rarely occurs, namely in dissecting the elephant which was burnt here in Dublin.[2]

Boyle was impressed by the young doctor from Dublin and he arranged for his admission to the Royal Society the following year. The physicist was interested in medical matters so he and Mullen undertook some experiments together. Boyle (1627–1701), who was born in Lismore Castle, County Waterford, was the most prolific writer of all the seventeenth-century scientists. He published original work on a wide range of subjects, including chemistry, physics, pharmacology, philosophy and medicine. In 1665 he received an MD *honoris causa* from Oxford University in recognition of his contributions to medicine. It was Boyle who, using an air pump to create a vacuum, first established that air was absolutely necessary for life. His *Memoirs for the Natural History of Extravasated Humane Blood*, which was published in 1683, was one of the first books to deal with the scientific analysis of blood and is regarded as marking the beginning of physiological chemistry. In this work he proved for the first time that sodium chloride is present in blood.

In 1685 Boyle recommended Allen Mullen to the Earl of Clarendon who had just been appointed Lord Lieutenant of Ireland. That same year Boyle's book *Of the Reconcileableness of Specifick Medicines* was published in London and he sent a copy to Mullen. Mullen read the book carefully and then sent a long letter to Boyle giving him his impression of the work and suggesting some additional remedies. Boyle's empiric use of 'specifick medicine' was a more scientific approach and a definite advance on the use of drugs according to their Galenic classification, which was common practice at the time.

THE FOUNDATION OF THE DUBLIN PHILOSOPHICAL SOCIETY

Mullen became one of the founders of the Dublin Philosophical Society in 1683. Among the original members were William Molyneux,

AN
Anatomical Account
OF THE
ELEPHANT
Accidentally Burnt in
DUBLIN,
ON
Fryday, June 17. in the Year 1681.

Sent in a LETTER
To Sir WILL. PETTY,
FELLOW OF
The Royal Society.

TOGETHER

With a Relation of new Anatomical Observations in the
Eyes of Animals: Communicated in another LETTER
to the Honourable R. Boyle, Esq; FELLOW of the same
SOCIETY.

(A. MULLEN)

By (A. M.) Med. of Trinity Colledge near Dublin.

London, Printed for Sam. Smith, Bookseller, at the Prince's Arms
in St. Paul's Church-Yard.   1682.

1.1   Title page of Allen Mullen's book on the elephant. (Courtesy of RCSI)

Narcissus Marsh and William Petty. Petty (1623–1687), who came to Ireland in 1652 as physician to the army, was a pioneer medical statistician. He was a founder fellow of the Royal Society of London and he became the first president of the Dublin Philosophical Society. The society was invited by Dr Huntington, provost of Trinity College, to meet in his lodgings. The new society received considerable support from the members of the Royal Society in London, which had been established twenty-three years earlier. Patrick Dun was another medical member of the society. In all there were ten doctors, comprising a quarter of the total membership. Petty drew up the original rules for the members, which placed an emphasis on statistics that was remarkable for the period:

> That they chiefly apply themselves to the makeing of experiments, and prefer the same, to the best Discourses, Letters and Books they can make or read, even concerning experiments.... That they annalise and divide complicate matters into their intigrall parts, and compute the proportions which one parte bear unto another.... That they provide themselves with Corrispondents in severall places, to make such observations as do depend upon the comparison of many experiments, & not upon single and solitary Remarques.[3]

Allen Mullen, William Molyneux and William Petty were the most able scientists in the new society. Of the papers read to the society during its first period of activity, forty-four dealt with medical matters, and over half of these were submitted by Mullen. Most of the medical presentations were concerned with human and animal oddities or monstrosities. There were also accounts of dissections, vivisections and experimental injections of animals, as well as a number of reports on patients' diseases. Among Mullen's papers were accounts of experiments which included the injection of fluids into the thoracic cavities of animals, the removal of a portion of a dog's lung and the ligature of the jugular vein in a dog. He also wrote on subjects as varied as ovarian disease, hydatid cysts, consumption, ague, peculiarities of the pulse, and the mineral waters of Chapelizod. He did not confine his contributions to medicine as he also wrote on archaeological subjects.

Mullen attempted to estimate the precise quantity of blood in humans. This he did by draining the blood from several animals, including a dog, a sheep, and a rabbit, and then calculating its weight in relation to the total weight of the animal in question. On the basis of his results and calculations, he estimated that a man weighing 160 pounds would contain about 128 ounces of blood. This work was very good for its time, but subsequent research showed that his calculations were too low as he did not appreciate that some blood remains in an animal's body even after a seemingly complete drainage.

On another occasion Mullen heard of a man suffering from severe thoracic pain who claimed that, if a small part of one of his lungs were removed, he would recover. Naturally his physicians were unwilling to comply with his request and he died. Mullen wondered if a thoracotomy could be carried out without the death of a patient, so he decided to try the operation on a dog. He removed part of the animal's lung and the dog made a complete recovery. Six months later he killed the animal and found that the wound had almost entirely disappeared. Mullen's scientific enthusiasm led him to perform several experiments on animals, many of which would be frowned upon today. His research also extended to non-medical matters; it was he who established that, contrary to popular belief, toads could live quite happily in Ireland.

In 1684 Mullen designed a laboratory for the Dublin Philosophical Society, to be used chiefly for chemical experiments. It was situated over an apothecary's shop at Crow's Nest off Dame Street. The society was following the precedent set by Boyle and Petty who had lodged with an apothecary at Oxford so that they could have easy access to his drugs and chemicals.

MULLEN LEAVES IRELAND

In 1686 Mullen was obliged to leave Dublin for England because of 'a scandalous love intrigue, of which he was ashamed'.[4] In London he frequented Jonathan's Coffee House in Exchange Alley, which was a favourite meeting place for fellows of the Royal Society. He took a keen interest in the work of Hans Sloane (1660–1753) who was also born in the north of Ireland. Sloane was a member of the Royal Society and a friend of Robert Boyle. He was a life-long collector of books and specimens, and the British Museum was eventually established to house them. In 1687 Sloane went to Jamaica as physician to the governor of the island, and after spending fifteen months there, he returned with 800 species of plants and with many fascinating observations on natural history. Mullen was very impressed by Sloane's achievements and he was delighted to be given the opportunity to travel to Jamaica with William O'Brien, Lord Inchiquin, when the latter was appointed governor of the colony. O'Brien was married to a niece of Robert Boyle's and so he had become acquainted with Mullen and was aware of his accomplishments.

The expedition set out for Jamaica in 1690 and on the way the ship put in at Barbados. There Mullen met some friends who apparently 'made him drink hard'. He subsequently developed a fever, became delirious and died. His last paper to the Royal Society was published posthumously. It contained a masterly description of the comparative anatomy of both the ear and eye in several varieties of birds and fish and it included a number of original observations. Mullen had an enquiring mind and a flair for original work. There can be little doubt that his death at an early age set back the development of medical science in Ireland.

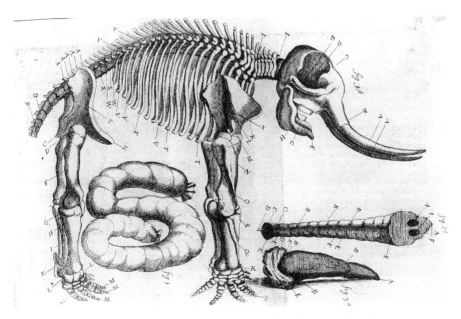

1.2   *The skeleton of the elephant dissected by Allen Mullen. (Courtesy of RCSI)*

A
SERMON

Preached in the Parifh Church of
St. *Giles* in the Fields.

At the FUNERAL of

Bernard Connor, *M. D.*

Who departed this Life, *Oct*.30.1698.

With a Short Account of his Life and Death.

By *William Hayley*, D. D. Rector of the faid
Church, and Chaplain in Ordinary to His
Majefty.

LONDON, Printed for *Jacob Tonfon*, at the *Judges-Head*,
near the *Inner-Temple Gate* in *Fleetftreet*; and at *Grays-
Inn Gate* in *Grays-Inn Lane*, 1699.

2.1   *Title page of sermon preached at the funeral of Bernard Connor in 1698. (Courtesy of
RCPI)*

2 A European reputation

Bernard Connor is the best known of several Irish doctors who gained European reputations during the seventeenth and eighteenth centuries. Connor was one of the first doctors to champion a scientific approach to the diagnosis and treatment of disease, and he was also the first to describe the disorder now known as ankylosing spondylitis. Very little is known about his early years other than that he was born in Kerry around 1666 and his father was also named Bernard. O'Hart in his *Irish Pedigrees* claimed that Connor was a member of a branch of the O'Connor Kerry family, lords of Kerry, whose seat was at Carrigafoyle. I have found evidence to suggest that, although a Catholic, he was educated by John Richards, the Church of Ireland Dean of Ardfert, County Kerry. At the age of twenty Connor went to France to study medicine. It is said that he spent some time at Montpellier before moving to Rheims, where he graduated as Doctor of Physic in 1693. His name was entered on the register there as O'Connor rather than Connor. He set up practice in Paris where he began to distinguish himself both as a teacher of anatomy and as a skilled physician. However, he did not stay long in the city as he was asked to accompany the sons of the chancellor of Poland on their return journey to their native country. They travelled on a circuitous

15

route, seeing Italy, Sicily, Germany and Austria on the way. Connor took advantage of this to visit the leading medical centres in Europe, exchanging ideas with scientific medical men such as Marcello Malpighi in Italy who first described the capillary system. Connor made a name for himself by treating sick members of the English community in each of the countries he visited. Many of these were aristocrats on the Grand Tour.

At Innsbruck he met the Earl of Carlingford who had recently inherited the title from his brother who was killed at the battle of the Boyne fighting for King James. Carlingford, the head of the Taaffe family, was in the Austrian army and when Connor met him he was establishing the political alliances which would make his descendants so powerful in the Austrian empire. He was kind to Connor and he introduced him to some of his aristocratic acquaintances. From Innsbruck Connor travelled into Bavaria and from there to Austria, proceeding down the Danube to Vienna, where he stayed for a while at the emperor's court.

PHYSICIAN TO THE KING OF POLAND

Connor travelled on through Moravia and Silesia to Cracow, and eventually to Warsaw where he arrived early in 1694. He was admitted to the court of John III, one of the most remarkable men to have ruled Poland. Connor impressed the king so much by his ability that he was invited to become his personal physician. It was an onerous post as the king did not enjoy good health; he was overweight, had intermittent oedema and respiratory problems, and he also suffered from gout. The king's sister, the Duchess of Radziwill, became very ill and Connor was asked to consult with the ten leading physicians of Warsaw on her treatment and prognosis. These physicians had already given a good prognosis but they had been treating her with Jesuit's Powder (quinine) for three months without improvement. Having examined the duchess, Connor diagnosed a liver abscess and said that the prognosis was hopeless. This caused a sensation and the king asked all the physicians to debate his sister's condition before him. The physicians were angered at Connor's impertinence in challenging their diagnosis and they were dismayed when the duchess died the following month. Connor later recalled that not one of the ten physicians came to the post-mortem:

> The Queen order'd her to be open'd, and three *Bishops* were present, but
> none of the Physicians would come but myself; we found not only an
> Abscess in her Liver, but likewise a great many square stones like Dice in
> her Gall Bladder....[1]

Although the king's respect for Connor grew as a result of this, other
members of the court began to resent him. His popularity was not
enhanced by the emphasis which he placed on the importance of
anatomy. Polish society considered that the practice of anatomy and
surgery was not an appropriate interest for a highly educated physician.
Connor not only antagonised the physicians, he also aroused the
displeasure of the bishops and clergy at the court. One evening when
the king was at dinner with some of Poland's leading clerics, he turned
to Connor and asked him in Latin where he thought the soul was
located in the body. Connor tried to avoid the issue by claiming that as
a physician he was only familiar with the body. However, the king was
insistent and Connor shocked the theologians present by arguing that
the soul was present in the brain and not in every part of the body, as
was the orthodox teaching of the time. The king agreed with the
physician and then he moved to another controversial subject by
announcing that he 'desir'd to know what was properly Death'. The
theologians said that death occurred when the soul left the body, but
Connor did not accept this view and argued:

> That the Death of the Body was the Cessation of the Motion of the
> Heart...which Cessation could not proceed from the Separation of the
> Soul...but it was occasion'd by some Defects in the Organs of the Fluids
> of the Body, which losing their Disposition, and their mutual
> Correspondence with one another, all their actions cease, which
> cessation is properly call'd Death....[2]

The debate continued for four hours and the clerics were even more
enraged when they perceived that the king was supporting Connor:

> Some of them had the boldness to tell the King, that his Majesty should
> not suffer such Heretical Opinions (as they called them) to be introduc'd

before such a great Assembly, contrary to the receiv'd Doctrine of the Church. [2]

The Royal Family offered Connor considerable inducements to stay in Poland. The king realised that his own health was not good and he was anxious to retain the services of the Irish physician. Connor, however, knew that he had several enemies in the court and he was anxious to leave Poland. Fortunately an opportunity presented itself which allowed him to leave Warsaw without seeming ungrateful to his royal patron. In August 1694 the king appointed Connor to care for his only daughter, the princess Teresa Cunigunda, who was to travel from Warsaw to Brussels following her marriage by proxy to the elector of Bavaria. The princess left Warsaw on 11 November 1694 with a retinue of 200 courtiers to accompany her on the long journey across Europe. Connor discussed Polish history and customs with his fellow travellers on their journey and he made careful notes which he would use later to write a history of Poland. He has left a detailed description of their reception and of the festivities at the courts of the different principalities through which they passed on their journey. Most of the princess's retinue left her at the Rhine and returned to Warsaw, and only five of her companions, including Connor, completed the last lap of the journey to Brussels, where they arrived on 12 January 1695.

OXFORD AND CAMBRIDGE

Having accomplished his task successfully, Connor spent some time in Holland, which was then becoming one of the leading scientific and medical centres in Europe under the influence of men such as Anton van Leeuwenhoek (1632–1723) and Herman Boerhaave (1668–1738). From there he crossed to England where he met many of the leading intellectuals of the period, including the Irish physician Hans Sloane. Sloane befriended Connor when he arrived in London. Within weeks he was present at a meeting of the Royal Society and he presented the society with seeds and minerals which he had collected in Poland. He became a regular attender at meetings of both the Royal Society and the Royal College of Physicians.

In the spring of 1695 Connor gave a course of lectures on medicine and natural philosophy at the University of Oxford. These were so successful that he was invited to give a course in Cambridge the following year. In these lectures he advocated an analytical approach to diagnosis and he emphasised the importance of research:

> Now the first step to this Method, is a good Insight by Chymical Experiments into the Nature, more especially the Figuration and Qualities of the Principles of mixt Bodies, and chiefly of the Blood; For want of such a Discovery (which is not impossible) has hitherto been a great Obstruction to the Improvement of Natural Philosophy, and the Practice of Physick. It is plain to me...that the Causes of Diseases, and the true use of Applications to cure them, can be render'd very intelligible; so that vulgar Axiom, *That there's no certainty in Physick* will be found most erroneous.[3]

During his lectures he described the discoveries of Marcello Malpighi, Lorenzo Bellini, Francesco Redi and other scientific men whom he had met abroad. Around this time he anglicised his name by dropping the prefix 'O' from O'Connor. He also became a member of the Church of England. Biographers generally refer to him as Bernard Connor, as this was the name he used in most of his publications. Whilst at Oxford he arranged for the publication of a book of four essays, entitled *Dissertationes Medico-Physicae*. Although Connor made friends in Oxford he also aroused suspicion, as revealed in two surviving letters from Dr Robert Gorge of St John's College to Sir William Trumball, a Privy Councillor and Member of Parliament for the university. In these letters Connor is described as a Jacobite sympathiser and a French spy whose real aim is to get Ireland out of the English hands'.[4]

Between his courses at Oxford and Cambridge, Connor also lectured in London, and he carried out chemical and anatomical experiments in the library of the Archbishop of Canterbury 'which his Grace, out of his wonted Inclination to serve the *Publick*, has been pleased to give me the use of for this purpose'.[5] In one of his letters, Connor gave Bow-Street in Covent Garden as his London address.

Connor's writings are a synthesis of the ancient views relating to philosophy and nature and the new scientific approach which was emerging in the seventeenth century. His tendency to voice critical opinions openly and candidly on different subjects was frequently

resented, despite pleas for tolerance: 'Since therefore Experience and
Reason are our only Guides, no Body is to take it amiss if I censure such
as wrote before me, with as much Justice as they did their Predecessors:
for I'm sworn to no Master.'[6] His work helped to pave the way for the
development of modern scientific medicine. In view of the current
emphasis on the importance of environmental factors in the
conservation of health, his approach appears particularly modern:

> But to have any accurate Knowledge of Man, we must not only have a
> distinct Account of his constituent Parts, but likewise of all the external
> Bodies which any way affect him, or contribute to his Preservation. Since
> therefore he cannot live without Earth to tread upon, Air to breathe,
> Animals and Vegetables to feed upon, Sun and Stars to afford him
> Warmth and Light, etc. we must by consequence examine the System
> and Elements of the World, and particularly as they concur to the
> Preservation or Destruction of Man.[7]

ORIGINAL OBSERVATIONS ON ANKYLOSING SPONDYLITIS

Connor wrote the original description of the skeletal changes found in
the condition now known as ankylosing spondylitis. This work resulted
from his study of the bones of the trunk of an adult skeleton which he
surmised had been found in some churchyard or charnel-house, as they
were very dry and dark red in colour. He made the observations in a
letter in French to Sir Charles Walgrave, which was published originally
in Paris in 1693. A translation of parts of the letter was published in the
Philosophical Transactions two years later:

> All of these Bones which Naturally are 38, each separate and distinct from
> another, were so straightly and intimately joyned, their Ligaments
> perfectly Bony and their articulations so effaced, that they really made but
> one uniform continuous Bone; so that it was as easie to break one of the
> *Vertebrae* into two, as to disjoynt or separate it from the other *vertebrae*, or
> the *Ribs*, or the *Os Sacrum* from those of the Ilia.... The Figure of this
> Trunk was crooked, making part of a Circle, the *Spine* making the
> Convex, and the inside of the *Vertebrae* the Concave part of this Segment.
> If the other *Vertebrae* of the Back and Neck had been preserved, and had
> bent in the same Curve, they would have made near the half of a Circle.[8]

Connor went on to remark that: 'It was a surprising sight to see the sport of Nature in the Fabrick and hardening of these Bones....'[8] He finished the letter by postulating how the condition might have occurred and the effects it might have had on the individual afflicted. Connor included a Latin version of his paper on the spondylitic skeleton in his book *Dissertationes Medico-physicae* which was published in Oxford in 1695. He dedicated this account to the physician John Radcliffe.

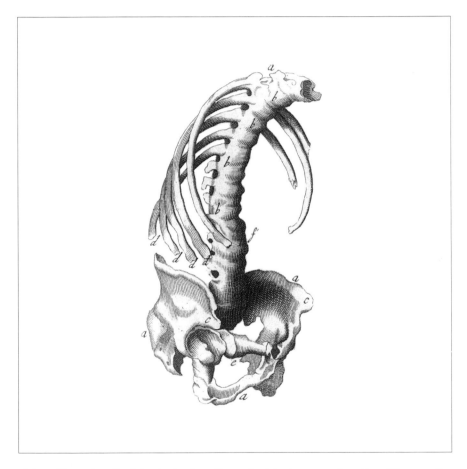

2.2   *Illustration of ankylosed spine from Connor's original paper on the subject. (Courtesy of RCSI)*

A CONTROVERSIAL PUBLICATION

One of Connor's principal works, *Evangelium Medici*, was published originally in London in 1697 and two years later in Amsterdam. In it he set out to explain all the phenomena of the human mind and body in health and disease by a few fundamental principles. The book caused a sensation because he appeared to suggest that the miracles in the Gospel could be explained by natural means. Many were outraged by the contents of the book, and the orthodoxy of the writer was called into question. Connor claimed that his intention was not to undermine belief in miracles but only 'to explain the *Mode* and *Mechanism* with which we may conceive how they might have been performed'.[9]

The publication of *Evangelium Medici* must have been very embarrassing for the Archbishop of Canterbury because the author had used his library during his studies. Connor wrote a long letter to the archbishop refuting the charges of heresy which were being levelled against him. As a further proof of his sincerity he received Communion in the church of St Martin-in-the-Fields. Despite this the Church of England was so alarmed by his views that they tried to limit the distribution of the book. In January 1698 Connor wrote a long letter to one of his former tutors, whom he addressed as Dean J R, justifying the book. This was almost certainly Dean John Richards of Ardfert in County Kerry. In the course of the letter he pointed out that at times supernatural claims are made for events which have a natural explanation:

> For Physicians may find sometimes that what the wilful Mistakes of some and the Ignorance of others take for supernatural, is the visible Effect of a Natural Cause, as I observ'd once at *Rome* some years since: passing by chance through the *Strada del Popolo*, I saw a multitude of People hurrying a Man to St *Mark's* Chappel, which belongs to the *Venetian* Embassadors; they told me that he was possess'd with the Devil, and that they were carrying him to be exorcis'd: I crowded thro' the Throng into the Church, and felt the Man's Pulse; I found him in a Fever, making hideous Grimaces and Motions with his Face, Eyes, Tongue, and all his limbs, which were nothing else but a fit of Convulsive Motions all over his Body.... The Clergy and People began very devoutly to fright the pretended Devil out of him, and in a little

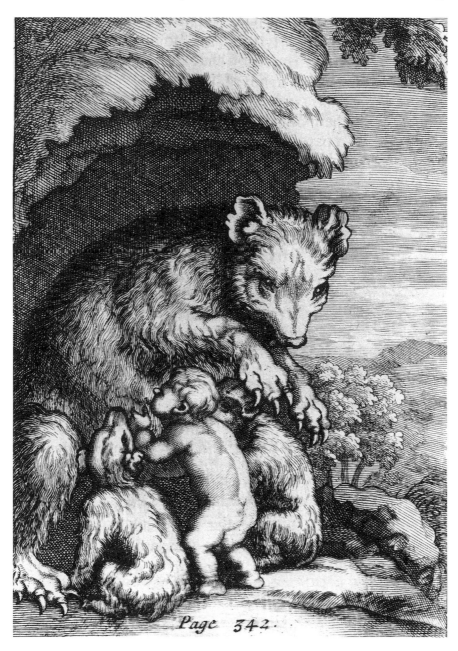

Page 342.

2.3 *An illustration from Connor's* History of Poland *depicting a child being reared by a bear in the woods of Lithuania. 'It was assur'd me often at Court and it is certainly believ'd all over the Kingdom that Children have been frequently nurtur'd by Bears, who are very numerous in these woods.' 1: 342. (Courtesy of TCD)* time his disorderly Motions ceased, which as they thought to be the miraculous Effect of their Prayers, I attributed to the natural abatement and usual cessation of such Fits.[9]

Connor found the whole controversy surrounding his book extremely uncomfortable and he finished the letter to his friend by observing: 'I am resolv'd not to meddle any more with Matters of this kind, but to apply myself entirely to the Practice of Physick.'[9]

CONNOR'S *HISTORY OF POLAND*

The time which Connor devoted to his experiments, his practice and the writing of *Evangelium Medici* left him little opportunity to edit his notes on Poland so that they could be published in book form. Moreover, the controversy following the publication of *Evangelium Medici* led him to take refuge in medical interests as 'being more suitable to my Temper and Profession than Historical ones'.[10] Rather than delay the publication of his Polish material he asked a friend to complete the editing of the work. This was a fortunate decision as Connor was not to live much longer.

The book is a substantial work of over seven hundred pages in two volumes. Apart from covering the history of the country, it gives a detailed description of contemporary Poland based on the first-hand observations of the author and of those he interviewed. Dalitz and Stone emphasised the importance of Connor's *History of Poland* in an article which they wrote in 1981: 'The book is the first of its kind in the English language, but its importance in the bibliography of Slavonic studies in Great Britain and as a source for the history of Poland in the seventeenth century has not been fully appreciated.'[4]

PREMATURE DEATH

Connor's European fame was remarkable considering the fact that he died when he was only thirty-two years old. In October 1698 he became very ill with fever and when he realised the seriousness of his condition he made his will. He left five pounds to the poor and he directed that all his property should be sold and the proceeds should go to his relations. He asked in particular that his largest diamond ring should be sold and the value be given to his youngest sister. He died on 30 October 1698. He was buried at St Giles-in-the-Fields and a funeral sermon was preached by William Hayley DD, who regarded him as 'a true and penitent member of the Church of England'.[11] Hayley attended him during his last illness and gave him Communion, but almost immediately afterwards a Catholic priest arrived and Connor accepted absolution. Hayley attributed Connor's act to confusion, but he has left us a graphic description of the event:

> A *Romish Priest*, came to the *Doctor's Lodgings*, and desired very earnestly to see him, declaring that he was his *Country-man*, his *Friend* and his *Relation*, those about him, looking upon him as near his departure, were unwilling he should be disturbed; but upon great *importunity* did at last grant the *stranger* admittance, who coming to the Bed side, call'd the Doctor by his name and saluted him in his *native* language *three* times before he regarded; but at the third time he cry'd out *for God's sake assist me*. Upon which the company was prevailed with to leave the room, but the Doctor's most intimate *friend* returned to the door and heard the Doctor repeating over his *Confiteor* in *Latin*, in a very *huddled* manner; upon which the *Priest* gave him *Absolution* and then asked him whether he would have *extream Unction*, and the Doctor said *yes*, after which it is suspected it was given him.[11]

The catalogue of achievements which Connor accomplished in his short life is astonishing. He was elected a fellow of the Royal Society, a fellow of the Royal College of Physicians and a Membre de l'Academie Française. An erudite scholar, he travelled widely throughout Europe, assimilating and imparting knowledge as he went. His observations were astute and he placed emphasis on the importance of experimental evidence. Despite his short life he made a definite contribution to the evolution of medicine and he played an important role in the interchange of new ideas on science and philosophy between the continent and these islands.

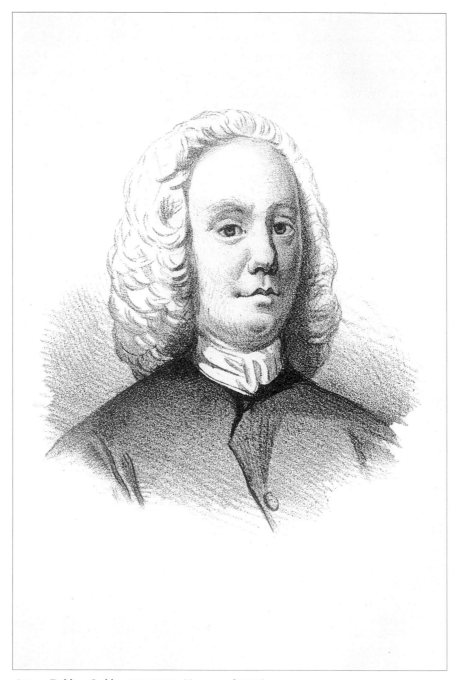

3.1   Fielding Ould c *1710–1789 (Courtesy of RCPI)*

FIELDING OULD
c 1710–1789

3 Significant contributor to obstetric practice

F ielding Ould is remembered today in obstetrics for his early accurate descriptions of the process of normal labour. He was born around 1710 in Galway. His grandfather, Colonel Ould, came to Ireland as commander of the Royal Regiment of Fusiliers in the army of King William. Colonel Ould commanded his troops at the Battle of the Boyne, and after the surrender of Dublin the leading officers of the conquering army were admitted freemen of the city. The names of Colonel Ould and his son, Captain Ould, are to be found on the Freemen's Roll. The Oulds took part in the Battle of Aughrim, after which the Welsh Fusiliers were quartered in Galway. There Captain Ould married a Miss Shawe, the daughter of a country gentleman. They had two sons, Abraham and Fielding.

When Fielding was a few years old his father was murdered at night in the streets of London. His mother then returned with her children to her father in Galway. Abraham subsequently studied law and Fielding decided to study medicine. He started work as a dissector in the Department of Anatomy in Trinity College Dublin. He spent five years dissecting and during that time he attended courses in natural philosophy, chemistry and botany. He later recalled that he 'spent that Time which others employ in their Improvement in polite Literature, in a more laborious Manner; namely in the Dissection of human Bodies, and a constant Application to Practice'.[1] He left Trinity, however, without a degree, a fact which was to have very serious consequences for the relationship between the College of Physicians and the university.

A CAREER IN MIDWIFERY

Ould decided to study midwifery in Paris, where Gregoire was a leading obstetric teacher. It was during this period that he made his first original contribution to obstetrics when he discovered the lateral position of the head during delivery. He returned to Dublin and having established a practice in Golden Lane he appears to have devoted himself largely to midwifery. In 1738 he obtained a licence in midwifery from the College of Physicians in Dublin. Four years later he published his famous book, *A Treatise of Midwifry*. It was dedicated to the president, censors and fellows of the College of Physicians in Dublin and it carried their imprimatur. The treatise contained many original observations and it was one of the first substantial obstetric works in the English language.

Until then it was universally taught and believed that the face of the baby should be directed towards the sacrum during normal labour. Many midwives rocked the head to and fro in order to get the face in this direction. The result was an agonising labour for the woman as the crown of the foetal head was pushed against the os pubis, leading often to a facial presentation with all its attendant dangers for the mother and baby. In his book Ould states quite clearly that the face is directed to one side of the pelvis during birth and not towards the sacrum, and he supported his contention with detailed anatomical observations. He introduced the subject in the preface of the book:

And here I will frankly acknowledge how this Discovery occurred to me. I was at a labour in Paris, which from all the Appearances promised to be very successful and speedy; the Water gathered and broke very advantageously, but as the Head approached towards the World, its Progress grew tedious, so that at the latter End, the Spectators saw it make its Appearance, and immediately return back out of Sight, and that several Times; whereupon seeing the Head in the above Direction with the chin on the Shoulder, it was unanimously declared, that the Child was in a preternatural Direction, which impeded the Delivery; I made a strict Inquiry with my Fingers, and found Space sufficient to give Passage to the Head, though in that Situation, and consequently, that some other Cause must retard the Operation. At length, by mere dint of the Patient's Efforts, who was strong and robust, the Head was thrust so far, that the Operator took hold of it, and with Difficulty brought it forth, and found the Funis (Cord) rolled several Times about the Child's Neck, which was the Cause of all our Trouble.

I at my Leisure reflected on the Circumstances of this Labour, and soon began to consider the Necessity of this Disposition of the Head; to confirm which, I made the strictest Examination of every Woman, which I either delivered, or saw delivered during my Continuance at Paris, which perfectly convinced me of the Truth of what I suggested.[2]

Ould also advocated that the foetus should be turned and delivered by the feet in cases where the cephalic presentation would be very difficult or impossible because of slight deformity of the pelvis. He used opium in prolonged labour, he allowed the placenta to be born by the expulsive efforts of the uterus and he recommended immediate delivery of the second twin. He also performed episiotomies, and he was familiar with the use of the forceps and with the technique of version.

Although Ould's textbook was certainly the most influential of its period, he was not the first to write an obstetrical book in Ireland. One of the earliest midwifery works in the English language, entitled *Speculum Matricis; or the Irish Midwive's Handmaid, Catechistically Composed*, was published in 1671. It was written by a Trinity graduate named James Wolveridge who was practising in Cork. Unlike Ould's work the content was not original, as the author had borrowed liberally from other obstetricians who had written in Latin during the previous century.

MASTER OF THE ROTUNDA

Ould became Master of the Rotunda in 1759, succeeding Bartholomew Mosse (1712–1759), the founder of that great institution. When Ould returned from Paris he pointed out that although excellent physicians and surgeons were being trained in Dublin, they had to go to France for knowledge of practical midwifery, as there alone they had the opportunity of 'ocular Demonstration of Women being delivered, both in natural and preternatural Labours; where, as well the external Parts of the Patient, as every Action of the Operator, are the whole Time in View; the Necessity of which Advantage, there is no Need of Arguments to prove'.[3]

The foundation of the Dublin Lying-In Hospital by Mosse in 1745 made the teaching of midwifery a practical proposition in Dublin, as well as providing excellent maternity facilities for the poor of the city. It was the first maternity hospital in Ireland and Great Britain and Mosse insisted on a grand design. The hospital was built to the plan of Richard Cassells, using the best materials which included hand-forged iron staircase rails, mahogany pews in the chapel and Adam ceilings and mantelpieces.

Much of the funding for the construction was raised through charitable means by Mosse, who made superhuman efforts to ensure the success of his brainchild. Ould had served as an assistant to Mosse and when he took over as master, after the latter's untimely death, he resolved to proceed with plans to build an impressive place of entertainment which would bring in funds for the hospital. John Ensor's plans for the Round Rooms were accepted in 1764 and the building cost £3000. After its completion the Lying-in Hospital became known as the Rotunda. The gardens of the hospital were also re-modelled and they became a meeting place for fashionable Dublin society.

Ould was knighted in 1760 by John Russell, Fourth Duke of Bedford, who was then lord lieutenant, and president of the Board of Governors and Guardians of the hospital. A Dublin wit penned the following poem to mark the occasion:

> Sir Fielding Ould is made a knight,
> He should have been a Lord by right;
> For then each lady's prayer would be,
> O Lord, good Lord, deliver me! [4]

Fielding Ould lived at 21 Frederick Street South. His house was later demolished and the site is now partially occupied by number 12 Nassau Street, which forms the east corner of this street and Frederick Street. Ould had a very large practice and he was present at the birth of a number of distinguished people. It was he who attended the Countess of Mornington at the birth of the Duke of Wellington.

Ould was the cause of a very serious dispute between Trinity College and the College of Physicians, two bodies which had been closely connected for over sixty years. In 1701 the Boards of both institutions had agreed that the fellows of the College of Physicians would be the examiners for the degree in medicine in Trinity College, and that only those who had graduated from Trinity would be admitted to the licence in physic and fellowship of the College of Physicians. The College of Physicians had a very narrow-minded attitude concerning the practice of midwifery, and in 1736 they passed a resolution stating 'that no man for the future shall have a licence to practise midwifery and physic together'.[5]

In 1756 Ould applied to both Trinity College and the College of Physicians for permission to be examined for a degree in medicine. The physicians adamantly refused to examine him, but this appears to have strengthened Ould's resolve. He was becoming an increasingly powerful figure in the city and the university considered that it could not continue to ignore such a distinguished candidate. Eventually he was examined without involving the College of Physicians and he received an MB on 27 January 1761. The physicians viewed this as a deliberate expression of contempt for their by-laws and they immediately severed all links with the university. They maintained their hard line for several years. Eventually they adopted a more enlightened approach and in 1785 several leading obstetricians, including Ould, were admitted licentiates in medicine. However the relationship between the College of Physicians and Trinity College would never again be as close as it had been before this dispute.

Ould's term as Master of the Rotunda came to an end in 1766. Bartholomew Mosse is justly famous for founding the first obstetric hospital in the world and the first practical school of obstetrics. Ould on the other hand, by his treatise on midwifery, laid the foundations for Dublin's subsequent fame in the science of obstetrics. He died on 29 November 1789 at his residence in Frederick Street.

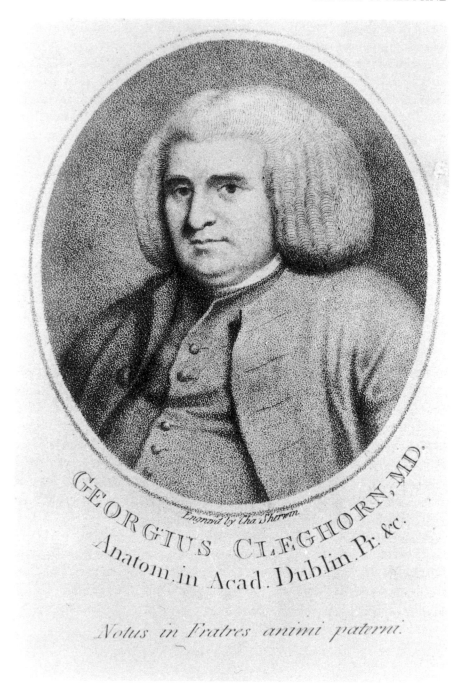

GEORGIUS CLEGHORN, MD.
Anatom. in Acad. Dublin. Pr: &c.

Engrav'd by Tha Sherwin.

Notus in Fratres animi paterni.

4.1   *George Cleghorn 1716–1789 (Courtesy of TCD)*

GEORGE CLEGHORN
1716–1789

4 Early progress in epidemiology

George Cleghorn, who was professor of anatomy at Trinity College, played a central role in eighteenth-century Irish medicine. He wrote one of the earliest works on epidemiology and he is credited with the first description of infectious hepatitis. He was born near Edinburgh in 1716 and when he was three years old his father died, leaving a widow and five children. He was educated in the local parish school and at the age of twelve he was sent to Edinburgh to study classics and modern languages. Three years later he began to study medicine. He was placed under the tuition of Alexander Monro, primus, the distinguished Scottish doctor, and he resided in his house for five years. Cleghorn formed a close friendship with John Fothergill and William Cuming, two fellow medical students. In 1734 the three of them, along with two other students, founded in Edinburgh the society which became known subsequently as the Royal Medical Society. At the third meeting of this society, Cleghorn delivered a paper on epilepsy.

RESEARCH IN MINORCA

In 1736 Cleghorn was appointed surgeon to the 22nd Regiment of

Foot, then stationed at Minorca. Apart from attending to his professional duties, Cleghorn collected material for a book on the diseases prevalent on the island. He also studied the comparative anatomy of the Barbary ape and man. His great industry brought him the admiration of his friends, as is apparent from a letter which Fothergill wrote to Cuming in August 1742:

> Thou wilt no doubt admire the industry of our friend Cleghorn; who, situated in a corner of the world, has made greater progress than any of us, who even do not want the proper aids of study. Let us therefore stimulate one another, that we may follow his footsteps, and become the worthy friends of so great a man.[1]

Fothergill sent him books from London during this period to help him with his studies.

Cleghorn travelled to Ireland in 1749 with his regiment, but he left shortly afterwards to oversee the publication of his book *Observations on the Epidemical Diseases in Minorca from the Year 1744 to 1749*, which was first published in London in 1751. It went through five English editions and in 1776 it was translated into German. The book, which has become a classic work on epidemic diseases, begins with a general account of the inhabitants, climate and natural history of the island, and then goes on to describe the diseases of the natives and of the British troops in chapters which contain many original observations. The book includes several descriptions of post-mortems carried out by the author and it also contains the first description of infectious hepatitis. Cleghorn describes fever patients whose skin was 'tinged with a deep yellow'.[2] He observes that 'The *English* in *Minorca* are more liable than the Natives to become yellow in these Fevers'.[3]

While in London, Cleghorn studied anatomy under William Hunter, thus gaining the experience for his future work as a lecturer in anatomy in Dublin. On his return to Ireland in 1751 he began to build up a practice which eventually became very successful. He also initiated private annual courses in anatomy. In 1753 he was elected as anatomist to the School of Physic at Trinity College. At that time Bryan Robinson was probably the most distinguished member of the staff. He was the regius professor of physic and he has been described as one of the most famous iatro-mathematicians of his time. His best known work, *Animal*

Œconomy, was first published in 1732 and was reprinted several times. He is remembered for a mathematical formula devised to calculate the velocity of circulating blood.

PROFESSORSHIP AT TRINITY

An unexpected development gave Cleghorn an opportunity for promotion early in his career. This was the row which arose between Trinity College and the College of Physicians over the former's decision to confer a degree on Sir Fielding Ould, the obstetrician. The decision of the Board of Trinity to go ahead and grant the MB degree despite the opposition from the College of Physicians caused great unhappiness amongst some of the staff in the School of Physic. The professor of anatomy, Robert Robinson, who was also a fellow of the College of Physicians, refused to co-operate with the university and he was dismissed from his post. Cleghorn was promoted in his place. He proved to be an able teacher, attracting many pupils to the school. Several young doctors came to him for career advice. Joseph Clarke, who was encouraged by Cleghorn to study obstetrics wrote that 'No man knew Dublin better, and few could so readily direct a professional man as to the manner by which its inhabitants were to be pleased'.[4] Cleghorn's judgement was obviously sound as Clarke became one of the most able Masters of the Rotunda.

On the death of his only brother, Cleghorn brought his widow Barbara and family of nine children to Dublin and settled them under his own care. Three of these nephews, William, James and Thomas, became doctors and one of his nieces married the obstetrician Joseph Clarke.

FRIENDSHIP WITH DAVID McBRIDE

David McBride (1726–1778), one of the founders of the Meath Hospital, was a close friend of Cleghorn's. McBride's book *Experimental Essays*, which was published in London in 1764, contained a detailed account of much of his scientific work. He was particularly interested in the treatment of scurvy, having worked in the Navy, but he also did experiments on fermentation and putrefaction and on the nature of carbonic acid. He wrote *A Methodical Introduction to the Theory and Practice of Physic* which was published in London in 1772. Cleghorn used his influence to help McBride with his research, particularly with his work on scurvy.

INVOLVEMENT WITH THE MEDICO-PHILOSOPHICAL SOCIETY

The Medico-Philosophical Society which was founded in 1756 was a meeting place for the doctors of this period. Its primary function was the pursuit of medical knowledge. Cleghorn was introduced to the society in September 1757. The following month he read the first of many papers to the society. This was entitled 'An account of an Hernia Dorsali — being a very rare species of rupture'. Earlier in the same year it was resolved that a book which would be called the *Repository* should be used to collect the original communications, thus avoiding the necessity of transcribing them. The *Repository* contains 230 articles by the leading Irish medical thinkers of the time, including George Cleghorn, David McBride, Samuel Clossy and John Rutty. In the first volume of the *Repository* Cleghorn laid out a detailed plan to bring the work of the new society up to international standards. He proposed that other able men should be encouraged to become members so that the research could be shared by more individuals. Members should be encouraged to develop an interest in a particular area of medical science so that high standards could be reached in these areas. He finished his presentation by telling his colleagues that:

> Many a Genius lurks among us, lost to the world and Ignorant of its own Powers, as it never had Occasion to Exert them. Let us endeavour to Rouse some of them into Action, and make them useful to themselves and the Rest of Mankind; and if we cannot do what we would wish, let us have the satisfaction of doing what we can to accomplish, so desirable an End.[5]

John Rutty (1698–1775) was one of the most regular contributors to the Medico-Philosophical Society. He had studied under Boerhaave in

Leiden, where he received his MD degree in 1723. For twenty years Rutty kept detailed records of the weather and the incidence of various diseases in Dublin. These observations, which included the first clear description of relapsing fever, were published in book form in 1770.

Cleghorn conducted an extensive correspondence with leading Irish doctors who lived outside Dublin and also with doctors in Great Britain. The more interesting of these letters were read to the Medico-Philosophical Society and incorporated into the minutes. For instance, there is a communication from Sylvester O'Halloran, the distinguished Limerick surgeon who wrote books on a number of subjects including cataract (1750) and head injuries (1793).

Cleghorn's energy and commitment re-established the fortunes of the School of Physic. His teaching attracted many pupils and he was the first to impress on the Board of the College the value of the medical school. It was Cleghorn who laid the foundation for the tradition of excellent anatomy teaching in Trinity. This reputation was built on in the next century by professors such as James Macartney, Daniel Cunningham (author of a famous anatomy textbook) and Alexander Macalister. In 1768 Cleghorn was given an honorary MD by the university, and at a meeting of the Medio-Philosophical Society in 1772 both he and John Rutty were made honorary members for life. He was nominated a fellow of the Royal Medical Society of Paris when it was established in 1777 and he was elected a fellow of the College of Physicians in 1784. In 1785 he took an active part in founding the Royal Irish Academy and became a member of its first council.

THE LAST YEARS

In 1781, at Cleghorn's request, his nephew William was appointed lecturer in anatomy at Trinity, but he died following a fever in 1783. Joseph Clarke, who was married to Cleghorn's niece, was appointed in a temporary capacity until another nephew, James, could complete his education on the Continent. Cleghorn had a very lucrative practice which allowed him to purchase several properties in the country, mainly in County Meath. In 1786, writing from his country home in Kilcarty, County Meath, he told his friend, the famous English physician John Coakley Lettsom, of his intention to retire:

....having learned by dearly-bought experience, that I was no longer able
to climb up two or three pair of stairs to bed-chambers and nurseries,
supporting a weighty corporation of nineteen stone and a half on a pair
of oedematous legs, and panting like a wind-broken horse, before I get
half way up. I thank God, that rural amusements, constant exercise in
the open air, in a carriage, and freedom from the cares of an anxious
profession, gradually removed all my pressing complaints.[6]

He enjoyed his time at Kilcarty, planting gardens and generally
improving the landscape.

Although Cleghorn was prepared to wait until his nephew would be
in a stronger position to apply for the professorship, he was against
outright nepotism. He prided himself on his integrity and honesty; he
once wrote that 'honesty is the best policy, and that a good name is
better than riches'.[7] When Joseph Clarke was applying for the
mastership of the Rotunda in 1786 he wrote to Cleghorn asking him to
use his influence with some of the governors of the hospital. Cleghorn
replied:

My stomach revolts against the usual mode of extracting promises and
engaging votes before the Governors can be sufficiently apprized of the
merits of the candidates. It is founded on a supposition that all men are
actuated by selfish motives, regardless of the public good, and that they
never consider whether their friend be fit for the place he wishes for,
provided the place be fit for him. If you gain the election I hope it will
be by means fair and honourable; I would rather hear you had lost it,
than that any others had been employed.[8]

Clarke was elected Master of the Rotunda but he also continued to run
the anatomy department for Cleghorn — an arrangement which cannot
have been too healthy for his patients. Cleghorn wrote to him from
Kilcarty: 'Nothing could draw me from this retreat, where I have every
convenience my heart could wish, but the ardent desire I have to
continue the anatomical lectures; but I must depend upon your taking
the chief part of the trouble upon your own shoulders, until James
returns.'[9] Cleghorn died on 22 December 1789. In his will he divided
his books, manuscripts and equipment between his nephews Thomas
and James. The latter succeeded him in the chair of anatomy.

SAMUEL CLOSSY
c 1724–1786

5 Founder of an American medical school

S amuel Clossy was a pioneer of American medical education and he also wrote one of the first pathology books to be based, along modern lines, on the different systems of the body. The exact date of his birth is unknown but it is thought that he was born in 1724. His father, Bartholomew Clossy, was a Dublin merchant who lived at 4 Suffolk Street. The name Clossy was an Anglicised version of the Irish Ua Clochasaigh, or O'Clohessy. As a child Samuel Clossy was sent to the preparatory school of the Reverend Alexander McDaniel in Cashel, County Tipperary. Here he received a sound classical education which was to be of value to him later when studying the medical works of Greek and Latin authors.

MEDICAL STUDIES

Clossy studied medicine at Trinity College Dublin, obtaining a BA in 1744 and an MB in 1751. The reason for the delay in taking his medical degree is uncertain, but Professor J B Lyons has suggested that it may have been due to family responsibilities imposed on him by the death of his father. Whilst an undergraduate Clossy came under the influence of Sir Edward Barry who was regius professor of medicine and William Stephens who had studied under Boerhaave in Leiden before becoming a university lecturer in chemistry in Trinity College and physician to Dr Steevens' Hospital. Barry was the author of *A Treatise on the Three Different Digestions* which was published in London in 1759. Clossy was also impressed by the work of George Cleghorn and the two men became friends.

When Clossy graduated William Stephens invited him to perform post-mortems on patients who had died at Dr Steevens' Hospital — an opportunity which was probably unique at that time. He would also have had access to the magnificent library of Edward Worth which was bequeathed to the hospital in 1733 for the use of the medical staff. Both George Cleghorn and William Stephens encouraged Clossy to study under William Hunter at Covent Garden. Clossy travelled to London on a number of occasions to attend Hunter's lectures and he worked at St George's Hospital for a time. He also continued his own studies at Dr Steevens' Hospital and he obtained his MD in 1755 by examination.

The fact that Clossy was given special permission to perform post-mortems at Dr Steevens' Hospital was a great advantage to him as at that time it was extremely difficult to obtain bodies for dissection. However, in 1756, after four years' work, he suddenly stopped performing autopsies at the hospital. He was at Dr Steevens' purely through a grace and favour arrangement and he may have antagonised some of the staff. On 29 April 1756 the Board of Governors of the hospital passed a resolution forbidding the dissection of bodies except 'By special direction of the Visiting Physician and the Visiting Surgeon'.[1]

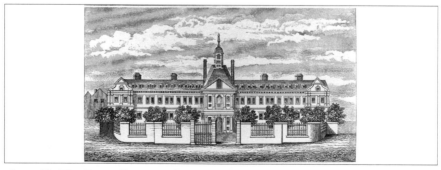

5.1   The West Front of Trinity College in 1728, from Brooking's map of Dublin. This was replaced by the present front later in the century.

SYSTEMATIC REVIEW OF PATHOLOGY

In 1761 Clossy became a fellow of the College of Physicians and a member of the Dublin Medico-Philosophical Society. One year later he was appointed physician to Mercer's Hospital and he also became a member of the Board of Governors of the hospital. In the meantime he was organising into book form the information which he had accumulated during his time at Dr Steevens'. The work was published in 1763 in London and was entitled *Observations on Some of the Diseases of the Parts of the Human Body*. This was one of the earliest attempts at a systematic review of pathology in the English language. In a reprint of the book published in 1967 the editor M M H Saffron emphasised the striking resemblance of his methodology in case presentation to the protocol of the modern clinico-pathological conference. The clinical presentation and post-mortem findings are presented and these are followed by a discussion of the case.

The book is divided into six parts, each one dealing with a different section of anatomy. According to Saffron the section dealing with the head is perhaps the best:

> Several of his observations in this area foreshadow knowledge of what has now become commonplace. For example he recognized that epidural effusions tend to be localized, whereas subdural effusions tend to become diffused over the brain.... Clossy knew the existence of the 'contrecoup' effect of cranial trauma, as well as convulsions resulting from 'splinters pricking the brain'.[2]

He describes the typical victim of stroke as someone addicted to 'full feeding, inactive life, want of due discharges, and sudden passions of the mind'.[3] Interestingly, in view of modern research he also describes exposure to cold as a predisposing factor to stroke.

EMIGRATION TO AMERICA

In 1763 Clossy must have surprised many of his contemporaries when he resigned his post at Mercer's Hospital and announced that he was going to emigrate to New York. The reasons for this decision remain

OBSERVATIONS

On some of the

DISEASES

Of the Parts of the

HUMAN BODY.

Chiefly taken from the Dissections of Morbid Bodies.

By SAMUEL CLOSSY, M. D.

LONDON:
Printed for G. Kearsly, in Ludgate-street.
MDCCLXIII.

5.2   *Title page of Samuel Clossy's book. When writing this book he used a format which closely resembles the approach used in modern clinico-pathological presentations. (Courtesy of RCPI)* unknown. Clossy had been married for four years at this stage and he had a young daughter. However, he left for America in September without bringing his family with him. Although Clossy was to stay in America for seventeen years, his family never joined him there. The reason for this is not known but we do know from contemporary records that his wife had a small independent income of about £40 per annum. He had hoped to obtain a post in a new military hospital which was planned for New York as a consequence of the French and Indian Wars, but when he arrived in the city he found that the plans for the hospital had been dropped.

Two months after his arrival in New York he wrote to George Cleghorn in Dublin informing him that he had started a course in anatomy. The local people, he said, suspected both him and his students of body snatching and they 'were so well known in the place that we could not venture to meddle with a white, and a black or Mulatto I could not procure'.[4] Towards the end of the letter Clossy mentions the Medico-Philosophical Society: 'Pray give my love to the Club, and if you think proper you may lay these observations before them.'[4] Cleghorn read the letter to a meeting of the Society on 4 August 1764.

FIRST PROFESSOR OF A MEDICAL SUBJECT

In 1763 Myles Cooper became the second president of King's College (later Columbia University) which had been founded ten years earlier. He invited Clossy to join him as his assistant. Clossy, the most scientific physician to reach America in his day, was skilled in mathematics and physics. He began a course in anatomy and he was appointed professor of natural philosophy, making him 'the first professor of a medical subject in North America'.[5] New York at the time had a population of approximately 20 000 but had no hospital. Clossy threw himself whole-heartedly into a scheme to establish a medical school at King's College. Cooper was very much in favour of the scheme but they made little progress at first because of the reservations of more conservative elements within the college.

In the summer of 1766 Clossy returned to Ireland on a visit and no doubt he brought his friends in the Medico-Philosophical Society up to date on developments in New York. When he returned to America he worked with renewed energy on the plans to establish a medical school in King's College. On 14 August 1767 the governors of the college, after considering submissions from Clossy and other doctors associated with the institution, decided to proceed with the project. Clossy was appointed as the first professor of anatomy. The following month he announced details of his anatomy course in the New York newspapers. He delivered a lecture on 'The uses of anatomy' at the opening ceremony of the new medical school on 2 November 1767. The following year the governors expressed their appreciation of Clossy's efforts by awarding him an honorary doctorate in medicine.

THE AMERICAN REVOLUTION

Clossy had a generous nature and he was popular with his students and colleagues, although some of the latter were jealous of his ability. A contemporary, John Wakefield Francis, recalled:

> At the vacation during the Christmas holydays he was annually supplied, like the old poet laureates, with a cask of wine by his friends. John Pintard told me he kept up the jollification with open house for all who visited him during the vacation. He became obnoxious to the British who held the city, because of his democracy....[6]

Clossy's brilliant career in New York was brought to an abrupt halt by the outbreak of the American Revolution in 1776. The students were by and large very anti-British and Clossy gradually became more openly supportive of their cause. He may have been influenced by reports of the distress caused in Ireland by the English laws which forbade the export of linen to America. However, Clossy's enthusiasm for the American cause was dampened when violence erupted on the streets of New York. His failure to join the rebels and his criticism of the loyalists gained him enemies in both camps. When George Washington and the rebel forces occupied New York in April 1776 they took possession of the college and converted it into a hospital. Clossy left the city for New Jersey. The British entered New York in September 1776 under Sir William Howe. The soldiers began to plunder the city; they broke into the college library where they destroyed many items of value. Five days after their arrival a fire swept through the city, destroying almost one-third of the buildings. When Clossy returned to New York in October 1776 he found the college buildings in a dreadful state and his instruments and books had been either stolen or destroyed. He inserted a notice in the New York newspapers offering a reward for their recovery.

Clossy commenced some lecturing and there were also plans to republish his book in America. However the latter scheme did not come to fruition. In 1777 his health began to deteriorate and he had to postpone anatomical lectures which he was due to give in November of that year. He was also very much out of favour with the British authorities who controlled New York at the time and he was given the menial post of 'surgeon's mate'. In December 1779 he wrote to General Clinton asking for promotion:

> Dr Clossy begs leave to signifie to your Excellency that he has been bred in the university of Dublin, that he has taken a Batchelor's Degree in Arts, a Batchelor's Degree in Physick, and a Doctor's Degree in Physick there, and is one of the Fellows of the College of Physitians in that City.
>
> Moreover that he has been several Years in London at the most approved places of Instruction there....[7]

Clossy did not receive a reply from Clinton and as a consequence he decided that there was little future for him in America. On 29 January 1780 he wrote again to the general asking him for permission to leave New York:

> It is with regret that I mention myself to your Excellency whose thoughts are engaged in matters of such vast importance, nor would I indeed were it not for Mrs Clossy and my Daughter who are in Ireland in very narrow Circumstances without my being able to service them in the Station I am in....[8]

RETURN TO DUBLIN

Clossy sailed for London in November 1780. One year later a ship carrying a cabinet and three chests filled with his personal belongings and teaching material sank off the French coast. Among the items lost were a double reflecting microscope, a large brass syringe, a silver catheter, several silver items including silver spurs and buckles and an inscribed silver cup which had been presented to him by his students. He also lost several items of furniture and many of his books. A later shipment carrying some other material arrived safely. Clossy maintained some connection with the army as he continued to receive military pay until 24 June 1784. He then received a pension of £80 per annum which allowed him to leave London and return to Dublin. Some of his former associates, such as George Cleghorn, welcomed him back to the city, and on St Luke's Day 1784 he was elected an honorary fellow of the Royal College of Physicians of Ireland. Two years later, on 22 August 1786, he died in Suffolk Street, the same street in which he was born over sixty years previously.

JOHN CRAWFORD
1746–1813

6 *The study of insects as carriers of disease*

John Crawford was the first physician to suggest that yellow fever might be transmitted by insects. He also argued that many diseases were caused by tiny organisms called animalculae, which multiplied within the bodies of their victims. He held these views at a time when it was generally believed that most diseases were 'chemical' in nature and that epidemics spread through the medium of foul vapours or gases. Crawford used his profound knowledge of nature, and particularly of the insect world, to support his argument. Sadly his ideas were ridiculed by many of his medical colleagues during his lifetime. Crawford was the son of a Presbyterian clergyman and he was born in the north of Ireland in 1746. When he was about seventeen years old he was sent to study medicine at Trinity College Dublin. However, he left before obtaining the MB degree to enlist as a ship's surgeon. His younger brother, Adair, also studied medicine and he became physician to St Thomas's Hospital, London.

PHYSICIAN IN BARBADOS

Crawford travelled twice to India and he also visited China in the service of the East India Company. He published his first book *An Essay on the Nature, Cause and Cure of a Disease Incident to the Liver* in London in 1772. In this book Crawford describes an illness which was almost certainly beriberi and which affected sailors under his care on a voyage between China and St Helena. It gives a graphic account of the hardships endured by sailors on long sea voyages.

Crawford married an O'Donnell of Truagh Castle, Limerick, around the year 1778, and he took his young bride with him to Barbados where he had been appointed physician-in-chief. He could have accrued considerable wealth in this post but he had other priorities. Even in 1780, when the island was devastated by a hurricane, Crawford refused to profit by the occurrence, although his property was the only one to escape without significant damage. He supplied medicine and help to those in need and he sought no compensation. In 1782 his health began to deteriorate and he decided to return to Europe with his wife and family. During the voyage his wife died under very distressing circumstances and he was left with two infant children.

When his health improved he returned to Barbados, but in 1790 he moved to Demerara as he had been appointed surgeon major to the colony, which was then in the possession of the Dutch. Here he had control of a military hospital, with sixty to eighty beds, and this afforded him great opportunities for observation and study. He performed a large number of autopsies. He was particularly interested in the role of parasites in the aetiology of disease and he was slowly formulating his own theories about the spread of infection.

In 1794 his health began to deteriorate again and he was obliged to return to Europe. He travelled to Holland to settle some business with the Dutch government, and whilst there he took advantage of the opportunity to obtain the degree of MD from the University of Leiden. He already had an MD from St Andrew's University in Scotland, which had been granted to him in 1791. Whilst in Leiden he discussed his ideas on infection with Professor Brugmans, the professor of natural history and botany, and he read the works of writers such as Athanasius Kircher, Jan Swammerdam and Francesco Redi who had previously suggested a possible link between micro organisms and disease. However their views had been condemned by such influential figures as Herman Boerhaave, Gerhard van Swieten and Giovanni Morgagni.

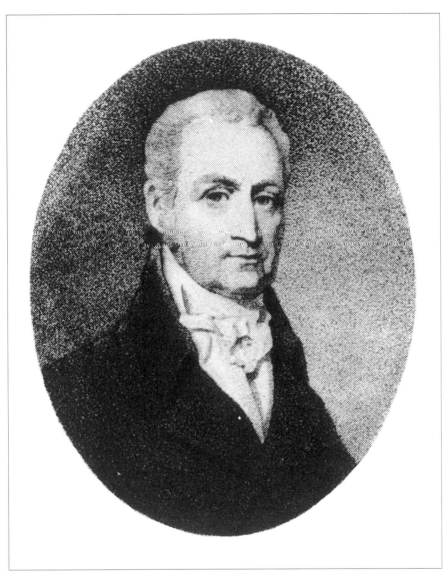

6.1   John Crawford 1746–1813 (From Aesculapius Comes to the Colonies *by M B Gordon. 1949. Ventnor, New Jersey. Courtesy of RCP, London.)*

FIRST BALTIMORE DISPENSARY

Crawford did not wish to return to the colonies and the United States appeared to offer better opportunities both for himself and for his family. His brother-in-law, John O'Donnell, was a merchant in Baltimore, and he encouraged Crawford to make the move, arguing that the climate in the United States would be beneficial for his health. Crawford also had medical links with the New World as he had been in correspondence with the famous American physician Benjamin Rush for some time. He travelled to Baltimore in 1796, the year that the city was granted its charter. He settled down very quickly in his new surroundings and he told Rush that he met more members of 'the Families amidst of which I was born, than I have ever seen since I left my native country....'.[1]

Crawford was appointed physician to the City Hospital and he soon became a leading figure in the medical and civic life of Baltimore. He continued to correspond with Rush and both men sought each other's advice on a regular basis. Among the topics which they discussed in their correspondence was the founding of a dispensary in Baltimore. The project came to fruition in 1801, largely due to Crawford's efforts, and it was the first of its kind in the city.

SMALLPOX VACCINATION

The previous summer Crawford had received a sample of Edward Jenner's vaccine from Dr John Ring of London. The latter mentions this in his *Treatise on Cow-pox*.

> In the summer of 1800, I sent some vaccine virus on cotton thread, rolled up in paper, and covered with a varnish which excluded air, to Dr Crawford, of Baltimore.... From the son of Dr Crawford, who is now pursuing in this metropolis, his studies in a profession which he is one day destined to adorn, I have received the pleasing intelligence, that when his father wrote to him, he could just discover, by the assistance of a magnifying glass, a vaccine pustule had taken place.[1]

Crawford began to use the vaccine around the same time as Benjamin

Waterhouse was experimenting with the new method of vaccination against smallpox in Cambridge, Massachusetts.

THEORIES ON INSECTS AND DISEASE

Crawford held views on the spread of infection which were regarded as very unorthodox by his colleagues. He claimed that insects acted as vectors for 'animalculae' so minute as to escape observation by the naked eye. He seems to have begun to entertain this concept as a cause of disease in 1790 when he went to Guiana and saw numerous patients with malaria and yellow fever. Relaxing after his day's work, he observed the myriads of insects which fluttered around the air and he thought to himself, 'If in the air, why not in my air tubes? Any why not thus the conveyors of disease?'[2]

Crawford was the first physician to express the theory of insect contagion in connection with yellow fever. He argued that all analogy showed that disease and decay were coincident with the presence of minute organisms. If the fly lays its eggs to develop later into worms, why may not minute insects, invisible to the naked eye, deposit their offspring in our bodies, where they subsequently develop and destroy the tissues? He pointed out that the geographical limitations of yellow fever were consistent with an insect-transmitted cause for the disease. In 'the herding together of insects', he wrote, 'will be seen the locality of disease.'[1] Crawford, giving practical application to these principles, insisted upon absolute cleanliness and perfect hygiene in the matter of water, air, food, clothing, sewerage, and mode of life. He also taught that persons with infectious diseases should be isolated, and he used remedies with the object of destroying pathogenic organisms.

In 1804 Crawford decided to found a weekly journal as a literary venture. It was entitled *The Companion and Weekly Miscellany* and he wrote for it under the pseudonym Edward Easy. After two years he found the duties of editorship too demanding, so he asked his daughter Eliza to take over from him. She changed the title to *The Observer and Repertory of Original and Selected Essays*. She became the second woman to edit a journal in the United States and she wrote under the rather formidable name of Beatrice Ironside. It was in this new journal that she published her father's paper 'Remarks on Quarantines' in 1807. The paper was serialised over a period of weeks and it was followed by a further paper 'Dr Crawford's theory and application to the treatment of disease', in which he developed his ideas on infectious diseases. It is quite likely that Crawford decided to publish his papers in his daughter's magazine because he may have surmised that a lengthy exposition of his theories would be unacceptable to a medical journal at the time. Crawford used his detailed knowledge of the insect world to support his theory that disease is caused by living organisms and, according to the microbiologist Raymond Doetsh, he presented his arguments in a way which 'reveals both depth and scope of learning, and he constructs a forceful, if unexpected, analogy between the silent, savage struggles among insects and the cause of human infectious disease. This exposition is logical, detailed, and closely knit, and there is nothing similar to it by even the most ardent contagionist preceding him'.[3] Crawford pointed out that the victims are usually unaware of the attack on them, and he argued that the same could happen to man as he was an integral part of the struggle for survival in nature. Some of his arguments anticipated the work of Darwin over fifty years later.

Although they were not published in a medical journal, Crawford's concepts were discussed by his medical contemporaries in Baltimore and Philadelphia. His ideas also merited editorial comment in the *Medical Repository* for 1807:

> He denies that the yellow fever is either the off spring of contagion or of gaseous effluvia. But in a long chain of reasoning, he labours to prove that distemper, and indeed all other epidemics, are consequences of ANIMALCULAR ACTION UPON HUMAN BODIES. When great swarms of these invisible creatures attack mankind at once, they excite diseases, which assume specific forms, according to the number and nature of the assailants. And as dropsy may be caused by the hydatid animal, and itch by the psoric animal, so may dysentery be caused by intestinal animals, and yellow fever and other fevers by their appropriate species of animalculae....
>
> For ourselves, who are believers in the chemical theory, we must refer such of our readers as wish further proofs of Dr C's learning and ingenuity, to his original dissertation.[1]

Some physicians used Crawford's unorthodox views on the transmission of infection to undermine his practice. His friend Benjamin Rush also disagreed with his hypothesis, but this did not damage their relationship. On 16 November 1808 Rush noted in his diary that he had received a visit from Crawford, and he added that the latter:

> had lost all his business by propagating an unpopular opinion in medicine, namely, that all diseases were occasioned by animalculae. He said he was sixty-two years of age and not worth a cent, but in debt.[1]

He did however receive some recognition from his colleagues as in 1809 his paper on contagion was published in the *Baltimore Medical and Physical Recorder*.

Seventy years were to pass before Crawford's views on insects as carriers of disease were vindicated. In 1878 Sir Patrick Manson (1844–1922) showed that *Wuchereria Bancrofti*, the cause of filiarial elephantiasis in man develops in, and is transmitted by, the Culex mosquito. This was the first proof that infectious diseases could be spread by animal vectors.

PUBLIC SERVICE

Apart from his interest in medicine, Crawford was very active in his community. He spent seventeen years in Baltimore and among the projects he helped to initiate were the Baltimore Public Library, the Maryland Society for Promoting Useful Knowledge, and the Maryland Penitentiary. He was an active member of the Hibernian Benevolent Society from the earliest period of its existence and he held several offices in it. A letter from a contemporary gives a vivid description of Crawford's house on Hanover Street in Baltimore:

> This house is miserably out of sorts, but it's so like the houses of men of Genius with whom I have been all my life more or less acquainted that everything appears right.... The dining room is very dirty and dark and has a stove in it. Dr Crawford's library is black with smoke, and covered with dust, cumbered with papers, and choked with books, bookcases and desks. In the midst of all this his giant figure sits on an easy chair. He is a true Milesian gentleman, his society and conversation is delightful, and

instructive, and he rides his hobby agreeably.[1]

Crawford was a keen bibliophile, and after his death in 1813 his daughter put the following advertisement in the paper:

> Those gentlemen who have been in the habit of borrowing books from the late Dr Crawford are earnestly solicited to examine their libraries, and if any belonging to him should be found to return them to the subscriber without delay.[1]

A significant portion of Crawford's library was sold after his death to the University of Maryland, and the collection has been preserved by the university. It numbers about four hundred items and is the oldest private medical library in continuous existence in the United States.

7 Outstanding surgeon of the nineteenth century

Abraham Colles was the most outstanding Irish surgeon of the nineteenth century. He was born in Kilkenny in 1773 and he received his early education at Kilkenny College, an institution which had many famous pupils, including Berkeley, Swift and Congreve. During his time in Kilkenny a flood in the river Nore severely damaged the house of a local doctor named Butler and swept a book of anatomy downstream where it was picked up by the young Colles in a meadow near his father's house. When he went to return the book the doctor presented it to him and the incident is said to have had a significant influence on Colles' choice of profession. In September 1790 he entered Trinity College Dublin, and at the same time he became an apprentice to Philip Woodroffe, surgeon to Dr Steevens' Hospital and the Dublin Foundling Hospital (which stood on the site of the present St James's Hospital). He also became a registered pupil of the Royal College of Surgeons in Ireland.

Colles was a bright student and Edmund Burke, who was a family acquaintance, is said to have suggested that he would make a good writer. However Colles did not seek honours in the Arts course at Trinity, where his brother William was elected a scholar in 1793. He gained most of his clinical experience at Dr Steevens' Hospital but in the

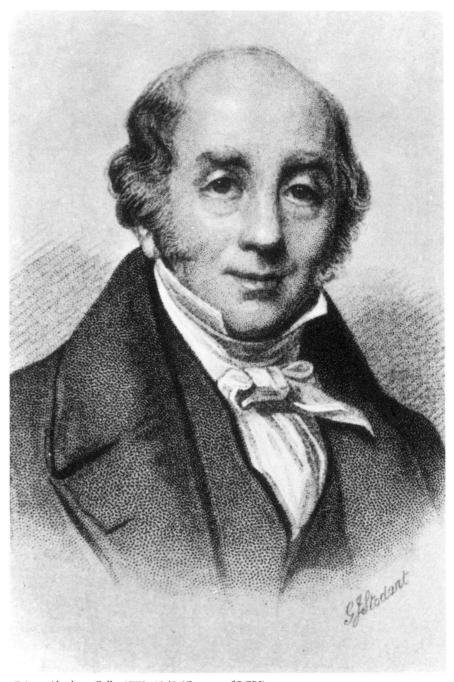

7.1   Abraham Colles 1773–1843 (Courtesy of RCPI)

winter session of 1793/4 he also attended the lectures of Stephen Dickson, King's professor of the practice of medicine, and Robert Perceval, professor of chemistry at Trinity College. In the spring of 1795 Colles graduated BA and in the summer of the same year he was granted Letters Testimonial by the College of Surgeons.

A STUDENT AT EDINBURGH

After graduating Colles decided to travel to Edinburgh where a school of medicine had been built up earlier in the century by Alexander Monro. It drew its inspiration from Leiden where all five of its original professors had been students of Herman Boerhaave. When Abraham Colles arrived in Edinburgh in September 1795 the medical school was at the height of its fame. Medical students were descending on the city from all over the world, particularly from Ireland. Colles soon settled into the routine in Edinburgh and in April 1796 he wrote:

> I must begin by telling you that I am much improved in point of personal appearance and accomplishments; for, having this day cast aside my winter clothes and put on my summer dress, my landlady could not be restrained, even by the dictates of female modesty, from telling me that I was a very 'spry buck', and recommending me very strongly to wear hair-powder. I need scarcely tell you that, strong as my pride is, it could not persuade me to go to the expense of six guineas a year.[1]

Colles graduated MD from Edinburgh in 1797, after defending a thesis on venesection. The MD was the basic degree of Edinburgh University as opposed to the MB degree of the Oxford, Cambridge and Dublin universities. This was an important factor in making Edinburgh so popular with students at that time. The majority of those qualifying with Colles were Irish. English students formed the next biggest group and the Scots formed the third. This was a persistent pattern during the last quarter of the eighteenth century. Colles realised that this pattern was damaging the prestige of medicine in Dublin and that it was a sad reflection on the medical schools in the city. However, the standards of medical teaching in Dublin would have to be markedly improved if the city were to compete successfully with Edinburgh. He was determined to play an active part in the great effort which would be required to remedy the situation.

REBELLION IN IRELAND

Colles spent a few months in London where he worked with the distinguished surgeon Ashley Cooper, before returning to Dublin in November 1797. It was a time of great upheaval in Ireland and the country was on the verge of revolution. Over the following twelve months Colles would watch the tragic events unfold as the 1798 rebellion was suppressed with ruthless efficiency. Several of the medical fraternity were either sympathisers or active members of the United Irishmen. William Dease, the leading surgeon of the time and first professor of surgery in the College of Surgeons, was warned that he was about to be arrested for treason. His sudden death, almost certainly by his own hand, must have grieved Colles as he had been one of Dease's pupils.

Colles did not become involved in the rebellion. His health was not very good and he spent some time in the country. He may have thought it unwise to stay in the city at a time when so many of his former associates were openly implicated in rebellion. In 1798 he gave his services free for a time to the Dispensary for the Sick Poor in Meath Street. He became a member of the Royal College of Surgeons in Ireland, and in 1802 he was elected president of the college at the age of twenty-nine.

DISPUTE WITH TRINITY COLLEGE

The chair of anatomy and chirurgery at Trinity became vacant in 1802 when James Cleghorn resigned. He had not been as successful a professor as his uncle, George Cleghorn, and the School of Physic had declined during his years in the chair. For some time before his retirement, his duties as professor were undertaken by William Hartigan, who had previously been professor of anatomy and surgery in the College of Surgeons. Hartigan did not have a university degree and Trinity had awarded him an honorary MD so that he could act as locum

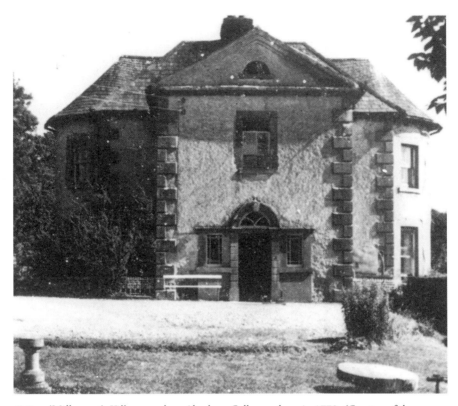

7.2   'Millmount', Kilkenny, where Abraham Colles was born in 1773. (Courtesy of the
Kilkenny People)

professor. He was popular with his students but he was rather eccentric.
He was very fond of cats and he frequently went out on his professional
visits with kittens ensconced in his coat pockets. Colles had been taught
by Hartigan in the College of Surgeons but now he challenged his old
teacher for the chair in Trinity College. Hartigan was appointed and the
aggrieved Colles took an action against the university, claiming that his
opponent was not qualified properly. The court found in favour of the
university and Colles never again applied for a post in Trinity.

ACADEMIC RECOGNITION

In June 1799 Colles' former teacher Philip Woodroffe died and Colles
was appointed to succeed him as resident surgeon to Dr Steevens'

Hospital. He was a very careful surgeon and from the outset of his career he had an analytical tendency. He was often critical of his own performance:

> This day I removed a cancer. My anxiety for my own character was the predominant sensation at the commencement of the operation: but this gradually wore off, and I soon felt for the success of the operation as if it had been a child of my own, or rather I felt as if I had performed some piece of mechanical work and was anxious for its success. My anxiety at the beginning of the operation was greater than I wish it to be on any future occasion, but on the whole I was well pleased that my state of mind had been such as it was.[2]

In 1804 his academic ability was recognised by his appointment to the chair of anatomy and physiology and to the chair of surgery in the College of Surgeons. Colles soon drew large crowds to his lectures and the college became so successful that it was necessary to expand the building on St Stephen's Green in 1825. His success helped to improve the status of the surgeon who was considered at the time to be inferior to the physician in social rank. Colles later recalled 'That at the commencement of his professional career in Dublin, when a consultation or any important case was held, the surgeon was not as a rule permitted to be in the room where the physicians held their deliberations, but after the consultation was over he was informed whether his services would be required or not'.[3]

Although he was now professor in a rival medical school, Colles did not lose his affection for his old university. He received an MA degree from Trinity College in 1832, and his five sons also graduated there, one of them eventually becoming professor of surgery in the university. During his lifetime Abraham Colles made several pleas for increased co-operation between hospitals and teaching institutions so that Dublin could attract more medical students from abroad. Unfortunately his advice fell on deaf ears. Seven years after his death a major dispute occurred between the College of Surgeons and Trinity College when the former refused to accept Trinity's certificates in surgery for its licence. Trinity responded by introducing its own licence in surgery in 1851, an MCh degree in 1858 and a BCh degree in 1872, thus becoming the first university to grant degrees in surgery.

In 1811 Colles published his first book *A Treatise on Surgical Anatomy*. This book earned him several eponyms, including Colles' Fascia in the perineum and Colles' Ligament in the inguinal area. The major significance of the work was the emphasis it placed on topographical anatomy, which deals with the precise positional relationship of the various structures within the body. Doctors now began to come from all over the world to see him operate at Dr Steevens' Hospital. He trained a number of men who subsequently became very distinguished, including the anatomist Benjamin Alcock, the eye surgeon Arthur Jacob, and the eye and ear surgeon William Wilde.

COLLES' FRACTURE

On 21 February 1814 Colles submitted his classical paper 'On the fracture of the carpal extremity of the radius' to the *Edinburgh Medical and Surgical Journal*:

> The injury to which I wish to direct the attention of surgeons has not as far as I am aware been described by any author; indeed the form of the carpal extremity of the radius would rather incline us to question its being liable to fracture. The absence of crepitus and of other common symptoms of fracture, together with the swelling which instantly arises in this, as in other injuries of the wrist, render the difficulty of ascertaining the real nature of the case very considerable.[4]

When he wrote this paper, Colles had not had the opportunity to check his observations by dissection, yet his description of the condition was so accurate that the many papers which have been written since then on the subject have added little to our knowledge. He described the impaction, the deformity, the ease of reduction and the difficulty of maintaining it, and he suggested a satisfactory method of treatment.

Colles did not gain immediate recognition for his description. His work was later rescued from oblivion by another Dublin surgeon, Robert William Smith, in his *Treatise on Fractures in the Vicinity of the Joints* (1847). When describing the fracture Smith remarked, 'It is certainly very extraordinary that although the pathology and treatment of this injury were fully and accurately described by Mr Colles so long back as April 1814 not a single British or foreign author who has written since has made the slightest reference to Mr Colles' name in connection with the subject, even when almost quoting his words.'[5]

WORK ON VENEREAL DISEASES

Colles wrote on syphilis and he published a book on the subject in 1837. In those pre-antibiotic days the treatment of syphilis, a disease which could cause horrible deformities, was a major problem. Mercury had been used as a treatment for the condition for many centuries. One of the effects of the drug was to stimulate the production of saliva, and physicians and surgeons judged the efficacy of the treatment by the amount of saliva produced. Large pewter mugs were kept in Dr Steevens' Hospital for the patients to spit into, and the dose of mercury was adjusted depending on the number of mugs filled during the day. Huge doses were frequently used and the side effects of the therapy were often worse than those of the disease being treated. Many who were cured were left without teeth and with permanently damaged kidneys.

Abraham Colles believed strongly in the efficacy of mercury treatment but he maintained that the best results were obtained with small doses of the agent. In a chapter on syphilis in infants he described what subsequently became known as 'Colles' Law'.

> One fact well deserving our attention is this: that a child born of a mother who is without any obvious venereal symptoms, and which, without being exposed to any infection subsequent to its birth, shows this disease when a few weeks old, this child will infect the most healthy nurse, whether she suckle it, or merely handle and dress it; and yet this child is never known to infect its own mother, even though she suckle it while it has venereal ulcers of the lips and tongue.[6]

The development of serological tests for syphilis has shown that the reason a mother did not develop the infection from her baby was due to the fact that she already had the disease in a latent form.

Colles' book on venereal diseases, which was also published in America and translated into German, was considered to be one of his best works. He was criticised by *The Lancet*, however, for not acknowledging the contributions made in this field by his contemporary William Wallace (1791–1837), who was on the staff of Jervis Street Hospital in Dublin. Between 1819 and his death in 1837 Wallace published five books and nearly thirty papers. His most successful work was *A Treatise on the Venereal Disease and its Varieties* which was published in 1833. This book contained the first description of the sexually transmitted infection 'lymphogranuloma venereum' which Wallace called 'indolent primary syphilitic bubo'. Wallace was the first to introduce potassium iodide as a treatment for syphilis and this therapy was used during the latter half of the nineteenth century. In a series of experiments he established beyond doubt that secondary syphilis was contagious. He published most of his original work in *The Lancet*, which probably explains why the journal attacked Colles for neglecting to give him credit.

Colles had retired from the chair of surgery because of ill-health shortly before the publication of his book on venereal disease. He had frequent attacks of gout and he suffered from troublesome dyspnoea. In 1840 he was treated for severe dyspnoea by William Stokes and he was advised to resign his hospital appointment and travel to Switzerland. He deteriorated on his return and he wondered if he had valvular heart disease and not, as Stokes had thought, bronchitis and a dilated heart. He developed marked oedema and hepatomegaly, and mercury appeared to relieve the symptoms. Before his death he arranged that a post-mortem examination of his body should be carried out by Dr Robert Smith. He thought it would be of benefit 'to ascertain by examination the exact seat and nature of my last disease. The parts to which I would direct particular attention are the heart and lungs, a small hernia immediately above the umbilicus, and the swelling in the right hypochondrium'.[7]

Colles died in 1843 and the post-mortem was performed as requested by Smith. The findings revealed a fibrotic left lung and a dilated heart without valvular heart disease, as Stokes had correctly diagnosed. Colles was a foundation president of the famous Pathological Society of Dublin and no doubt the members were very conscious of this when Smith read out his post-mortem findings to the society at their meeting on 9 December 1843.

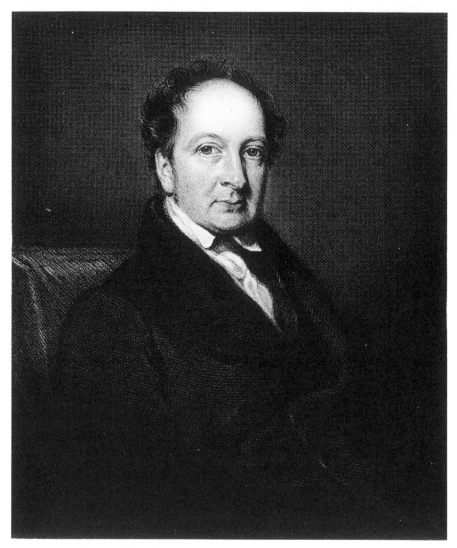

8.1   John Cheyne 1777–1836 (Courtesy of RCPI)

JOHN CHEYNE
1777–1836

8 A founder of the Irish school of medicine

The Battle of Vinegar Hill marked the end of the 1798 rebellion in Wexford. Government troops defeated the poorly organised Catholic rebels and they exacted a terrible revenge by slaughtering thousands in cold blood. It cannot have been a pleasant sight for the army medical officers present on the field of combat. One of these was John Cheyne, a twenty-one-year-old Scotsman from Leith near Edinburgh, who is now remembered for the historical role which he played in the development of medicine in Ireland. Medicine had been in his family for many generations and his father, grandfather and great-grandfather had been members of the Edinburgh College of Surgeons. According to T J Pettigrew, one of Cheyne's early biographers, his mother was: 'An ambitious woman, of honourable principles, constantly stimulating her children to exertion, and intently occupied with their advancement in life.'[1]

In his thirteenth year Cheyne began to assist his father in his practice. Three years later he enrolled as a medical student at Edinburgh. He qualified in 1795 and immediately joined the Royal Regiment of Artillery at Woolwich as assistant surgeon. In 1797 he was promoted to the rank of surgeon and dispatched to Ireland with a brigade of horse artillery. Although he was present at the main actions with the Irish rebel forces, he spent most of his time shooting game, playing billiards and reading books supplied through a circulating library. He found the lifestyle unfulfilling and so he resolved to undertake some further postgraduate studies.

WORK WITH CHARLES BELL

In 1799 he returned to Scotland where he was placed in charge of the Leith Ordnance Hospital. He also became an assistant in his father's practice. He worked with the famous surgeon Sir Charles Bell whose name is associated with facial paralysis:

> At this period I formed a friendship with Mr. afterwards Sir Charles Bell, who was occupied in the study of pathology, laying the foundation of future eminence. He opened most of the bodies which I obtained permission to dissect, taught me many things which I might not otherwise have learned, and confirmed my taste for distinction. As an example of diligence in study he could not be surpassed, and it was already manifest that he was a man of genius.[2]

Cheyne took a particular interest in the cause and management of fever and in children's diseases.

SERIES OF APPOINTMENTS

Cheyne never lost his interest in Ireland and after nine years he decided to revisit Dublin. Another factor which almost certainly had a major influence on his decision to investigate the possibility of a career in Ireland, was his marriage to Sarah Macartney, the daughter of the vicar of Antrim. Sarah stayed with her father in Antrim while Cheyne explored the medical scene in Dublin. He found that the Irish physicians relied chiefly upon symptomatology and that they largely ignored pathology. Because of this, much of the purely medical practice was in the hands of surgeons. Cheyne concluded that there were good prospects for a physician and so he decided to commence practice in the city. He became a licentiate of the College of Physicians in 1811 and in the same year he was appointed physician to the Meath Hospital. Two years later he was appointed professor of medicine in the College of Surgeons. He was the first to fill the chair, which had been established at the request of the British Army Medical Board, and he occupied it for six years. His lectures were mainly on military surgery and medicine and they were attended by army and naval surgeons as well as regular pupils of the college. In 1815 he resigned his position in the Meath on his appointment as physician to the House of Industry Hospitals (The Richmond Hospital) in Brunswick Street:

> I had there to visit daily upwards of seventy patients in acute diseases, most of these labouring under fever, of whom probably eight or ten demanded careful examination. As I had experienced and well trained sick-nurses, who allowed nothing to escape their observation, the rest of the patients required only a glance of the eye; so that the visit was always finished in little more than an hour. But I have ever experienced great fatigue from that stretch of mind which arises from going the round of an hospital. Then the walk to and fro occupied more than an hour, and I invariably reached home much exhausted; I therefore felt it necessary to resign my professorship at the College of Surgeons, as well as my charge of the Meath Hospital, that my private practice, which in 1816 yielded £1,710, might not suffer by the extent of my official duties.[3]

PROLIFIC WRITER

In collaboration with others, Cheyne launched the *Dublin Hospital Reports* in 1815. However, as William Wilde has pointed out:

> The main projector of the undertaking was Cheyne, who to his great sagacity and vast medical acquirements united that activity of mind and untiring energy and perseverance, as well as the art of eliciting the knowledge and bringing forth the powers and acquirements of others, together with a stern honesty of purpose, and a suavity of manner — qualities rare, but very essential in the editor of a periodical.[4]

The papers which he wrote for this journal set the standard for the subsequent famous work of the physicians and surgeons who would form the Irish school of medicine. William Stokes described these papers as models of clinical observation, presented with both accuracy and clarity. One of his most masterly papers was on the subject of fevers and it was published in the *Dublin Hospital Reports* in 1817. It is apparent from this report that Cheyne paid particular attention to his nurses, whom he trained and supervised himself. Each nurse carried a printed card of Cheyne's own instructions on patient care. According to the historian J D H Widdess, this is the first recorded attempt at nursing education in these islands.

Cheyne was a prolific writer and he published several books. *Essays on the Disease of Children* (1801) was produced in collaboration with Charles Bell, who illustrated the work. *Essays on Hydrocephalus Acutus* (1808), which contained the first detailed description of the condition, was published in Edinburgh and was dedicated to Charles Bell. Seven years later he published *A Second Essay on Hydrocephalus Acutus* in Dublin, and this was dedicated to Abraham Colles by his 'obliged colleague and friend'. *The Pathology of the Larynx and Bronchia* (1809) was also illustrated by Bell and it is an important early monograph on laryngology. In 1812 he published a work entitled *Cases of Apoplexy and Lethargy, with Observations of Comatose Diseases*. It was 224 pages long and contained five plates. The most widely read book today on the same subject is *Diagnosis of Stupor and Coma* by the American neurologists Fred Plum and Jerome Posner. They honour Cheyne by using the title page of his book on coma as a frontispiece for their own work.

Cheyne is chiefly remembered for his description of the respiratory pattern observed in patients with cerebrovascular disorders and other conditions which lead to a lowering of the sensitivity of the respiratory centre. Cheyne published his description in a paper entitled 'A case of apoplexy, in which the fleshy part of the heart was converted into fat', which appeared in the *Dublin Hospital Reports* in 1818:

A.B. sixty years of age, of a sanguine temperament, circular chest, and full habit of body, for years had lived a very sedentary life, while he indulged habitually in the luxuries of the table....

His appetite being remarkably keen, he ate more than usual, and took at least a pint of port wine or Madeira daily, as was his habit, and this notwithstanding a hard frequent cough, which came on after I was consulted by him....

On the 10th of April he was found in bed flushed, speechless, and hemiplegiac. How long he had been in that state could not be ascertained, as he had peremptorily ordered his servant not to remain in the chamber with him, and not to come to him in the morning till called. All attempts to relieve him were unavailing; his right side continued powerless, and his attempts to articulate were vain. The only peculiarity in the last period of his illness, which lasted eight or nine days, was in the state of the respiration: For several days his breathing was irregular; it would entirely cease for a quarter of a minute, then it would become perceptible, though very low, then by degrees it became heaving and quick, and then it would gradually cease again: this revolution in the state of his breathing occupied about a minute, during which there were about thirty acts of respiration.[5]

This phenomenon was described again by William Stokes in 1846 and it is now known throughout the medical world as 'Cheyne-Stokes Respiration'. The patient described by Stokes was also about sixty years old:

For more than two months before his death, this singular character of respiration was always present, and so long would the periods of suspension be, that his attendants were frequently in doubt whether he was not actually dead. Then a very feeble, indeed barely perceptible inspiration would take place, followed by another somewhat stronger, until at length high heaving, and even violent breathing was established, which would then subside till the next period of suspension. This was frequently a quarter of a minute in duration.[6]

DEPRESSION AND DECLINE

In later years Cheyne lost much of his youthful enthusiasm for academic distinction and instead concentrated his efforts on securing a substantial income from his private practice in Ely Place. He had a large family of sixteen children and this must have helped to concentrate his mind on financial matters. In 1825 when Cheyne was in his forty-eighth year, he began to suffer from depression:

In the Autumn of that year dysentery proved fatal to many of the inhabitants of Dublin; disappointment often attended the means which

I employed for their relief, and a pretty constant depression of spirits was the consequence of unsatisfactory practice: at the same time my mind was harassed by anxieties not connected with my profession. I became so weak that I was not able to dress in the morning till I had had coffee, and when I returned from a day of toil at seven or eight o'clock in the evening, I was obliged to go to bed to obtain rest before I was able to dine. After a struggle of two months, I went to England, where I recovered some strength, and thought I was again able for business, to which I returned too soon. I found one of my most-esteemed professional friends, the father of 15 children, labouring under a disease which ultimately proved fatal. He had awaited my return, in order to put himself under my care. His sufferings proved an incubus on my spirits, which strangled every cheerful thought.[7]

He reduced his commitments but by 1831 he was finding his medical practice an intolerable burden and he resolved to retire to England. When it became apparent that Cheyne did not plan to return to Dublin, forty-five eminent physicians signed a letter asking him to reconsider his decision:

We cannot but deeply lament the absence of one who, whilst occupying for many years the first rank in his profession, equally maintained its respectability and protected our interests. In you we have witnessed the enlightened practitioner and experienced the disinterested friend. Faithful alike to your patients and your colleagues, you became pre-eminent without exciting jealousy. Your extensive information and sound practical judgement, the candour and kindness which you have ever shown to your brethren, and the sterling integrity and dignified deportment which have always been conspicuous in your intercourse with every member of the profession, have so fully commanded our highest esteem and unlimited confidence, that we should hail with sincere pleasure your return to that important station amongst us which you have so long and so deservedly occupied.[8]

Cheyne decided not to yield to their entreaties and he settled in the village of Sherrington in England. During his retirement he became increasingly preoccupied with religious subjects. He wrote a number of medical articles and his last book was entitled *Essays on Partial Derangement of the Mind.* He wrote this book during a period when one of his sons was very seriously ill. He also wrote an autobiographical sketch which he finished in 1835. His health began to deteriorate seriously soon after he had completed this and he died on 31 January 1836. He left very specific directions in his will:

> My body, attended only by my sons, is to be carried to the grave by six of the villagers, very early on the fourth or fifth morning after my decease. I would have no tolling of bells, if it can be avoided. The ringers may have an order for bread, to the amount usually given upon such occasions; if they get money they will spend it in the ale-house; and I would have them told, that in life or death I would by no means give occasion for sin. My funeral must be as inexpensive as possible: let there be no attempt at a funeral sermon. I would pass away without notice from a world which, with all its pretensions, is empty.[9]

It must have been very sad for Cheyne's relatives and friends, who had known him at the height of his abilities, to witness his last years being darkened by depression and a growing sense of personal worthlessness. It is clear from statements made by men such as Graves and Stokes that he had an enormous influence, through the high standards which he demanded of himself, in establishing the ground rules which ultimately led to the great success of the Irish school of medicine in the last century.

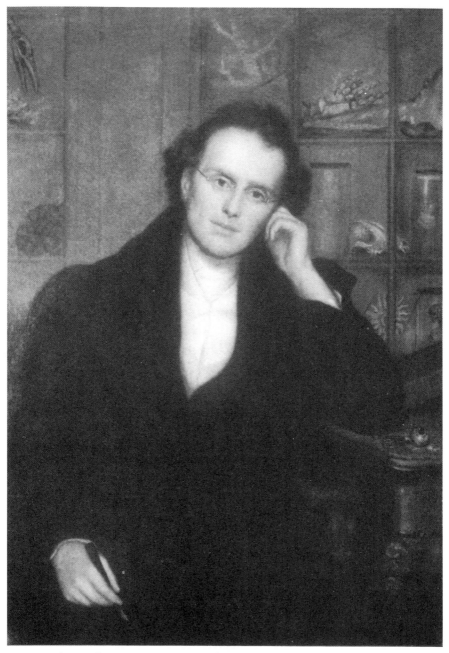

9.1   Arthur Jacob 1790–1874 (Courtesy of RCSI)

ARTHUR JACOB
1790–1874

9 Medical researcher and reformer

rthur Jacob was the first to discover the delicate membrane in the retina of the eye which contains the cellular structures upon which we depend for both colour and black and white vision. Jacob was born at Knockfin near Portlaoise on 13 June 1790. His father, John Jacob, was surgeon to the Queen's County Infirmary, and his grandfather, Michael Jacob, was also a surgeon. Arthur Jacob began his medical education when he was indentured to his father in 1808. Three years later he entered the College of Surgeons and became a pupil at Dr Steevens' Hospital under Abraham Colles. After qualifying he left Dublin in 1813 to continue his studies in Edinburgh where he graduated MD one year later. He then moved to London where he worked with some of the great medical men of that city, including Benjamin Brodie and Astley Cooper. He travelled to Paris to do some further postgraduate training but his visit was cut short by the political upheaval caused by Napoleon's escape from Elba.

OPHTHALMIC RESEARCH AND DISCOVERY

When Jacob returned to Dublin, Professor James Macartney invited him to lecture in his department at Trinity College on the anatomy, physiology and pathology of the eye, and to assist him at the dispensary which he had opened in 1814 for skin and eye problems. Macartney had already carried out some research on the anatomy of the eye and Jacob continued this work. Jacob's research was rewarded in 1819 when he published a paper describing his discovery of the bacillary layer of the retina. The work appeared in the *Philosophical Transactions* and the layer became known as Membrana Jacobi:

> I cannot describe it better, than by detailing the method to be adopted for examining and displaying it. Having procured a human eye, within forty-eight hours after death, a thread should be passed through the layers of the cornea, by which the eye may be secured under water, by attaching it to a piece of wax, previously fastened to the bottom of the vessel, the posterior half of the sclerotic having been first removed. With a pair of dissecting forceps in each hand, the choroid coat should be gently torn open and turned down. If the exposed surface be now carefully examined, an experienced eye may perceive, that this is not the appearance usually presented by the retina; instead of the blue-white reticulated surface of that membrane, a uniform villous structure, more or less tinged by the black pigment, presents itself. If the extremity of the ivory handle of a dissecting knife be pushed against this surface, a breach is made in it, and a membrane of great delicacy may be separated and turned down in folds over the choroid coat, presenting the most beautiful specimen of a delicate tissue which the human body affords.[1]

The layer which he identified was later recognised as that containing the light-sensitive cells known as rods and cones. In 1827 Jacob described 'an ulcer of peculiar character which attacks the eye lids and other parts of the face'.[2] This ulcer, which became known as Jacob's ulcer in the last century, is now called a rodent ulcer. Jacob was proud of his description and he never failed to draw it to the attention of subsequent writers who failed to mention his work:

> The characteristic features of this disease are the slowness of its progress, the peculiar condition of the edges and surface of the ulcer, the comparatively inconsiderable suffering produced by it, its incurable nature unless by extirpation, and its not contaminating the neighbouring lymphatic glands.[2]

He condemned local and general treatment and he emphasised that early surgical removal was the only hope of cure. This remained true until the advent of radiotherapy.

JACOB'S TREATMENT OF CATARACT

Jacob was particularly adept at the removal of cataracts by a process known as 'needling'. For this purpose he used an ordinary round sewing needle bent at the point. He has left us a vivid description of his technique:

> I seat the patient in a chair and make him sit straight up or inclining, according to his height. If very tall, I raise myself by standing on a large book or two, or on anything which answers the purpose to be found at hand. In my own place of business I find old medical folios answer the purpose well; operating chairs, although very imposing and calculated to produce effect, I have not adopted, not finding myself at ease with such things. When he is seated I lay the patient's head against my chest, and placing the middle finger of my left hand on his lower and the forefinger on his upper eyelid, and gently holding the eye between them, I strike the point of the needle suddenly into the cornea, about a line from its margin, and there hold it until any struggles of the patient, which may be made, cease.[3]

Jacob broke up the cataract by this needling technique and he claimed that absorption took place remarkably quickly, patients sometimes being able to read within ten weeks. Speed and skill were critical in an operation such as this as it was performed in the pre-anaesthetic era.

HOSPITALS AND MEDICAL SCHOOLS

Jacob founded his own eye hospital in Kildare Street South in 1817. It was known as the Charitable Institute for the Cure of Diseases of the Skin and of the Eye. After four years he closed the hospital so that he could devote his energies to founding the Park Street School of Medicine. However, six years later he opened another ophthalmic hospital in Pitt Street (now Balfe Street) where he worked until he moved his practice to the new Royal City of Dublin Hospital in Baggot Street. He lived at 23 Ely Place with his wife Sarah and five sons.

In 1824 Jacob joined with James Cusack, Samuel Wilmot, Robert Graves, Henry Marsh and James Apjohn to found the Park Street School of Medicine. It is said that Cusack recommended that the school should be erected in the style of a Methodist meeting-house so that, in the event of the venture failing, the buildings could be sold for religious purposes. The building consisted of a large lecture theatre, a small one for chemical lectures, a dissecting room, a museum and some other rooms. Jacob lectured on anatomy and physiology at the Park Street School and Benjamin Alcock was one of his demonstrators. Robert Graves lectured on the institutes of medicine and toxicology and James Apjohn lectured on chemistry. William Stokes joined the school in 1828 to lecture on medicine. From 1837 John Houston lectured on anatomy, physiology and surgery and he built up an excellent museum which was subsequently sold to Queen's College, Belfast, for £250. The anatomist Hugh Carlisle became the principal proprietor of the school and in 1849, when he was appointed professor of anatomy in the newly established Queen's College, Belfast, the school was closed. It was then acquired by William Wilde and refurbished as an eye hospital. The building is still standing and it now houses the genetics department of Trinity College. This department, under the direction of Professor David McConnell, takes a major interest in the scientific aspects of medical genetics. Professor Peter Humphries and his team recently located two genes responsible for autosomal dominant retinitis pigmentosa. It appears that the condition is due to mutations within the genes for the light receptor protein rhodopsin and the structural protein peripherin, which are present in the membrane first described by Arthur Jacob.

The satirical writer who used the pseudonym Erinensis (now thought to be Dr Hennis Greene) has left us a description of the opening of the Park Street School. The inaugural lecture was to have been given by Samuel Wilmot, but he became ill and Jacob had to substitute for him. He gave the lecture in an amphitheatre which was crowded with some of the leading citizens of the city. Erinensis described Jacob as he appeared on the day:

He was harnessed in a pair of spectacles, so admirably fitted to the prominences and depressions of the orbitary processes that one might have mistaken the whole optical apparatus as a natural production of the parts, or an expansion of the cornea spread out upon a delicate frame of silver wire.[4]

After apologising for Wilmot's absence, Jacob proceeded to give a lecture on comparative anatomy. Under the cloak of anonymity, Erinensis gave free vent to his wit in his description of the lecture:

He principally trusted to his memory for what he had to say, but the treacherous jade betrayed him in almost every sentence.... The great excellence, however, of this *spree* prelection consisted in the minute fidelity with which the speaker gave practical illustrations of animal locomotion. With the albatross, he seemed about to take wing and leave us all behind him; the penguin soon brought him down again to the very depths of the ocean; with the snail, his fingers crept along the wall, ... but we confess, when he came to illustrate the fantastic tricks of the monkey tribe, he looked the character to such perfection, that we could not help considering it, of all the characters he assumed, as his *forte*.[5]

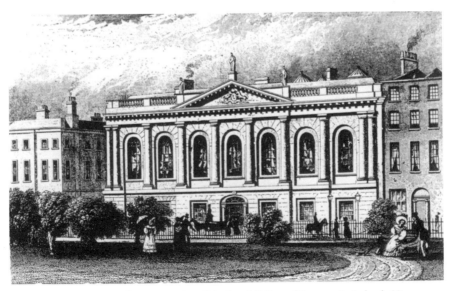

9.2   *An early nineteenth-century print of the Royal College of Surgeons in Ireland. (Courtesy of RCSI)*

In 1826 Jacob was appointed professor of anatomy and physiology at the College of Surgeons, and in 1828 he was nominated in the Second Charter granted in that year by George IV as one of the six censors of the college. Jacob was to occupy the chair of anatomy and physiology in the College of Surgeons for no less than forty-one years. He served as president of the college on two occasions, in 1837 and 1864.

CAREER AS EDITOR

For a short period in 1836 Jacob joined Graves and Stokes to edit the *Dublin Journal of Medical Science*. The relationship appears to have been an unhappy one and his connection with the journal was discontinued. However, he realised that there was a need for a medical newspaper, so he decided, with Dr Henry Maunsell, to establish the *Dublin Medical Press* in 1838. Maunsell occupied the chair of midwifery at the College of Surgeons. He had already published a book on obstetrics, *The Dublin Practice of Midwifery*, in 1834, and two years later in conjunction with Richard Evanson, a lecturer in the Park Street School, he wrote *Treatise on the Diseases of Children*, which went into several editions both at home and abroad.

Jacob and Maunsell were reformers who were determined to improve the lot of the Irish doctor; they planned to use the *Dublin Medical Press* to unify the medical profession. They worked with Richard Carmichael towards the establishment of a medical association which would represent the views of Irish doctors. Carmichael chaired the first meeting of the Medical Association of Ireland in 1839 at the Royal College of Surgeons. The *Dublin Medical Press* under Jacob's leadership maintained a constant campaign to improve the working conditions of doctors, particularly the poorly paid dispensary doctor. It was quick to condemn abuses within the medical profession and it highlighted the practice of fee splitting and nepotism in appointments. It also drew attention to the appalling conditions of the Dublin slums.

In 1848 Jacob published his only book, *A Treatise on Inflammation of the Eye Ball*, which drew attention to social conditions among the poor as a major cause of ocular inflammation. Jacob also carried out research and published work on comparative anatomy. One summer he set off for the west of Ireland on hearing that a dead whale had been found floating off the coast. Although it had probably been dead for six weeks, he dissected it while it was floating and brought the specimens back to his museum. On another occasion he bought a whale that had been washed ashore on Killiney Strand near Dublin and dissected it there.

Two of Jacob's contemporaries, Joseph O'Ferrall and Samuel Bigger, also contributed to the development of eye surgery. O'Ferrall was the first doctor on the staff of St Vincent's Hospital when it opened in 1835. In 1841 he wrote a paper for the *Dublin Journal of Medical Science* in which he advocated the enucleation of the eyeball for diseases confined to it, instead of the risky operation of emptying the entire orbit, which had been the mode of operation up to that time. Samuel Lennox Bigger, who qualified from Trinity College in 1834, was a pioneer in corneal grafting. In 1835, while a prisoner of a nomadic tribe of Arabs 'about twelve or fourteen days journey from Cairo', he operated successfully on a blind pet gazelle.[6] He obtained the donor cornea from another gazelle which was brought in badly wounded but not quite dead. Forty years were to elapse before the real significance of Bigger's achievement was appreciated, namely, that to be successful a transplant must be homologous.

MAN OF HUMILITY

Jacob was one of the founders of the City of Dublin Hospital, Baggot Street, in 1852. He devoted all his time to his professional and editorial duties and to his research. He had no time for hobbies or festivities and he had an ever-present fear of showing the smallest indication of self-aggrandisement. When his colleagues decided to honour him by presenting him with a gold medal, he told them, 'I cannot accept of this or any other testimonial, but if at my death you shall think that I deserve it, you may nail it on my coffin.'[3] However he subsequently changed his mind and was persuaded to accept the honour. He was granted the honorary degree of Doctor of Medicine by Trinity College in 1863. Six years later Jacob resigned his professorship and retired to Barrow-in-Furness in Lancashire, where he died on 21 September 1874, aged eighty-four.

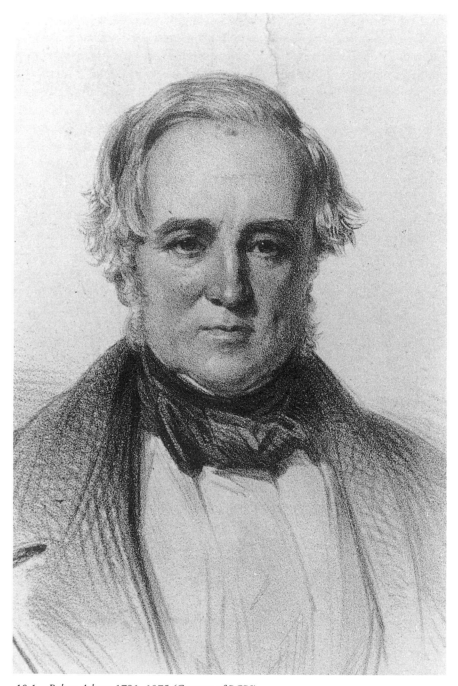

10.1   *Robert Adams 1791–1875 (Courtesy of RCPI)*

ROBERT ADAMS
1791–1875

10 *Surgeon and cardiologist*

Although Robert Adams was a surgeon he is remembered today primarily for the major contributions which he made to the development of cardiology. He was born in 1791 and was the son of a Dublin solicitor. He studied at Trinity College and at the College of Surgeons. He was apprenticed to William Hartigan, and when the latter died he transferred to George Stewart, surgeon-general to the Forces in Ireland. He graduated BA in 1814 and in 1815 he became a licentiate of the College of Surgeons. He then went on a tour of the Continent, visiting the hospitals of the best surgical teachers of the day. When he returned to Dublin he was appointed to the staff of the Charitable Infirmary and he became a member of the Royal College of Surgeons. He did not take his MB degree until 1842, and in the same year he received an MD from Trinity College.

Adams established a medical school in the stable of his home near Marlborough Street, but this came to an untimely end when it was attacked and burnt by an irate mob objecting to the practice of body snatching. After the destruction of Adams' school another young Dublin doctor, O'Bryen Bellingham, rented him his coach house and stable in Eccles Street and both men collaborated in developing a new school.

81

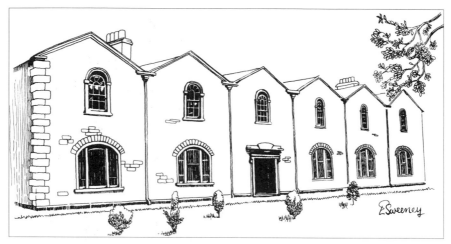

10.2   *The medical school built by James MacCartney in Trinity in 1825. Part of this building still survives, although it is surrounded by more recent structures.*

Bellingham, the son of a baronet, had a distinguished career ahead of him. He joined Joseph O'Ferrall on the staff of St Vincent's Hospital and he developed an international reputation for his treatment of aneurysms by compression. He also wrote a book entitled *Diseases of the Heart* which he dedicated to his life-long friend Arthur Jacob.

Adams was apparently very fond of horses and always had a good one to draw his chaise. He was very sociable and had a great store of anecdotes, even his intimate friends could scarcely recall him ever telling the same story twice. He lived at 22 St Stephen's Green, next door to Abraham Colles, and over a period of time he built up a very successful surgical practice. A large part of his success in surgery was attributed to his remarkable sense of judgement.

THE RICHMOND SCHOOL OF MEDICINE

In 1827 Adams, in association with Richard Carmichael, founded the Richmond School of Medicine and Surgery in a large old house in Channel-row, opposite the Richmond Hospital. This school became known as the Carmichael School of Medicine later in the century and it eventually amalgamated with the Royal College of Surgeons. Adams gave the introductory lecture on 'The History of Medicine' at the opening of the teaching year at the Richmond School in 1828. Dr Hennis Greene (Erinensis), the satirical correspondent of *The Lancet*, was in the audience and he was not very impressed. The weather was dull on the day of the lecture so Green stretched himself on the bench and dozed whilst waiting for Adams:

> A gentleman, of rather short stature, with black bushy hair, a degree of affrighted expression in his looks, a few of what we call in Ireland 'grog-blossoms' scattered over his face, and dressed in a suit of seedy black, entered the theatre, and proceeded to read from a paper certain sentences, the import of which the unparalleled rapidity of their recital entirely prevented us for some time from learning. Exercising that faculty of seeing and hearing while asleep which the constant habit of critical vigilance has endowed us with, we endeavoured to catch the tenor of discourse, but all in vain, until the announcement of the name of Hippocrates warned us of the approach of a history of medicine for about five-and-twenty centuries, and of the propriety of indulging ourselves in the luxury of insensibility to so terrible an infliction, through the means of sound sleep.[1]

STOKES-ADAMS SYNDROME

Adams was a prolific writer and he wrote about many subjects which would have been considered to be in the domain of the physician. He made more than one hundred contributions to medical literature. He published his most famous paper in the *Dublin Hospital Reports* in 1827, entitled 'Cases of diseases of the heart accompanied with pathological observations'. In this paper he described a patient suffering from blackouts associated with a pulse rate of thirty beats per minute. The patient was a sixty-eight-year-old revenue officer whom Adams saw just as he was recovering from an episode of unconsciousness. He got an interesting history from the patient's own medical attendant:

> He had been in almost continual attendance on this gentleman for the last seven years; and that during that period he had seen him, he is quite certain, in not less than 20 apoplectic attacks. Before each of them he was observed, for a day or two, heavy and lethargic with loss of memory.

He would fall down in a state of complete irreversibility and was on several occasions hurt by the fall. When they attacked him, his pulse would become even slower than usual his breathing loudly stertorous.[2]

Adams made the connection between the slow pulse and the loss of consciousness and he was the first to appreciate that cerebral symptoms may be caused by disorders of the cardiac rhythm. Nearly twenty years later William Stokes published further observations on this condition, which included a careful analysis of Adams' case. The names of both men are now linked together as the condition is known as Stokes-Adams syndrome.

William Stokes spoke highly of Adams in his famous book *Diseases of the Heart and Aorta* which was published in 1854:

Among the contributions to our knowledge upon this subject which have appeared since the time of Laënnec, the researches of Dr Adams are to be placed first in rank of importance, as they are in time of publication. His memoir, which appeared in 1827, may be held to mark a period midway between that of the discoverer of auscultation and of the investigators of the present time. In this memoir, ... he shows the effect of mitral obstruction in causing enlargement not only of the left auricle but of the right ventricle. Again the doctrines as to the pulsation in the jugular veins, synchronous with the ventricular systole, and the natural insufficiency of the tricuspid valves are here fully developed; and the special modifications of the form of the heart, according to the predominance of the disease in the auriclo-ventricular, or the aortic valves, are accurately described. Lastly, the mechanism and effects of the regurgitant diseases of the mitral valves are detailed and exemplified; and if all were wanting to establish Dr Adams' character as a philosophical observer, it is the dignified silence which he has maintained, while subsequent writers have laid claims to discoveries of facts which he long before had announced.[3]

Stokes-Adams syndrome was the first Irish cardiac eponym. In recent times two Irish doctors, Conor Ward and Frank Pantridge, have also gained eponymous fame for work relating to disorders of cardiac rhythm. In 1963 Ward, formerly professor of paediatrics at University College Dublin, described a serious arrhythmia in children, which is associated with episodes of loss of consciousness (The Romano-Ward syndrome). Pantridge, who worked as a cardiologist in Belfast, introduced pre-hospital coronary care in 1965 and he also developed a portable defibrillator (the Pantridge defibrillator) to treat life-threatening arrhythmias. Clinical contributions such as these maintain the high standards in Irish cardiology which were originally established by Adams and Stokes.

SURGICAL APPOINTMENT

In 1838 a vacancy arose on the staff of the Richmond Hospital and Robert Adams and John McDonnell competed for the position. Both candidates were very able and the Board had great difficulty in deciding which one to appoint. In a generous gesture, Richard Carmichael resigned his post as surgeon to the hospital so that both men could be appointed. The new surgeons made major contributions to the development of the hospital in subsequent years. In was John McDonnell (1796–1892) who performed the first operation under anaesthesia in Ireland at the Richmond Hospital on New Year's Day 1847, within a few months of the first public demonstration of anaesthesia at the Massachusetts General Hospital in Boston. Rather appropriately, he asked Richard Carmichael and Robert Adams to assist him during the historic operation. Apart from his appointment to the Richmond Hospital, Adams also served on the consultant staff of the Rotunda and Sir Patrick Dun's Hospitals.

JOINT DISEASE AND SYNOVIAL CYSTS

Adams had a special interest in joint pathology and was the first to describe a synovial cyst. This he did at a meeting of the Dublin Pathological Society in 1840, when he was demonstrating some arthritic knee joints. Sir Philip Crampton was in the chair:

> The enlargement observed at the posterior surface of the joint is chiefly owing to the increased size of the bursa which lies under the internal head of the gastrocnemius. Mr Adams exhibited several specimens in illustration, and said that the attention of the Profession was now, for the

first time, directed to the enlarged bursa as a sign of this disease. This enlarged bursa is normally situated beneath the inner head of the gastrocnemius, and communicates with the joint by a species of valvular opening.[4]

The cyst which he described extended from the knee joint into the popliteal space. Many years later an English doctor, William Baker, reported his own observations on synovial cysts, giving rise to the common eponym Baker cysts for popliteal cysts.

In 1857 Adams published a book on rheumatoid arthritis entitled *A Treatise on Rheumatic Gout, or Chronic Rheumatic Arthritis, of all the Joints*, which went into a second edition in 1873. In the preface he acknowledged the help of his friend and colleague Robert Smith, who shared his interest in joint disease. Adams wrote that Smith had been associated with him in most of the post-mortem examinations described in the book.

Eight years later, at the age of seventy-four, Adams travelled to France to present his work on rheumatic diseases to the Surgical Society of Paris, despite the fact that he was suffering from severe arthritic problems himself. The president of the society received him with great honour, according to a short report of the meeting in the *British Medical Journal*.

A DISTINGUISHED CAREER

Adams became regius professor of surgery at Trinity College in 1861, when he was seventy years old. He was an enthusiastic teacher and was very proud of the achievements of the Dublin school of medicine. In an introductory lecture at the Richmond Hospital in 1860 he told his students:

And here let me mention, which I do not do in any spirit of ostentation, but as an incitement to young beginners to take advantage of their present opportunities, that there is not one of my colleagues who has not, from distant climes and colonies, from the seat of war itself, received letters expressive of the deepest gratitude from their pupils for the instructions afforded to them when within the walls of these hospitals, the value of which instructions they confessed they had not significantly estimated until they had been tested by the realities of disease and accident they had to encounter alone, and without colleague or consultant, in distant regions of the globe.[5]

When the new Queen's Colleges were established, Adams occupied a seat on the senate. In 1861 he was appointed surgeon to Queen Victoria. He served as president of the Royal College of Surgeons on three occasions, and he was also president of the Dublin Pathological Society. He was president of the College of Surgeons in 1867 when the British Medical Association visited Dublin, and he presided at the conferring of an honorary fellowship on William Bowman, the distinguished English surgeon and physiologist. The latter, in expressing his gratitude, mentioned a period when as a young student he had studied in Dublin:

> I found Colles, Cusack, yourself, sir, Carmichael, Porter; with Graves and Stokes in medicine, laboriously and richly turning to the best uses of science and of instruction the great opportunities you possessed — exhibiting yourselves to your students as students yourselves in the great field of nature, and imbuing them thus with your noble spirit as well as with your doctrines.... I am conscious that no reward which so humble an individual as myself can possibly receive for professional labours could be more flattering than the spontaneous and honourable testimony of the good opinion of such a corporation as yours. I may be permitted to say that its value is enhanced by the circumstance that in receiving it I stand by the side of one of the most distinguished men that any age of great surgeons had produced.[6]

Adams died in 1875 at the age of eighty-four. According to his obituary in the *British Medical Journal* he died in harness, working up to a short time before his death. The famous American cardiologist James Herrick paid him the following tribute in 1942: 'He was of greater brilliancy than has been generally recognised. He had in him the elements of the true clinical investigator and deserves more honourable mention in any history of cardiology.'[7]

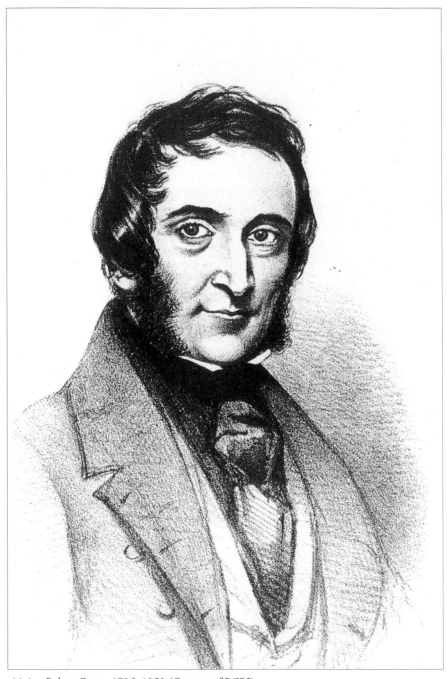

11.1   Robert Graves 1796–1853 (Courtesy of RCPI)

11 *International reputation as physician and teacher*

Although most doctors and medical students around the world would associate the name of Robert Graves with disease of the thyroid gland, few are aware of the key role he played in the development of bedside clinical teaching. He was the youngest son of Richard Graves DD, Dean of Ardagh, and he received his early education from the Reverend Ralph Wilde, an eminent scholar of Trinity College and an uncle of William Wilde. Graves obtained first place at the entrance examination to Trinity College in 1811 when he was just fifteen years old, and he maintained this place throughout his undergraduate career. He was equally gifted both at science and at classics. As a student he came under the influence of James Macartney, professor of anatomy and surgery, and as a result he became proficient in anatomy, which at that time was unusual for someone intending to be a physician.

POSTGRADUATE TRAINING

Graves graduated in 1818 and then studied in London for a short period before proceeding to the Continent where he spent the following three years. During this time he visited the most distinguished medical schools in Europe and met their leading professors. He studied under Stromeyer and Blumenbach at Göttingen, Cohlston in Copenhagen, and Hufeland and Behrend in Berlin. He also visited medical schools in France and Italy. Graves was very impressed by the emphasis placed on bedside teaching in Berlin and he decided that he would introduce this method of teaching on his return to Dublin. He spent a few months in Edinburgh on his homeward journey. During his travels on the Continent, Graves wrote regularly to Robert Perceval, the professor of chemistry at Trinity College, to whom he was related. Perceval had considerable political influence and he was largely instrumental in the building of Sir Patrick Dun's Hospital as a teaching hospital for Trinity College.

BEDSIDE TEACHING

Shortly after his return to Dublin, Graves was involved with others in founding the Park Street School of Medicine in 1824. When the institution opened Graves lectured on medical jurisprudence but he later taught pathological anatomy and the practice of physic. In the same year he was appointed physician to the Meath Hospital. Here he began to organise bedside teaching and his approach had a major influence on the development of clinical teaching throughout the English-speaking world. There were two elements to the radical changes which he introduced. The first involved the distribution of the care of patients to a larger number of advanced students than had previously been the case. Maurice Collis, a medical student in the Meath, recalled later that in the period immediately before Graves arrived, the number of clerks used to average around ten, but a few years later it had risen to seventy. The second element involved changing the scene of instruction from the lecture room of the hospital to the bedside of the patient. These changes developed the perceptive faculties of the students, encouraged careful habits of observation, and ensured that errors in clinical judgement were corrected on the spot. Graves encouraged the students to think carefully about medication and he stressed the importance of ensuring that the patient was able to afford the medication prescribed. The following extract from his first introductory lecture in the Meath Hospital in 1821 gives some of his philosophy on medical education:

> Students should aim not at seeing many diseases everyday; no, their object should be constantly to study a few cases with diligence and attention; they should anxiously cultivate the habit of making accurate observations. This cannot be done at once; this habit can only be gradually acquired.[1]

Graves also appreciated that if a teacher is to maintain the credibility of his students he must keep up to date with modern advances. The demands of his practice, teaching commitments, reading and research placed great pressure on Graves' time. One of his students, Arthur Guinness, a member of the famous brewing family, later recalled those early days:

> As he had a very large practice he used to come in winter time, when I was resident, about 7.00 o'clock in the mornings when it was quite dark to visit the wards, and many a time have I walked round with the clinical clerk, Hudson, and often carried a candle for Dr Graves....[2]

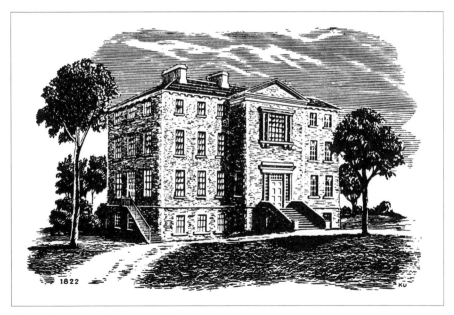

11.2   The Meath Hospital in 1822

REVOLUTIONARY IDEAS ON THE TREATMENT OF FEVER

In 1822 the west of Ireland was in the grip of famine and many people were dying from typhus fever. The local doctors struggled to contain the disease against great odds. However, in their exhausted condition they themselves began to fall victim to the epidemic. The doctors began to die and this increased the fear among the population. The government responded by sending six volunteer doctors to the fever-stricken area. Robert Graves was one of these and he was greatly affected by the suffering which he witnessed. It awakened in him a great interest in the treatment of fever. He wrote frequently on the subject and eventually he was to revolutionise the management of fever patients by advocating that they should be encouraged to eat. Up to then these patients had been placed on a very sparse diet. Graves pointed out that patients needed adequate nutrition if they were to survive the illness. He told his students:

> You may, perhaps, think it unnecessary to give food, as the patient appears to have no appetite, and does not call for it. You might as well think of allowing the urine to accumulate in the bladder because a patient feels no desire to pass it. You are called upon to interfere where the sensibility is impaired, and you are not to permit your patient to encounter the terrible consequences of starvation because he does not ask for nutriment.[3]

KING'S PROFESSOR, AUTHOR AND EDITOR

Graves was appointed to the King's professorship of the Institutes of Medicine in Trinity College in 1827. This professorship covered physiology, pathology and therapeutics. He was a prolific writer and his work covered many subjects. He wrote several papers for the *Dublin Hospital Reports*, a journal which had been established by John Cheyne. There was a total of five volumes of this publication and Cheyne thought so highly of Graves that he asked him to edit the fifth volume. Graves became the first Dublin physician to publish his lectures regularly in the *London Medical and Surgical Journal* and in the *London Medical Gazette*. These lectures were read widely and they had a major influence on clinical practice. In 1832 Graves, together with Robert Kane, founded the *Dublin Journal of Medical Science*. This provided a forum for Irish medical writing and it kept its readers abreast of medical progress on the Continent. It also brought the work of Irish doctors to the notice of investigators abroad. This journal is still published today as the *Irish Journal of Medical Science.*

GRAVES' DISEASE

Graves' most famous paper 'Newly observed affection of the thyroid gland in females' was published in the *London Medical and Surgical Journal* in 1835. This was his classic description of Graves' Disease and it was based on a lecture which he gave at the Meath Hospital.

> I have lately seen three cases of violent and long continued palpitations in females, in each of which the same peculiarity presented itself, viz. enlargement of the thyroid gland; ....One of these ladies, residing in the neighbourhood of Black Rock, was seen by Dr Harvey and Dr William Stokes, another of them, the wife of a clergyman in the county of Wicklow, was seen by Dr Marsh, and the third lives in Grafton Street. The palpitations have in all lasted considerably more than a year, and with such violence as to be at times exceedingly distressing, and yet there seems no certain grounds for concluding that organic disease of the heart exists.... The enlargement of the thyroid, of which I am now speaking, seems to be essentially different from goitre in not attaining a size at all equal to that observed in the latter disease. Indeed this enlargement deserves rather the name of hypertrophy....[4]

He went on to describe the eye signs which he observed in a twenty-year-old woman with the condition:

> It was now observed that the eyes assumed a singular appearance, for the eyeballs were apparently enlarged, so that when she slept or tried to shut her eyes, the lids were incapable of closing. When the eyes were open, the white sclerotic could be seen, to a breadth of several lines, all around the cornea.[4]

THE FIGHT AGAINST CHOLERA

Graves wrote extensively and indeed passionately on cholera. In 1832 a major epidemic of the disease reached Ireland, having spread gradually across Europe. At that time several medical authorities disputed the infectious nature of the disease. By meticulously tracing the origin of the epidemic, its subsequent progress along lines of communication and trade, and its spread up rivers, Graves demonstrated clearly that the condition was infectious and he called on the government to implement appropriate measures to stop its propagation. His appeals to the authorities fell largely on deaf ears, but a number of doctors around the country followed his advice and they had some success in limiting the impact of the epidemic.

INFLUENCE EXTENDING TO NORTH AMERICA

The form of bedside teaching which Robert Graves and William Stokes developed at the Meath Hospital spread from there throughout the English-speaking world. Daniel Reisman, professor of clinical medicine at Philadelphia, acknowledged this when addressing the Section of Medical History of the College of Physicians of Philadelphia in 1921:

> Graves, as well as Stokes,... while not the first to make use of bedside teaching — Boerhaave had done it 100 years earlier — did it so consistently and so successfully that it was adopted by clinical teachers elsewhere and especially in this country where the lectures of Graves had been published in repeated editions and had been read with avidity. Moreover, the Americans who studied in Dublin brought back with them the methods of bedside teaching, to learn which had been, as Moreton Stille states, their chief motive for going to Ireland.... The practice of Graves and Stokes of having the students examine and follow the cases in the hospital became the American method. It is the one obtaining everywhere in this country today.[5]

Graves' clinical lectures were first published in book form in 1838 by Robley Dunglison, professor of medicine in Philadelphia and editor of the *American Medical Library*. The book had a major influence on the development of medical thinking and teaching in North America. In a letter to Dunglison from his home at 9 Harcourt Street in 1837, Graves wrote:

> It is a great satisfaction to us here, to observe the progress our brethren in the States, are making in all the Sciences and especially the Medical. I always feel much pleasure in paying attention to physicians and surgeons of your country who visit us and, lately, have had the pleasure of seeing two eminent men, Dr Warren of Boston and Dr Ludlow of New York.
>
> When any of your friends visit Dublin, I shall be glad to have an introduction from you by them.[6]

Another American visitor, William Gibson, who was professor of surgery in Philadelphia, visited Dublin in August 1839 and he later described Graves in his book *Rambles in Europe*.

> I had heard nothing, it so happened, of the appearance or manners of Dr Graves, and, therefore, when ushered into his presence in his own parlour, was startled at finding myself looking up to the face of a very tall, slender, handsome, and well-dressed man, whom, if I had met by chance in the street, I should have turned round to look at and inquired of some passer-by who he was.... After this I saw as much of Dr Graves as a fortnight in Dublin would allow. That is, I saw him every day, either at his own house, or at my lodgings, or the Meath Hospital, where he may be found, every morning, peeping and prying into every hole and corner of the building, cracking jokes with the patients or pupils, or old women, or poring over, intently, some medical production, or volume of natural history, or book of travels: for he is very fond of such studies, and took great delight in asking all sorts of questions about our Indians, and lakes, and trees and prairies, and cataracts and great rivers, and buffaloes. And, for all I did see of him, I felt justified, I thought, in jumping to the conclusion, that he is a man of very extraordinary abilities.[7]

James Bovell of Toronto and Palmer Howard of McGill University, Montreal, teachers of the great American physician William Osler, both spent time with Graves in Dublin when they were young doctors. At the bicentenary meeting of the School of Physic in Dublin's Mansion House in 1912, Osler acknowledged the influence which the teachings of Graves and his colleague Stokes had on him: 'I owe my start in the profession to James Bovell, kinsman and devoted pupil of Graves, while my teacher in Montreal, Palmer Howard, lived, moved and had his being in his old masters, Graves and Stokes.'[8]

A SYSTEM OF CLINICAL MEDICINE

In 1843 Graves published his *magnum opus, A System of Clinical Medicine,* in Dublin. The first edition was sold out within a few months and a second edition was published five years later. The book clearly demonstrated that Graves was many years ahead of most doctors of the period in both the theory and practice of medicine. There are several original clinical observations in the work, including first descriptions of peripheral neuritis, scleroderma, erythromelalgia, the pin-point pupil in pontine haemorrhage and cough fracture. He also describes angioneurotic oedema, thus pre-dating Heinrich Quincke's description by forty years. There can be few, if any, other single author books on clinical medicine with a similar wealth of original observations on so many different conditions. The book was subsequently translated into French, German and Italian. In the preface to the French edition, the famous physician Armand Trousseau wrote:

> For many years I have spoken of Graves in my Clinical Lectures; I recommend the perusal of his work; I entreat those of my pupils who understand English to consider it as their breviary; I say and repeat that, of all the practical works published in our time, I am acquainted with none more useful, more intellectual, and I have always regretted that the Clinical Lectures of the great Dublin practitioner had not been translated into our language.[9]

Recognition of his stature and worth now began to bring Graves several honours. He was elected president of the College of Physicians in 1843 and a fellow of the Royal Society in 1849. He also received several European honours, including honorary diplomas from Berlin, Vienna, Tubigen, Hamburg and Bruges.

NON-MEDICAL INTERESTS

Graves' had wide-ranging interests outside medicine and Stokes drew attention to these in his biography of his friend:

> Many important writings, to which his name is not attached, were contributed by him as leading articles in the public press, all distinguished by a careful preparation and a singular knowledge of the history, topography, the political condition and material resources of various countries. Among the events of the time which most interested him may be mentioned the Hungarian Revolution, and the war in Afghanistan. His history of the latter event is a good example of his powers of investigation and arrangement.[10]

Graves was also interested in painting. As a young man he sketched with the English painter John Mallard Turner in Italy.

THE LAST DECADE

Graves resigned from the Meath Hospital in 1843. In his letter of resignation he said he found that he could no longer discharge his duties to his patients and pupils in a satisfactory manner. He remained until his death consultant physician to the Adelaide and Coombe Hospitals, and Peter's Parish Dispensary. It was not uncommon at that time for a physician to resign from some or all of his public commitments when he was at the height of his powers. For instance, Patrick Harking, Graves' predecessor as physician to the Meath, resigned in 1821 at the age of forty-two. Cheyne also gave up some of his public commitments and his teaching when he found it difficult to cope with these and his private practice. Consultants did not receive any remuneration for their public work at that time.

Graves had several personal tragedies in his life. His first wife died in 1825, four years after their marriage, and their daughter died in 1831. Graves had married again in 1826 but his wife died a year later, leaving a daughter who also died in childhood. When he was thirty-three he married his third wife, Anna Grogan of Slaney Park, Baltinglass. She had expensive tastes which must have placed some stress on his finances, making it necessary for him to concentrate on private practice. In 1852 she persuaded Graves to buy Cloghan Castle, an estate near Banagher in the west of Ireland.

Unfortunately Graves did not survive to enjoy the life of a country gentleman. In the autumn of 1852 he began to show the first signs of an abdominal tumour. The following February he started to deteriorate and he also suffered from severe bouts of pain. He lingered on for a year, with occasional periods of ease during which, according to Stokes, 'he showed all his old cheerfulness and energy'.[11] On 19 March 1853 it was obvious to his family that he was sinking rapidly and as they gathered around his bedside he asked them to recite some of the prayers which his father had said with him when he was a child. He gradually slipped into a coma and he died peacefully the following day.

A statue of Graves was unveiled in the hall of the College of Physicians in December 1877. Of the four statues that now stand in this hall, that of Graves was the last to be placed in position, the others being of William Stokes, Dominic Corrigan and Henry Marsh. It is a mark of the great confidence of Irish medicine at that time that even though the college was over two centuries old, they chose from their own generation when selecting the men whose statues would adorn the magnificent hall of their new building in Kildare Street.

FRANCIS RYND
1801–1861

12 *The first hypodermic injection*

The first hypodermic injection was administered by an Irish surgeon named Francis Rynd. He was the son of James Rynd of Ryndville, County Meath. He was born in Dublin in 1801 and was educated by a Dr Burrowes before entering Trinity College at the age of sixteen. He received his early medical education at the Meath Hospital where he was apprenticed to Sir Philip Crampton. He was not a diligent student as he was passionately fond of hunting and when he ought to have been attending his hospital he was out on horseback following the hounds. Crampton recognised the potential of his pupil and he asked William Porter (1790–1861), one of the younger surgeons in the hospital, 'to take charge' of him. Porter responded by taking Rynd into his house and treating him with great kindness. Porter was a distinguished surgeon who wrote a number of works, including *Surgical Pathology of the Larynx and Trachea* which was published in 1826. He discovered the pre-tracheal fascia known as Porter's Fascia. He also described Porter's Sign, a tracheal pulsation seen in conditions such as aortic aneurysm and mediastinal tumours.

Rynd settled down and made rapid progress under Porter's guidance. After qualifying he established his practice at 19 Ely Place and then moved to 14 Hume Street where he resided until the time of his death.

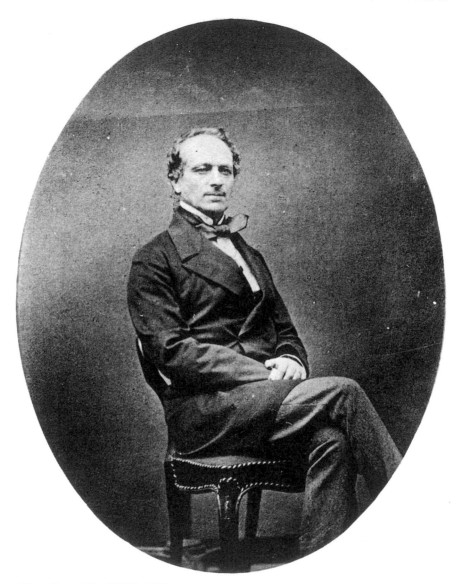

12.1   Francis Rynd 1801–1861

He became a fellow of the Royal College of Surgeons in Ireland in 1830. He had most of the nobility in Ireland as his patients and he was one of the few doctors admitted to the exclusive Kildare Street Club. A great favourite with women, he was a sought-after guest at fashionable dinners. Not surprisingly he was not popular with his colleagues in the city, probably because he appeared to court public rather than professional appreciation.

Rynd was elected surgeon to the Meath Hospital in 1836 where he became a colleague of Robert Graves, William Stokes and Sir Philip Crampton. Crampton (1777–1858), who was a fellow of the Royal Society, was probably the most flamboyant Irish surgeon of the nineteenth century. He was known as 'flourishing Phil' because of his love of good company and fine clothes, yet he was a very skilled surgeon and published several papers on different aspects of surgery. Ormsby tells us in his history of the Meath Hospital that all through life Rynd 'was bound to his old master with the strongest ties of affection and regard — in fact it was Sir Philip Crampton who helped him in early life to get into the large and fashionable practice he afterwards enjoyed'.[1]

THE FIRST SUBCUTANEOUS INJECTION

On 18 May 1844 a woman with a five-year history of severe facial pain came under Rynd's care at the Meath Hospital. He recalled the first episode quite vividly:

> She thought her eye was being torn out of her head, and her cheek from her face; it lasted about two hours, and then suddenly disappeared on taking a mouthful of ice. She had not had any return for three months, when it came back even worse than before, quite suddenly, one night on going out of a warm room into the cold air. On this attack she was seized with chilliness, shivering, and slight nausea; the left eye lachrymated profusely, and became red with pain; it went in darts through her whole head, face, and mouth, and the paroxysm lasted for three weeks, during which time she never slept. She was bled and blistered, and took opium for it, but without relief. It continued coming at irregular intervals, but each time generally more intense in character, until at last, weary of her existence, she came to Dublin for relief.[2]

He decided to treat her by injecting morphia beneath the skin and for that purpose he invented a special instrument. This instrument was the predecessor of the modern hypodermic syringe and with it Rynd gave the first subcutaneous injection. The instrument developed by Rynd did not have a plunger and the fluid entered the tissues by the force of gravity alone. He described his technique in the *Dublin Medical Press* on 12 March 1845:

> On the 3rd of June a solution of fifteen grains of acetate of morphia, dissolved in one drachm of creosote, was introduced to the supra-orbital nerve, and along the course of the temporal, malar, and buccal nerves, by four punctures of an instrument made for the purpose. In the space of a minute all pain (except that caused by the operation, which was very slight) had ceased, and she slept better that night than she had done for months. After the interval of a week she had slight return of pain in the gums of both upper and under jaw. The fluid was again introduced by two punctures made in the gum of each jaw, and the pain disappeared.[2]

Rynd also treated a twenty-eight-year-old man with intractable sciatic pain in his right lower limb:

> He is unable to sleep from the pain, and quite unable to walk. He is much emaciated, and the muscles of the limb are attenuated and wasted. He has been ill for three years, during which time he has been almost always confined to bed. He has been frequently treated for the disease with calomel, to produce salivation, cupping, blistering, leeching, &c., all without any salutary effect. Exposure to cold and wet is assigned as the cause of the disease.
>
> On the 13th of November the fluid was introduced, ten grains acetate morphiae to the drachm of creosote, one puncture behind the trochanter, and one half-way down the thigh. He was instantly relieved from pain, and walked steadily through the ward without any pain or difficulty; before, walking increased the pain.[2]

Following these initial successes Rynd used his technique extensively to relieve pain. He had a small instrument for injecting superficial nerves and a larger one for those nerves lying deeper within the tissues. However, he pointed out that 'It is not necessary to introduce the fluid to the nerve itself to ease pain, still the nearer to the seat of pain it is conveyed, the more surely relief is given'.[3] Rynd used large doses of morphine, very little of which can have been absorbed. The dramatic relief from pain which he observed in his patients was almost certainly due to the local effect of the creosote, which is composed of a mixture of

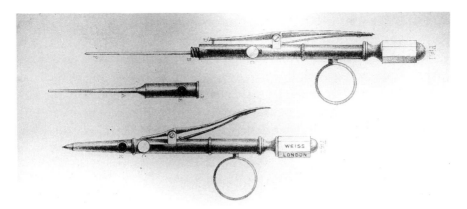

12.2   Rynd's hypodermic instruments

highly neurotoxic phenolic compounds. The injection of the creosote along the course of the nerve would interfere with conduction and in this way give rapid pain relief.

In 1853 Dr Charles-Gabriel Pravaz designed a syringe with a plunger for the purpose of giving intravenous injections. The Pravaz syringe was subsequently adopted by Alexander Wood, a Scottish physician, and Charles Hunter, a London surgeon, for giving subcutaneous injections. Wood used the term 'subcutaneous' to describe his method of injection, and Charles Hunter introduced the term 'hypodermic'. Wood and Hunter subsequently entered into a long correspondence in the *Medical Times and Gazette* over priority of discovery. Rynd stayed aloof from this debate but he did publish a short paper in 1861 at the height of the dispute describing the technique which he had used when giving the first subcutaneous injections in 1844.

OTHER COMMITMENTS

Rynd worked for a time as a medical superintendent of Mountjoy Prison. However, his main commitment was to the Meath Hospital where he was a popular teacher as well as an able surgeon. He wrote several papers on various subjects for different medical journals. In 1849 he published a book entitled *Pathological and Practical Observations on Stricture and some other Diseases of the Male Urethra* which he dedicated to Sir Philip Crampton. He served as honorary secretary to the Medical

Board of the Meath Hospital for many years, and in this capacity he received a letter of resignation from Robert Graves in October 1843. Rynd went immediately with Stokes to try to persuade Graves to change his mind, but to no avail. In 1857 Rynd resigned his position as medical superintendent at Mountjoy Prison, having served in the post for ten years. He accumulated a large fortune through his private practice, but he invested unwisely in securities and as a result he lost a considerable sum of money.

TRAGIC DEATH

Rynd's death in 1861 occurred under unfortunate circumstances following an unpleasant altercation near the crescent on the Clontarf Road. The tragic events were witnessed by a medical student named Hans Powell who saw Rynd pass him driving his phaeton, a light four-wheeled open carriage. He then heard the surgeon shout two or three times as if to warn someone to get out of the way, and on looking he saw a man lifting a woman from the road. Rynd having satisfied himself that the woman was not seriously hurt attempted to go on but his carriage was stopped by some men and a dispute ensued. When Rynd ordered his servant to get the police the men attempted to go away and Rynd turned his horse to follow them. He was then seen to slump forward over the reins and the horse bolted. When the vehicle was eventually stopped Rynd was found to be comatose. He was driven to the house of a Dr Faussett who lived locally but he died on the way.

A black-bordered obituary notice appeared at the beginning of the November issue of the *Dublin Quarterly Journal of Medical Science*. The obituary not only highlighted some of Rynd's achievements and expressed regret at his death, but it also gave the findings found at his post-mortem:

> His death was the result of fatty disease of the heart, there never having been any but the slightest symptoms, on one or two occasions, of its existence; and on the day of his death he went through his usual professional avocations.... Post-mortem examination revealed commencing disease of both liver and kidneys, in addition to the affection of the heart.[4]

Ironically the same issue of the journal carried two papers from his pen, the proofs of which he had just corrected before his death. One paper was on 'Remedying deformities of the lips', the other bore the title 'Description of an instrument for the subcutaneous introduction of fluids in affections of the nerves'. The latter was a short illustrated description of the instrument which he had used to give the first hypodermic injections nearly twenty years previously. 'For this invention alone', wrote his first biographer, 'his name can never be forgotten, as the hypodermic needle is now so extensively used.'[5]

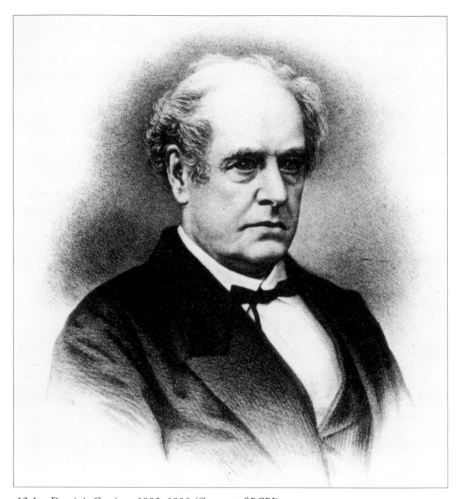

13.1   Dominic Corrigan 1802–1880 (Courtesy of RCPI)

13 *Fundamental observations in cardiology*

Duríng his lifetime Dominic Corrigan gained an international reputation in medicine, he played a prominent part in national politics and he accumulated considerable wealth from his large practice. These achievements are all the more remarkable when one considers that Corrigan did not have the type of patronage often thought essential for professional advancement in Victorian Ireland. He was born in 1802 in the heart of the old city of Dublin. His father was a merchant in Thomas Street and his house stood on a site where an Augustinian church stands today and where, in the past, Dublin's medieval hospital of St John the Baptist was situated. This hospital was suppressed by Henry VIII in the first wave of religious persecution. In subsequent years the enactment of a whole range of penal laws made it virtually impossible for the native Catholic Irish to play an active part in the professional life of the country. Towards the end of the eighteenth century these laws were relaxed and the new, more liberal approach by government opened up opportunities for young Catholics like Corrigan.

MAYNOOTH AND TRINITY

Corrigan received his early education in a lay college which was linked with the new ecclesiastical college in Maynooth. The local practitioner and medical attendant to the college, Dr O'Kelly, recognised Corrigan's talent and gave him some training in medicine. Corrigan was also influenced by one of his teachers, Dr Cornelius Denvir, who later became Bishop of Down and Connor and by whom he was taught mathematics and experimental physics. Corrigan used this training to advantage later in his career when investigating the subject of aortic incompetence. After leaving Maynooth he commenced the study of medicine at the School of Physic in Trinity College. There he came under the influence of Macartney, the dynamic professor of anatomy, who had also made such a great impact on Graves.

Macartney, who was from Armagh, was elected professor of anatomy and surgery at Trinity College in 1812 to succeed William Hartigan. His great energy and enthusiasm inspired several of his students to strive for excellence and in this way he made a fundamental contribution to the development of the Irish school of medicine. One of Macartney's greatest difficulties in the school of anatomy was the shortage of bodies for dissection. In his diary he tells us that he and his demonstrator were obliged to undertake 'the resurrection of bodies' with very little assistance. 'On one occasion, I was taken prisoner and not liberated before morning and treated with the greatest indignity....'[1] Corrigan took an active part in body snatching when he was in Macartney's department and in later life he published a vivid description of his experiences in *The Lancet*.

APPOINTMENTS AND PUBLICATIONS

Corrigan also studied in Edinburgh before he graduated MD, with William Stokes, in 1825. When Corrigan returned to Dublin he became a physician to the Sick Poor Institution in Meath Street. This was the largest dispensary in the city and although it was not attached to a hospital Corrigan had the satisfaction of knowing that the post had once been held by Abraham Colles. Two years after this appointment Corrigan published papers in *The Lancet* on aneurysm of the aorta and on systolic heart murmurs. They were followed by several other papers, and Corrigan's hard work was rewarded in 1831 when he was appointed physician to the Charitable Infirmary.

The following year Corrigan's classic paper 'On permanent patency of the mouth of the aorta or inadequacy of the aortic valves' appeared in the *Edinburgh Medical and Surgical Journal*. This paper contains a description of Corrigan's Sign, that is, the visible pulsation in the neck of patients with aortic incompetence:

> When a patient affected by the disease is stripped, the arterial trunks of the head, neck, and superior extremities immediately catch the eye by their singular pulsation.... The pulsations of these arteries may be observed in a healthy person through a considerable portion of their tract, and become still more marked after exercise or exertion; but in the disease now under consideration, the degree to which the vessels are thrown out is excessive. Though a moment before unmarked, they are at each pulsation thrown out on the surface in the strongest relief. From its singular and striking appearance, the name of visible pulsation is given to this beating of the arteries....[2]

Corrigan also recognised that the hypertrophy of the heart which accompanies this condition is compensatory in nature. Although he was not the first to describe the pathology of aortic incompetence, his paper was the most lucid on the subject up to that time. Soon physicians around the world, including Armand Trousseau in Paris, began to speak of Corrigan's Disease, and the eponym first appeared in print in 1839 in *La Lancette Française*. Corrigan made another very significant contribution to cardiology in 1838 when he published his paper 'On aortitis, as one of the causes of angina pectoris'.

It is of interest that the first comprehensive account of aortic regurgitation was written by a physician named Thomas Cuming, who was born in Armagh in 1798. His paper entitled 'A case of diseased heart, with observations' appeared in the *Dublin Hospital Reports* in 1822. Cuming, who had studied for three years as clinical clerk with John Cheyne, was the first to make the distinction between the full volume pulse of aortic regurgitation and the small volume pulse of aortic stenosis:

Although the shrivelled and contracted state of the aortic valves prevented them from completely closing the ventriculo-aortic aperture, and they allowed a reflux of blood from the artery into the ventricle, there was no diminution of the aortic aperture itself, and therefore a full stream of blood was thrown into the artery at each stroke of the ventricle; whence arose the full, hard and vibrating pulse,.... Had there been actual diminution of the aortic aperture, the smallness of the stream of blood, which would have passed from the ventricle into the artery, must have given rise to a small, feeble, and thready pulse....[3]

Sir David Barry, FRS, from Roscommon was another Irish doctor who, like Cuming and Corrigan, wrote on cardiac problems. In a series of experiments Barry demonstrated the contribution of intrathoracic negative pressure in assisting the return of venous blood to the heart. Laënnec described Barry's work as being 'most remarkable' in the second edition of his famous classic *On Mediate Auscultation*.[4]

OBSERVATIONS ON FIBROSIS OF THE LUNG

In 1837 Corrigan was appointed physician to the Cork Street Fever Hospital and three years later he joined the staff of the House of Industry Hospitals (Richmond Hospital). There were several very able doctors already on the staff of this hospital, including Robert Adams. At an evening meeting of the College of Physicians in March 1838, Corrigan read a paper on 'Cirrhosis of the lung' during which he described a disease process whereby 'Contraction of the fibres of the fibro-cellular tissue obliterates the small air-vesicles'.[5] This was published subsequently in the *Dublin Journal of Medical Science* and it contained a number of original observations on pulmonary fibrosis. He described the condition as cirrhosis, preferring, he said, to add an additional fact rather than a new name to the science of medicine. Corrigan was the first to question the generally accepted view that lung fibrosis was secondary to bronchiectasis. He pointed out that the reverse may be the case. He also claimed that fibrosis of the lungs could occur in patients who were not suffering from tuberculosis. His new ideas formed the basis of subsequent work on pulmonary fibrosis and bronchial dilatation.

INVENTIONS

Corrigan invented a number of items of equipment including an inhaler and a special bed for immobilised patients. The bed worked on the same basic principle as the modern ripple bed. The base of the bed was formed by a series of leather straps which could be released and tightened as required, so that one could alternate the areas of the body taking the pressure. He designed an instrument known as Corrigan's Button, which was a small circular metal plate with a handle. It was heated before use, then run along the course of the sciatic nerve as a counter irritant in the treatment of sciatica.

REJECTION BY THE COLLEGE OF PHYSICIANS

In 1843 Corrigan sat the examination for membership of the Royal College of Surgeons of England. The first and only question asked of him was, 'Are you the author of the essay on the patency of the aortic valves?' His reply in the affirmative admitted him to the college. Corrigan was black-balled, however, at an election for an honorary fellowship of the Royal College of Physicians of Ireland in 1847. Around this time he had been criticised by Graves because he was a member of the government's Board of Health. Graves was furious over the Board's miserly attitude to the dispensary doctors who worked in such dangerous conditions during the height of the famine epidemics. It was an unfortunate rift between the two great men as it would appear that inadequate government measures lay at the root of the problem, and Corrigan himself had been very critical of the authorities. However, it is almost certain that it was Graves' censure which lost Corrigan the fellowship.

ELECTION TO HIGH OFFICE

The decision was probably regretted and in 1849 Corrigan received an honorary MD from Trinity College. Six years later, in 1855, Corrigan submitted himself for examination to become a licentiate of the Royal College of Physicians of Ireland and he was successful. A year after this

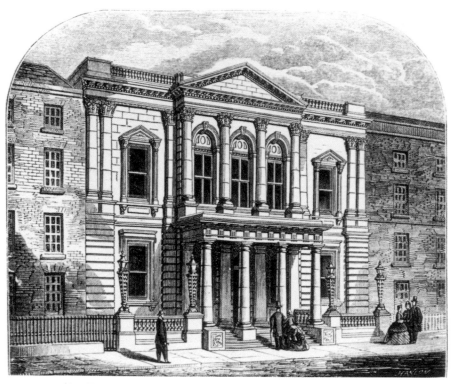

13.2   Royal College of Physicians of Ireland in Kildare Street. (Courtesy of RCPI)

courageous act he proceeded to the fellowship, as there was now no academic bar since he possessed a Trinity MD. In 1859 he was elected to the office of president of the College of Physicians. He was a dynamic president and during his five-year term of office the college acquired its fine premises in Kildare Street, where it is still based today. Corrigan introduced legislation removing the restrictions which limited entry to the fellowship. It became possible for the college to elect as fellows, graduates of any university in Ireland or Great Britain or any foreign university, and licentiates who might not have university degrees but who merited the fellowship by other distinction. During his presidency the college also became the first in these islands to admit women to the licence examination, thus enabling them to be entered on the medical register. Corrigan also promoted the interests of the Pharmaceutical Society of Ireland, of which he was the first president. He commanded the respect of many of his colleagues:

Success was obtained by him, not by the patronage of wealth or power, servility, or affectation. He had no faith in any such wretched extrinsic influences. The only patron he looked to for advancement was his own professional character. Such a man naturally exercised an influence that was almost marvellous on all with whom he came in contact; and there were few subjects on which you could converse with him on which he did not throw a new ray of light, which clearly illuminated that which perhaps before had been in obscurity.[6]

During his early and difficult years Corrigan had been encouraged by reading *The Lives of British Physicians, from Linacre to Gooch*. In later years he referred to it as proving that 'There is but one road to excellence and success in our profession and that is by steady, sturdy and hard labour'.[7]

PRIVATE PRACTICE

Corrigan had the most lucrative private practice in Dublin. He lived in Merrion Square and he rode every day to the Richmond on horseback. He was very much aware of the dignity of the physician and he objected once during a domiciliary consultation when he and the patient's practitioner were shown into a cold room without a fire after seeing the patient. On another occasion a nervous woman with a minor gastric complaint asked her surgeon, Mr Charles Coppinger, to bring Sir Dominic Corrigan with him in consultation:

> When Sir Dominic, after examining the patient and having had a short consultation with Coppinger, returned to her room, she asked him to tell her exactly what he thought was the matter with her. 'Oh! the matter with you, madam,' said Sir Dominic, and having paused and looked through the window for some seconds he pointed to the region of her stomach and said: 'You've got a little em-porium there.' The lady thanked him and seemed quite satisfied. On his way to his carriage he said to Coppinger: 'It is a great mistake to give that kind of person too much information.' On going back to take farewell of his patient, Coppinger, happening to look through the window, saw a painter putting the finishing touch to the word 'Em-porium' on a shop front at the opposite side of the street.[8]

FOREIGN TRAVELS

In 1862 Corrigan published a book entitled *Ten Days in Athens with Notes by the Way.* It is a journal of a visit to Greece the previous year when he was accompanied by his daughter. As well as describing the antiquities of the countryside, Corrigan took the opportunity to visit hospitals. He was in Athens in early September and he visited the Military Hospital where he discussed therapeutic problems with the medical officers:

> 'Among all the gratifications of life,' he wrote in his diary that evening, 'I know of none greater than learning some new mode of curing diseases or relieving pain. It is a pleasure unalloyed by any other consideration, and sought for itself alone.'[9]

The travellers returned through Florence and again Corrigan took the opportunity to make a detailed study of the hospital system of the city. He was impressed by the clinical school of medicine where the salaries of some of the doctors were being defrayed by the state, thus allowing them time to concentrate on teaching. Although the city was well provided with beds, he was critical of the care and he was not reticent about voicing his disapproval whenever he thought the situation demanded it:

> A gentleman accompanied me in my visit who was connected with the government of the hospital. He asked me was I not greatly pleased with the floors, the cleanliness, &c. My reply was, passing my foot across a ventilator under the head of a patient's bed, and lifting it for his inspection, with a large, thick cobweb covering my shoe. I could not sacrifice candour to politeness.[10]

CORRIGAN ENTERS POLITICS

In 1866 Corrigan was made a baronet, and four years later he was elected to Parliament at Westminster as a Liberal. In an address to the British Medical Association in 1867, urging higher standards in medicine, he gave an insight into his own philosophy when he said,

'And among the bonds that unite the three divisions of this our kingdom together, there are none stronger than those of our profession, soaring in its exercise above all sectarian discords. We know no difference of race, or creed, or colour, for everyman is our neighbour.'[11]

As a politician he championed non-denominational education and he opposed Home Rule for Ireland. He served as president of the Royal Zoological Society and in 1871 he became vice-chancellor of the Queen's University. He devoted much of his energy to medical reform, he fought to improve the working conditions of dispensary doctors and he was an original member of the General Medical Council.

Corrigan retired from active politics in 1873 and began to spend more time at the magnificent country residence which he had built in Dalkey. The Tudor-style house, which he called Inniscorrig, was erected right on the shore, with its own private slip-way.

Corrigan became seriously ill at his residence in Merrion Square on 30 December 1879. He was seen by Dr Francis Cruise who diagnosed a stroke. Although incapacitated, Corrigan survived another month, during which time Cruise slept in an adjoining room so that he would be in a position to render immediate assistance. Corrigan finally succumbed on 1 February 1880. Later in the same year the surgeon Sir William Stokes gave the customary introductory address to the students in the Richmond Surgical Hospital at the opening of the teaching session. During his address he recalled the deaths of Adams and Smith some six years earlier and then went on to say:

> To-day we have another loss to deplore, one sustained more recently, that of Corrigan — three men who had all passed the line that separates eminence from greatness, who in any walk of life would have been distinguished; men who in disposition and tastes widely differed from one another, as widely as it is possible for men to differ, but, at the same time, similar in one respect, similar in having one great motive, one noble aspiration, one goal that was their ambition to reach, and that was to elevate and advance in these hospitals, by original research and philosophical electicism, the sciences of medicine and surgery, sciences to which almost from their very boyhood they were devoted.[12]

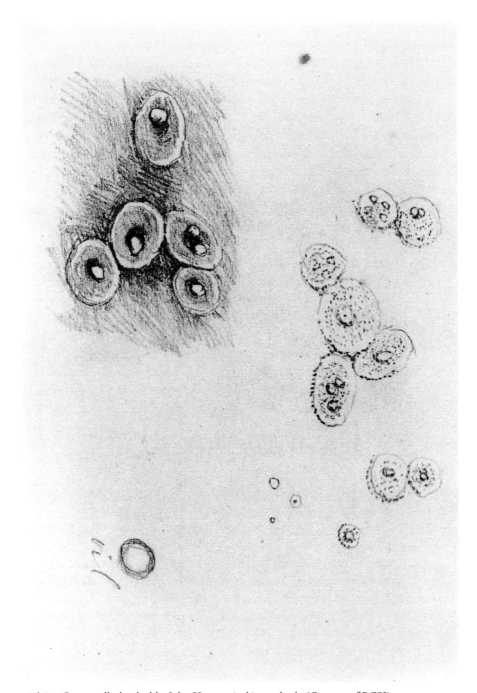

14.1   *Cancer cells sketched by John Houston in his notebook. (Courtesy of RCSI)*

JOHN HOUSTON
1802–1845

14 *Introducing the microscope to medicine*

John Houston is associated today with the rectal valves which bear his name, but he was also a pioneer in the use of the microscope in medicine and he could be said to be Ireland's first investigator in the field of cancer research. He was the son of a Presbyterian clergyman and was born in the north of Ireland in 1802. When a boy he was adopted by his maternal uncle, Dr Joseph Taylor, who was then physician to the forces. Taylor financed his nephew's education and he hoped to place him in the medical department of the army. Houston was apprenticed to John Shekleton in 1819 and began his studies in the Royal College of Surgeons.

Shekleton was a dynamic young surgeon who built up a pathological museum in the college. Unfortunately he died from the effects of a dissecting wound in May 1824 in his twenty-ninth year. A close relationship had developed between Shekleton and Houston, and when the latter's uncle died leaving him in a difficult financial situation, Shekleton had come to the rescue. Houston's apprenticeship finished in 1824 and he successfully sat the examination for licentiate of the College of Surgeons. The day of the examination was a particularly stressful one for him as it was on that day that Shekleton was buried; Houston attended the services at the graveside before proceeding to the examination hall.

Houston became a demonstrator of anatomy in the College of Surgeons in 1824, and two years later he graduated MD at Edinburgh. He was active in the project to build the City of Dublin Hospital in Baggot Street as a teaching hospital for the Royal College of Surgeons, and he began clinical work in the hospital when it opened in 1832. He built up a very busy practice and according to the surgeon Richard Butcher, who had been one of Houston's pupils, he was 'not only an acute observer of disease, but an admirable operator, and an excellent clinical surgeon in every respect'.[1] When William Gibson, professor of surgery at Philadelphia, visited Dublin in 1839 he met Houston at the home of Robert Graves. In his book *Rambles in Europe* Gibson described Houston as one of 'the most intelligent and enterprising young surgeons of Dublin'.[2]

Houston was appointed a lecturer in surgery in the Park Street School of Medicine in 1837. It was common practice at the time for individuals to lecture in a number of different hospitals. There appears to have been a particularly close relationship between the College of Surgeons and the Park Street School, although the latter also shared staff with the School of Physic. Apart from Houston, a number of other excellent anatomists such as Arthur Jacob and Benjamin Alcock served on the staff of the Park Street School. Alcock, who subsequently became the first professor of anatomy at Queen's College, Cork, is still remembered today for his description of the pudendal canal.

CURATOR OF THE PATHOLOGICAL MUSEUM

Before his death Shekleton had built up a substantial pathological museum in the College of Surgeons. At the end of 1822 there were 600 pathological specimens, of which 300 had been placed there within the year. Apart from pathological specimens, the museum had some unusual exhibits. Richard Carmichael presented the tattooed head of a New Zealand chief in 1821 and this excited considerable curiosity. A large number of heads of New Zealand natives were imported into Europe and placed in various museums around this time. It was said that several natives were murdered for the purpose of acquiring their heads for the export industry. Eventually the British government stopped this trade by banning the importation of heads. After Shekleton's death, John

Houston was appointed curator of the museum and he remained in the post for seventeen years. The museum attracted many donations of material from the leading surgeons and physicians of the time and it was necessary to construct a new museum in 1828 to cope with all the extra material. There were also some unusual acquisitions during Houston's period as curator, including the skull of a hippopotamus, the fossil of an Irish elk, the skeletons of an elephant and a giraffe, a Peruvian mummy and a collection of skulls from India.

Houston had the distinction of performing the second post-mortem examination on Jonathan Swift which took place in unusual circumstances ninety years after the great writer died. The river Poddle is now one of Dublin's underground streams but during Swift's life, and for many years after, it was the cause of regular floods. As St Patrick's Cathedral stood near its banks, religious services were frequently disrupted and the constant dampness was causing structural problems. In 1835 steps were taken to prevent the regular inundations and during the work it was necessary to expose several coffins, among them those of Swift and Stella, lying two and a half feet beneath the aisle, below the monuments to their memory. William Wilde tells us in his book *The Closing Years of Dean Swift's Life* that when a few scientific gentlemen became aware of the exhumations they decided to ask John Houston to examine Swift's remains. It was the enthusiasm for phrenology at the time rather than pathology which motivated these investigations. However, it was fortunate that Houston was asked to carry out the examination because he used his anatomical skills to write a detailed description of Swift's skeletal remains. These details have been quoted ever since in the battles which have raged in medical literature over the exact cause of the dean's death.

PIONEER OF THE MICROSCOPE AS A DIAGNOSTIC AID

Houston introduced the microscope into Irish medicine with a paper entitled 'On the microscopic pathology of cancer', which was published in 1844 in the *Dublin Medical Press*. He ranks as one of the pioneers of early microscopic research in medicine. Johannes Müller's famous book *On the Minute Structure and Form of Morbid Tumours* had been published just six years prior to Houston's paper. Müller was one of the first to use the microscope to study pathology, and his students Theodor Schwann, Jacob Henle, Albert von Kölliker and Rudolf Virchow built on his work. Theodor Schwann formulated the cell theory in 1839 and Henle earned eponymous fame with his kidney loop. Kölliker wrote the first textbook of histology in 1852 and Virchow introduced the concept of cellular pathology in 1858.

Houston was fascinated by Müller's work and he was given the opportunity of entering this field of research himself when he acquired an 'achromatic microscope of high magnifying power'. He was the first to use the microscope in medicine in Ireland, although another medical graduate, George James Allman, FRS, also became an enthusiastic microscopist around the same time. However Allman's interests lay in the field of botany and he became professor of that subject in Trinity College. Houston used his microscope to study tumours which he had removed from patients at Baggot Street Hospital or which had been supplied to him by colleagues who were interested in his work. He presented his observations to the Surgical Society of Ireland in 1844, and because his research was so new he had to begin with a basic description of the structure of a cell.

Houston concluded from his observations that it should be possible to stage tumours on the basis of their microscopical appearances, and that the microscope could play a key role in the accurate identification of malignant tumours and in differentiating them from benign lesions:

So far as these investigations have gone, they appear to warrant the inference that .... the cells seen in a cancer are only monstrosities of the normal cells. The amount of deviation in these cells from the natural condition would appear, also, to indicate the amount of degeneracy in the tumour, and its consequent distance from under the healthy controlling influence of the system, as illustrated by a comparison of carcinoma medullare with carcinoma simplex, in respect of their organisation and results. To the question, whether primary cancer be originally a local or a constitutional affection, no positive answer has yet been given. But circumstances, as they stand, would appear to favour the opinion that there is a stage, in many cases of cancer in which the disease is strictly confined to the part, and in which it may be removed effectually by operation; but that when once, from a continuance of the affection, the system becomes influenced by it, a cure by such means is hopeless.[3]

The library of the Royal College of Surgeons in Ireland possesses one of Houston's notebooks, dated 1844 to 1845. It contains original drawings of cancer cells and urinary deposits, with notes concerning the patients. Unfortunately many of Houston's colleagues did not share his views on the importance of microscopy. This is strange considering that two decades earlier the leaders of the Dublin school of medicine embraced the stethoscope with great enthusiasm. Part of the difficulty may have been the time-consuming nature of medical microscopy in the early days. It often took several hours to study one small piece of tissue, as the modern techniques of fixation, embedding, automatic sectioning and staining were unknown. 'Some sneer at it', wrote Richard Butcher, Houston's student and biographer, 'because they do not wish the trouble of studying it; and others lay it aside because it sets at naught some previously conceived views in relation to pathology.'[4]

RESEARCH AND PAPERS

Houston's name is remembered today for his paper describing the rectal 'valves', the permanent folds in the wall of the rectum. In this paper, which he wrote in 1830, he emphasised the practical importance of recognising the presence of the folds, as many patients were being placed at risk by surgeons attempting to dilate non-existing strictures with instruments known as bougies. Houston pointed out that as a result 'Many have brought on the very malady which these instruments were intended to remove'.[5]

Houston published widely on many surgical topics and he was a corresponding member of several learned societies, including the Institute of Washington and the Society of Naturalists of Heidelberg.

Houston was also interested in natural science. One of the subjects most hotly disputed at the time by anatomists and physiologists was the mechanism by which the chameleon rapidly projects its tongue to strike a fly or insect on which it feeds. Some scientists, including Sir Philip Crampton, argued that air was forced into the tubular cavity of the tongue. In a careful anatomical study which was published in the *Transactions of the Royal Irish Academy*, Houston correctly argued that erectile tissue in the tongue played an important role in the mechanism. He followed this work with another paper entitled 'An account of two newly-discovered muscles for compressing the dorsal vein of the penis in man and other animals, and also of a similar provision for compressing the vein of the chameleon's tongue'. Houston illustrated these papers with his own beautiful drawings. He was elected a member of the Royal Irish Academy in 1829.

UNTIMELY DEATH

In April 1845, at the age of forty-three, Houston collapsed with a violent headache, probably due to a cerebral haemorrhage, whilst giving a clinical lecture in Baggot Street Hospital. He died two months later on 30 July, and it was generally thought at the time that he had 'overworked' his brain. In 1846 the *Dublin Quarterly Journal of Medical Science* published a short biography of Houston by Richard Butcher. Butcher had been taught microscopy by Houston and he held his teacher in great esteem. He wrote a detailed biographical sketch, which unfortunately the editor of the *Dublin Quarterly Journal of Medical Science* felt 'of necessity obliged to abridge considerably'.[1] Sadly Houston did not attract another biography as his importance was not appreciated in his own time. Although his name has been perpetuated in anatomy, it is only in fairly recent years that he has been given appropriate recognition for being the first to introduce the microscope into Irish medicine. In 1958 the Royal College of Surgeons in Ireland honoured Houston and his teacher Shekleton by inaugurating the Shekleton research fellowship in microbiology and the Houston research fellowship in medicine, surgery and pathology.

WILLIAM STOKES
1804–1877

15 A founder of modern cardiology

Members of the Stokes family have not only made major contributions to medicine over the years, they have also made significant contributions to science, literature and art. William Stokes, who is considered one of the founders of modern cardiology, is the most famous member of this remarkable medical dynasty. His grandson Adrian Stokes is the subject of a separate biography, and his great granddaughter Barbara Stokes received international recognition for her work in the field of childhood mental handicap in 1990 when she was presented with the Kennedy Award in the United States.

William Stokes was born in Dublin in 1804. He was the son of Whitley Stokes (1763–1845), a physician in the Meath Hospital who succeeded John Cheyne as professor of surgery in the Royal College of Surgeons in 1819. Whitley Stokes subsequently became regius professor of physic at Trinity College. He wrote a number of books, including a treatise on contagion, and is credited with the first description of ecthyma terebrans (pemphigus gangrenosa), an eruptive skin disease of children. Whitley Stokes left the Established Church to follow the teaching of the 'Walkerite' sect, named after the Reverend John Walker. The latter resigned his fellowship of Trinity College because he

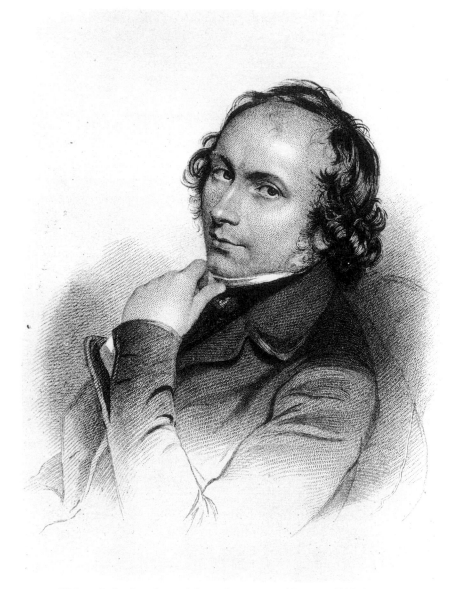

15.1   William Stokes (1804–1877) by Frederic Burton. (Courtesy of TCD)

considered the beliefs and practices of his associates to be unscriptural. William Stokes spent much of his childhood at his father's country home in Ballinteer and he was tutored privately in classics and mathematics by John Walker. Because of Walker's views William never entered Trinity College as an undergraduate, but he was a pupil of Robert Graves at the Meath Hospital and he also assisted his father in many of his scientific pursuits.

THE EARLY YEARS

In 1822 William enrolled for the course of anatomy in the College of Surgeons. He became interested in chemistry, a development fostered by his acquaintance with James Apjohn, who became a noted chemist and professor of chemistry in Trinity College. Apjohn devised a formula for calculating the dew point, which became known as the Apjohn formula. Stokes decided to study chemistry in Glasgow and he spent two years there before going to Edinburgh on his father's advice to continue his medical studies. He was very impressed by the work of the Frenchman René Laënnec, the inventor of the stethoscope, and he was one of the first to recognise the value of this work. While still a student Stokes wrote a book of two hundred and sixty-nine pages on the use of the stethoscope. He achieved this at a time when most senior physicians completely underestimated the potential of the instrument.

PHYSICIAN AT THE MEATH HOSPITAL

In 1825 Stokes obtained the degree of MD from the University of Edinburgh, and one year later he joined Robert Graves as a colleague at the Meath Hospital. Together they would work to make the Meath one of the great teaching hospitals of that period and they would both make a major contribution to the development of clinical medicine. It was an uphill struggle, particularly in the early years, as Stokes' son later recalled: 'My father has often related to me how, when he was a young man, and when he introduced into the Dublin School, along with Graves, the methods of physical diagnosis advocated by Laënnec and Louis, he was ridiculed, satirized, and even caricatured, by his contemporaries.'[1]

The famous American cardiologist, Herrick, has written about the remarkable relationship between Graves and Stokes:

In reading of the beautiful friendship between these two eminent physicians, one feels that they must have been activated by a spirit far purer than that of ordinary mortals, a spirit that had no room for envy, much less enmity. One involuntarily contrasts their mutually helpful attitude with the acrimonious debates of Laënnec and Broussais, the none too friendly relations between Skoda and some of his colleagues, the frictions and bitter jealousies of Traube and Schönlein in Berlin.[2]

Shortly after Stokes' appointment there was a major outbreak of fever in the city and many huts and tents had to be erected in the grounds of the Meath Hospital to cope with the crisis. In the spring of 1827 Stokes himself contracted fever and almost died. In the same year Graves and Stokes wrote a short book entitled *Clinical Reports of the Medical Cases in the Meath Hospital*, based on their clinical experience. The book was written primarily for their students and they dedicated it to John Cheyne.

Stokes became a very able lecturer and he illustrated his talks with his own original research. His lectures were published over several volumes in the *London Medical and Surgical Journal*. They were subsequently edited by John Bell and published in Philadelphia in 1840 under the title *Clinical Lectures on the Theory and Practice of Medicine*. This served as a textbook for many years in the American schools of medicine. Meanwhile Stokes continued his research on the stethoscope and in 1837 he published his book *The Diagnosis and Treatment of Diseases of the Chest*. This made a major impact and within a year it was translated into German. It contained many original observations and a masterly description of emphysema.

Stokes was now emerging as one of the leading physicians in the city, however the College of Physicians was prevented by its Constitution from making him a fellow. He had not graduated in arts, something he would always regret, and his MD was from Edinburgh rather than Dublin, Oxford or Cambridge as the charter required. There were also other eminent physicians in the city who could not become fellows for the same reason. Perhaps both institutions had learnt from the Fielding Ould controversy years before, as the College of Physicians was now helped out of its difficulties by Trinity College when the latter agreed to confer an honorary MD on any six licentiates nominated by the physicians. Stokes was one of those honoured and immediately

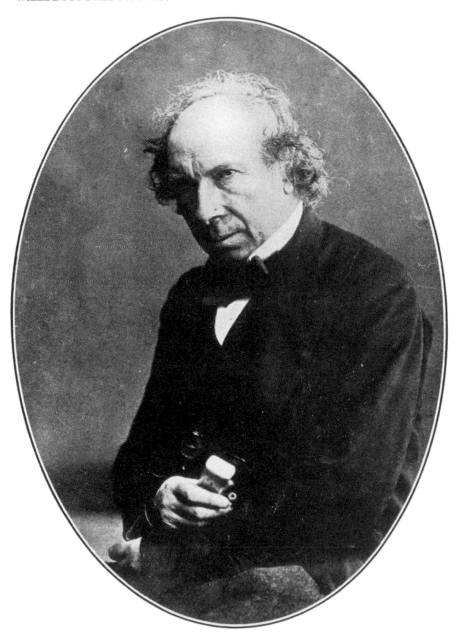

15.2   William Stokes in old age. (Courtesy of RCPI)

afterwards he was admitted to fellowship of the college. In 1838 Stokes founded the Pathological Society of Dublin with Dr Robert Smith, his brother-in-law. Both men were the first joint secretaries of the new society.

THE EFFECTS OF FAMINE

Stokes was deeply affected by the tragedy of the Irish Famine. He strove to improve medical services for the poor and he was appalled by the high death rate amongst the doctors who were engaged in the Poor Law services, many of whom were his former students. With Graves, Wilde and Cusack, he helped to establish a small voluntary group called the Medical Temporary Relief Committee. They distributed money to the families of medical men who were experiencing hardship. He also travelled to London with Cusack to give evidence on behalf of the dispensary doctors to a Select Committee of the House of Commons.

CLINICAL OBSERVATIONS AND PUBLICATIONS

After the publication of his work on diseases of the respiratory system in 1837, Stokes concentrated his clinical research on diseases of the heart. During the following years he published several papers on cardiology in the *Dublin Quarterly Journal of Medical Science*. One of his most famous papers 'Observations on some cases of permanently slow pulse' was published in 1846. In this paper he acknowledged the previous work by Robert Adams on the same subject which appeared in the *Dublin Hospital Reports* in 1827. The first case which Stokes described was that of Edmund Butler, a sixty-eight-year-old man who was admitted to the Meath Hospital on 9 February 1846:

> He stated that his health had been robust, until about three years ago, at which time he was suddenly seized with a fainting fit, in which he would have fallen if he had not been supported. This occurred several times during the day, and always left him without any unpleasant effects. Since that time he has never been free from these attacks for any considerable length of time, and has had, at least fifty such seizures....

Pulse twenty-eight in the minute, of a prolonged, sluggish character; the arteries pulsate visibly all over the body, but no bruit is audible in them....

He says he has had two threatenings of fits since his admission, both occurring in bed, *and both warded off by a peculiar manoeuvre: as soon as he perceives symptoms of the approaching attack, he directly turns on his hands and knees, keeping his head low, and by this means, he says, he often averts what otherwise would end in an attack.*[3]

He was discharged from the hospital in March but he was re-admitted in June:

The cardiac phenomena remain as before, but a new symptom has appeared, namely, a very remarkable pulsation in the right jugular vein. This is most evident when the patient is lying down. The number of the reflex pulsations is difficult to be established, but they are more than double the number of the manifest ventricular contractions. About every third pulsation is very strong and sudden, and may be seen at a distance....[3]

The syndrome which Stokes and Adams described, syncope resulting from sudden reduction of cardiac output, became known as the Stokes-Adams syndrome. The same paper contained a description of the respiratory pattern now known as Cheyne-Stokes respiration.

All this work formed the basis of his most famous book *Diseases of the Heart and the Aorta* which was published in 1854. This book was, in many aspects, far ahead of its time and it was translated into several languages. Stokes was always generous in acknowledging the achievements of his colleagues and the book contains several references to the work of Irish physicians and surgeons, thus enhancing the reputation of the Irish school of medicine. In a modern analysis of the book, the distinguished Irish cardiologist Professor Risteard Mulcahy wrote that:

Even a short review of some of these pages will confirm one's impression of his extraordinary gifts of observation and deduction. The text is alive with his personality, and his intellectual powers are immediately apparent to the reader. He shows a truly scientific approach to his subject; this is well exemplified by his objective and critical examination of established teaching, and by his constructive and logical reasoning on physiological matter.[4]

In this book Stokes stressed that many heart murmurs are benign. This was very important as at that time people were being invalided unnecessarily just because their physician heard a heart murmur. Instead Stokes placed emphasis on the functional condition of heart muscle and he also advised exercise in certain forms of heart disease. The book contains an excellent description of pericarditis and the first account of paroxysmal tachycardia. There is also an interesting early description of aortic sclerosis:

> The phenomena arise from the extensive ossific disease of the aortic opening, which is rendered not only rigid, but singularly irregular, from the deposit of great quantities of earthly matter in the form of intersecting and irregular plates, stretching downwards into the ventricle, as well as into the aorta, for an inch above the sinuses. In one of these cases the appearance of the opening might be aptly compared to that of the mouth of a shark in miniature; all traces of the valves had disappeared.[5]

The book was largely instrumental in gaining for him the Order of Merit of the German emperor, William I, an honour never previously conferred on a medical writer.

Stokes and other members of the Dublin school of medicine, such as Adams, Smith and Bellingham, wrote extensively on fatty degeneration of the heart. However none of them developed as clear an understanding of the subject as their fellow countryman Richard Quain, FRS, who worked in London. Quain was born in Mallow, County Cork, in 1816 and, like Stokes, he was a member of an outstanding medical family. He used the microscope to assist him in his studies and he published his classic paper 'Fatty degeneration of the heart' in 1850. In this paper he recognised that degenerative softening of the myocardium was sometimes preceded by obstruction of the coronary artery and that angina may be associated with the condition. H A Snellen in his *History of Cardiology* stated that Quain was 'an early pioneer in bringing together most, if not all, of the important aspects of coronary heart disease'.[6] Stokes was aware of Quain's work and he referred to it in his *Diseases of the Heart and the Aorta*. However Stokes, and indeed Quain himself, did not appreciate the full significance of the latter's observations and it was not until the work of the American physician James Herrick earlier this century that the implications of coronary artery obstruction were finally understood.

Stokes was appointed regius professor of medicine in Trinity College in 1845 and he became president of the College of Physicians in 1849. He had ideas on social and preventive medicine which were far ahead of his time and he was largely responsible for introducing the first university diploma in this subject.

BROAD CULTURAL INTERESTS

Stokes' home in Merrion Square was a Mecca for the cultural life of the city. Oscar Wilde's mentor, John Pentland Mahaffy, was very impressed by Stokes as a conversationalist and he quoted him in his book *The Art of Conversation*. Stokes was a very close friend and biographer of the antiquary and artist George Petrie. Whenever he travelled abroad Stokes wrote regularly to Petrie describing the ancient monuments and churches he had seen. Stokes went on a number of expeditions throughout Ireland to view archaeological remains, accompanied by friends such as George Petrie, Samuel Ferguson, William Wilde and the Earl of Dunraven. On occasion he was besieged by the local people when they became aware that the famous doctor was in their area. He was in Donegal in the autumn of 1864 at a time when the weather was very bad and the crops had suffered as a result. Lady Ferguson recalled accompanying Stokes on his visits to the poor families who had requested his attention:

> The sufferers were generally aged peasants. 'A weakness about the heart,' an 'oppression on the chest,' and rheumatic pains, were the ills of which they chiefly complained. Dr Stokes's manner was full of sympathy. He listened, with his hand on the pulse, to all they had to say, with the utmost patience. Then he prescribed, invariably, the same remedy. With the pills — which were to be taken at stated intervals — he produced half-a-crown, with strict instructions to apply it to the purchase of mutton-chops, one of which was to be eaten daily.[7]

Stokes realised that the real problem was poverty and malnutrition. Lady Ferguson was very impressed by 'the depth of his sympathy for the suffering and sorrowful'.[7]

FAMILY MAN

Despite his many commitments, Stokes always made time for his family and he enjoyed playing with his children:

> William used to arm himself with a large wet sponge and hide. The children hunted for him in a pack and when they found him they fled pursued by their father who generously applied the sponge to any child he caught.[8]

The care and attention which Stokes and his wife gave to the intellectual development of their children were reflected in their later achievements. Three of them became leaders in their chosen field: Whitley became a Celtic scholar with an international reputation, Margaret became a writer and authority on Irish antiquities, and William became a surgeon.

Stokes was consulted during his last years by an old family friend who thought he had cancer:

> Stokes examined the patient carefully and he then moved away without saying anything. He stood by the fireplace with his elbow on the mantelpiece and he seemed to be lost in thought. His friend was naturally becoming very agitated as he thought that Stokes was hesitating before giving him bad news. But this was not the case as Stokes suddenly stopped day dreaming and said 'I think my son Willie will be a great surgeon'.[9]

Stokes, having assured himself that his friend was not seriously ill, had ceased to think of him as a patient, but rather as someone who took a great interest in his family. Stokes was right about his son as he became an eminent surgeon who was knighted for his achievements. Sir William Stokes was professor of surgery at the Royal College of Surgeons and his name is associated with the Gritti-Stokes amputation of the lower limb.

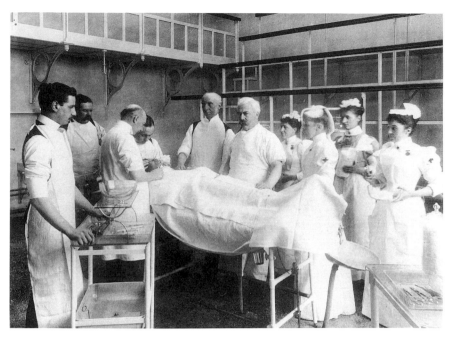

15.3   An operation in the Meath Hospital in the late nineteenth century. Sir William
Stokes, son of the physician William Stokes, is the second surgeon from the right, facing the
camera. (Courtesy of RCSI)

THE LAST YEARS

Stokes was elected president of the Royal Irish Academy in 1874, the
first practising physician to be honoured in this way. He received many
international honours, including the degree of LL D from the
universities of Cambridge and Edinburgh and the degree of DCL from
Oxford. He continued to practise medicine until he was injured whilst
travelling to see a patient in Wicklow when he was over seventy years of
age. He died three years later, in 1877, at his country home, Carrig
Breacc, at Howth on the Dublin coast.

During an address to the medical school at Trinity College's
tercentenary celebrations in 1892, Professor Stockvis, rector of the
University of Amsterdam, spoke of the achievements of Graves and
Stokes:

I congratulate you with all my heart on being students of that same university in which Graves held his celebrated clinical lectures in that Meath Hospital which is known by all the world through his fame. His lectures, even to this day, are a model of clear, scientific, eloquent and elegant writing, ... you may name as yours that renowned and skilful physician, William Stokes, the author of the classic 'Diseases of the Heart' and 'Diseases of the Chest'. He was the first to follow Laënnec, and understand all the significance of the great Frenchman's discovery; he was the first to find out all the use that could be made of percussion and auscultation for the exact diagnosis of the circulatory and respiratory organs. The history of medicine is proud of these men. They are not national, they are international glories; and so long as human suffering shall be relieved by medicine, so long will the names of Graves and Stokes be honoured all over the world.[10]

16 *Reducing maternal mortality in childbirth*

R obert Collins was the most distinguished master of the Rotunda Hospital in the last century. He graduated in medicine in Glasgow in 1822 and two years later was admitted licentiate of the College of Physicians. He worked as a student in the Rotunda and subsequently became assistant to the master, John Pentland, in 1822. When Pentland died in office in 1826, Collins was elected to take his place. This was a remarkable promotion for the young doctor who had been qualified for only four years. The fact that Collins had married a daughter of Joseph Clarke, a former distinguished master of the hospital, may have had a bearing on his meteoric promotion.

OUTSTANDING WORK ON PUERPERAL FEVER

It was in any case one of the best appointments ever made to the post. After taking up the position Collins found the hospital in a very unhealthy condition. There was a significant maternal death rate, particularly from puerperal fever. At that time more women died in childbirth from puerperal fever than from any other cause. In an effort

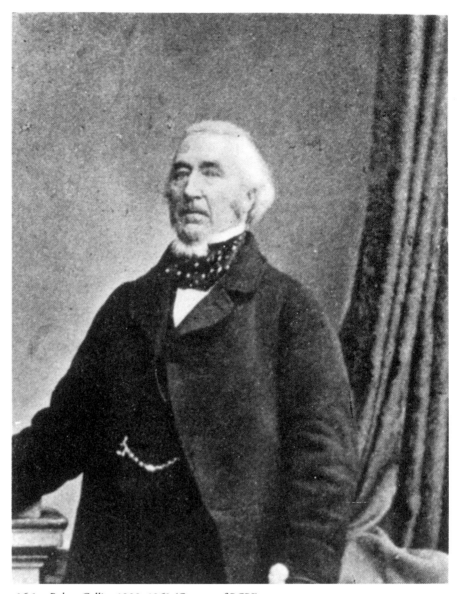

16.1   *Robert Collins 1800–1868 (Courtesy of RCPI)*

to control the incidence of the disease, Collins reduced admissions by
encouraging women to remain in their own homes and he supplied
them with gruel, whey and medicine. He emphasised principles first
introduced during the mastership of his father-in-law, Joseph Clarke.

The latter stressed the importance of cleanliness and adequate ventilation in the hospital. He also introduced the practice of disinfecting wards and using them in rotation so that each ward in turn was out of use for periods of one to three weeks. In 1790 he published his ideas in 'Observations on the puerperal fever, more especially as it has of late occurred in the Lying-In Hospital of Dublin'.

Collins used a number of wards in rotation as labour wards. There was a midwife in charge of each ward, and both midwives and patients were forbidden to move away from the ward. When the ward was full, no further admissions took place until all the mothers had been discharged. Following this the floor of the empty ward was treated with chloride of lime:

> In this way each ward was washed every ten to twelve days, the solution being left on for 24 hours, during which time the blankets, quilts, linen, &c., were suspended, so as to be exposed completely to the chlorine gas, which is copiously disengaged from the preparation mentioned. The chloride of lime was then carefully washed off, and the boards when dry, polished with a brush. It may appear strange that a process, such as stated, should be considered advisable in an establishment which is at all times kept in the most perfect state of neatness and cleanliness, in every respect; so much so, that few private houses would bear comparison; yet the result consequent on such a practice will fully justify our having had recourse to it.[1]

If any of the mothers developed fever:

> The bedding is instantly scoured and stoved; the wood-work and floor washed with the chloride of lime solution, and the entire whitewashed. This is readily effected, as the sick are invariably placed in a small ward, apart from the healthy. To this precaution too much attention cannot be paid; I am satisfied the instant separation is of vast importance to both.[2]

His approach to prevention was so successful that there was not one case of maternal death from puerperal fever during the last four years of his mastership. He did not accept the commonly held belief that puerperal sepsis was transmitted through miasmata or foul air: 'The facts here detailed are strongly calculated, not only to lead us to suspect, but even to prove, that this fever derived its origin from some local cause, and not from anything noxious in the atmosphere.'[3] He demonstrated clearly that the incidence could be reduced dramatically by a regime of cleanliness and fumigation. However, he found it difficult to reconcile his observations with the fact that puerperal fever also occurred in the 'houses of the affluent'.[3]

In 1835 Collins published his *Practical Treatise on Midwifery*, which contained a description of his work on puerperal fever. He outlined in the preface his reasons for writing the book:

> My object in the publication of the present volume is to give a minute and faithful detail of what actually passed under my observation in the Hospital, during the seven years it was intrusted to my care, so as to enable the reader to form his own conclusions, and thus avoid the error into which so many have been drawn, of remaining satisfied with assertions made by men no wiser than themselves, and whose opinions often rest on the same foundation.[4]

The book came to the notice of Ignacz Semmelweis in Vienna, and he resolved to travel to Dublin to work with Collins. He began taking English lessons but in March 1847 he was appointed as an assistant in a Vienna Hospital and as a result he changed his plans. However, his thinking on the aetiology of puerperal sepsis was certainly influenced by the work of Robert Collins. Semmelweis proved statistically that regimes of cleanliness markedly reduced the incidence of puerperal fever. These ideas were eventually accepted and it was realised that puerperal fever was caused by infection of the birth canal. It was first treated successfully with antibiotics earlier this century.

PROMOTER OF THE STETHOSCOPE IN OBSTETRICS

Robert Collins was one of the first obstetricians to recognise the importance of the stethoscope in obstetrics. John Creery Ferguson (1802–1865) introduced him to foetal auscultation which he had learned from Jacques de Kergaradec, who pioneered the technique, during a visit to Paris in 1827. Ferguson used the technique when he established his practice as a physician in Dublin and he was the first to

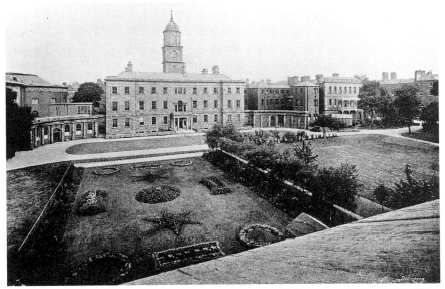

16.2   The Rotunda Hospital and gardens in the early years of this century. (Courtesy of RCPI)

hear the foetal heart in Ireland and Great Britain. He published his observations in a paper which appeared in the *Dublin Medical Transactions*. His first case was a twenty-two-year-old woman whom he saw at the Dublin General Dispensary in November 1827, complaining of indigestion:

> She told me her menses were regular and that her abdomen which I observed to be enlarged was so only occasionally. Indeed such was the excellent arrangement of the dyspeptic symptoms which she stated herself to labour under that she completely blind-folded me. However, on her third visit....I employed the stethoscope.... The patient received the news with extreme indignation.[5]

Both Kergaradec and Ferguson were physicians and not obstetricians. Ferguson's main interest in the foetal heart was its value as a method which would allow a physician to make a definite diagnosis of pregnancy, where doubt might otherwise exist. French obstetricians had either ignored or ridiculed Kergaradec's work on foetal auscultation, but Collins appreciated its great potential. By 1830 the stethoscope was being used almost daily in the Rotunda to detect the foetal heart. *The*

Lancet contains a report from the Rotunda by David Nagle on the diagnosis of twins using the new instrument in November 1830. Nagle heard two distinct foetal heartbeats in the abdomen of a thirty-year-old woman:

> In order to draw a diagnosis, I compared, with as much accuracy as I was capable, the pulsations on both sides with each other, and then each separately with the impulse at the chest, and the pulsations at the wrist, of the mother. The diagnosis was, that there were twins; and I may add, that auscultation induced me to predict that the head of the second child would present.
>
> The announcement of this discovery was received with considerable interest by some whom I took to examine the case; and Dr Collins, the highly respectable master of the Hospital, was so satisfied of the accuracy of the diagnosis, that he declared 'he could no longer repose confidence in the stethoscope in the practice of midwifery if the case did not prove to be twins.'[6]

Happily for Nagle the diagnosis proved to be correct. Collins encouraged his assistant masters, Evory Kennedy and William O'Brien Adams, to become adept at foetal auscultation, and both men published on the instrument within a short period. In 1833 Evory Kennedy (1806–1886) published his classic work *Obstetric Auscultation* in which he described his experiences of the new art of foetal auscultation at the Rotunda. Collins praised his assistant's book in his own *Practical Treatise* which was published just two years after Kennedy's work. Kennedy stressed the value of monitoring the foetal heart during labour so as to detect foetal distress. His book had considerable influence on the development of British obstetric theory and practice in relation to the well-being of the foetus. Collins' other assistant master, O'Brien Adams, published his 'Observations on mediate auscultation as a practical guide in difficult labours' in the *Dublin Journal of Medical Science* in 1833. O'Donel Browne summarised the significance of this paper in his history of the Rotunda Hospital:

> Several cases of obstructed labour were described in detail, and, while the advantages of accurate observation of the foetal heart were fully realised and stressed, O'Brien Adams and Collins laid emphasis on the fact that if the foetal heart were inaudible it would be wrong to conclude that the

foetus was dead. They recognised that the position of the child, the presence of tumours or of excessive fat of the mother's abdominal walls, could cloak the foetal heart sounds.... They were impressed by the fact that cessation of previously audible foetal heart sounds was strongly suggestive of intra-uterine death of the foetus.[7]

Another significant achievement in Irish obstetrics around this time was the publication of William Montgomery's classic book on pregnancy. Montgomery graduated from Trinity College in 1822 and was the first to fill the chair of midwifery when it was established in the School of Physic five years later. His book, *An Exposition of the Signs and Symptoms of Pregnancy, the Period of Human Gestation and the Signs of Delivery*, contained a description and illustrations of Montgomery's tubercles, small glands in the areola surrounding the nipples which become more prominent during pregnancy.

The imaginative and innovative approach to obstetrics championed by Collins was continued by others over the years, as witnessed by the work of Lombe Atthill on antisepsis, of Ernest Tweedy on eclampsia and the collaborative work of Ninian Falkiner and James Brontë Gatenby on the human ovum. Dublin obstetricians have been noted for their contributions to the design of obstetrical instruments, and a number, including Robert Collins, devised their own modifications of the obstetrical forceps.

Collins lived and practiced at 2 Merrion Square, next door to William Wilde, and he also had a country residence 'Ardsallagh' at Navan. He was elected president of the Royal College of Physicians of Ireland in 1847 and in the same year he was awarded the MD of Trinity College, *honoris causa*. Collins died on 10 December 1868.

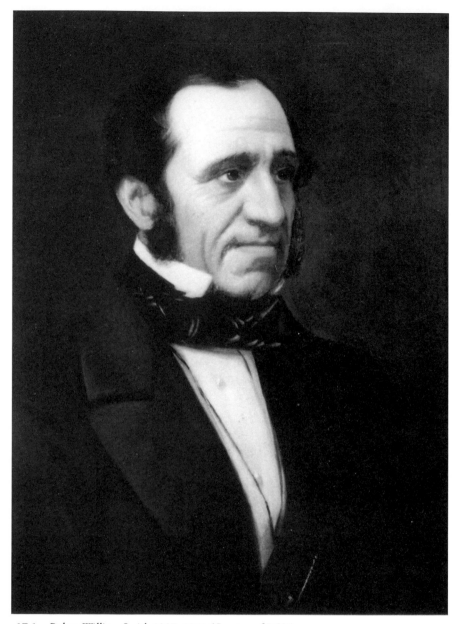

17.1   Robert William Smith 1807–1873 (Courtesy of RCSI)

ROBERT WILLIAM SMITH
1807–1873

17 A major contributor to pathology

Although Robert Smith is remembered in medical literature primarily for the fracture of the wrist which bears his name, he deserves greater recognition for the part he played in the development of modern pathology. He was born in Dublin on 12 October 1807. His father died when Smith was a child, but despite this loss his mother was determined that he should receive a good education. He studied at Trinity College, taking his BA in 1828 and his MA in 1832. He also studied at the Royal College of Surgeons, and he was apprenticed to Richard Carmichael. In October 1832 he obtained the Letters Testimonial of the College of Surgeons and in 1838 he was appointed surgeon to the House of Industry Hospitals. In 1842 he obtained his FRCS and he also received an MD from Trinity College. Smith lectured initially on forensic medicine and afterwards on surgery at the Richmond Hospital Medical School.

THE PATHOLOGICAL SOCIETY OF DUBLIN

Smith played a key role in establishing the Pathological Society of Dublin in 1838. Both he and William Stokes were the first joint secretaries, and they were also married to sisters. The object of the new society was to cultivate the study of pathology and to advance the diagnosis and treatment of diseases by relating pre-mortem symptoms and signs to post-mortem findings. The great strength of the society lay in the fact that it brought surgeon, physician and obstetrician together, thus encouraging a spirit of mutual co-operation in the pursuit of knowledge.

At the inauguration of the society, six presidents, two vice-presidents, two secretaries, a treasurer and a council of members were elected. Four surgeons, Richard Carmichael, Abraham Colles, Philip Crampton and James Cusack, and two physicians, Robert Graves and Henry Marsh, were the first presidents. Robert Adams and William Montgomery were vice-presidents and Dominic Corrigan was on the council.

These outstanding men formed the nucleus of the society which was to become very famous and was the forerunner of many similar societies around the world. The members met at 4 o'clock every Saturday afternoon, when pathological specimens were presented. The proceedings of the society demonstrate the high standards of clinical observation and pathological description achieved by its members. The first clinical meeting of the society took place on 10 November 1838, when Robert Graves took the chair. Eight years after the foundation of this society, William Wilde wrote the following in an editorial on Irish medical societies in the *Dublin Quarterly Journal of Medical Science:*

> Of these, the Pathological Society merits more than a passing notice, having achieved more for the healing art in this country, than all its predecessors together. It was established in 1838, by Dr Stokes, and Dr Robert Smith, two of the most distinguished pathologists in this country: for its results, we refer with no small degree of pride to the pages of our own Journal, which, when there was no other medical periodical in Ireland, devoted a large space to the transactions and reports of this body; and its beneficial effects have extended even beyond our island, this society having since been initiated in nearly every large city in Great Britain.[1]

Senior students from the various schools of medicine in Dublin were encouraged to attend meetings of the society. Here they became familiar with the pathology of a wide range of conditions, and in later years microscopic changes were also demonstrated to them. A gold medal was awarded to the student who was the author of the best essay on some pathological subject, as chosen by the council of the society:

> To the students who were permitted to attend, the advantages were manifold; first of all there was the exceptional opportunity they were afforded of studying microscopic pathology, and what perhaps was a still greater advantage, the moral one, derived from witnessing so many distinguished men such as Corrigan, Gordon, Hutton, Mayne, Adams, Banks, McDowell, Law, R.W. Smith, and others whose names were 'familiar as household words,' not only attending the meetings from beginning to end with praiseworthy regularity, but also taking an active part in the exhibition of morbid specimens, the description of which was always accompanied with a graphic account of the clinical features of the case from which the specimen was obtained.[2]

Robert Smith continued to serve as secretary of the pathological society from its establishment until his death in 1873, a period of thirty-five years.

TREATISE ON FRACTURES

In 1847 Smith published *A Treatise on Fractures in the Vicinity of the Joints*. This book established his reputation and is one of the classics of surgical literature. It was a substantial work of 314 pages, with 200 fine illustrations. The book contains the first description of the wrist fracture now known as Smith's Fracture. This fracture is also known as the Reversed Colles' Fracture, as the deformity is the opposite to that which occurs in a Colles' Fracture. Smith's Fracture:

> ....generally occurs in consequence of a fall upon the back of the hand, and the situation of the fracture is from half an inch to an inch above the articulation.....[3]

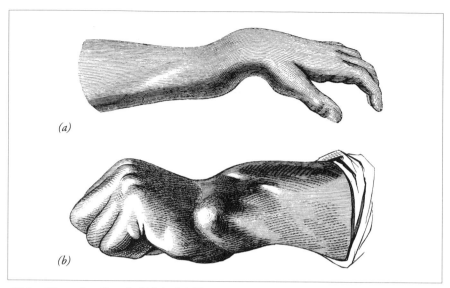

17.2   *Illustrations from Smith's book* A Treatise on Fractures in the Vicinity of the Joints *showing (a) Colles' Fracture, (b) Smith's Fracture. In a Colles' Fracture the distal portion of the fractured radius is displaced backwards, whereas in a Smith's Fracture it is displaced forwards.*

NEW APPOINTMENTS

In 1847 the Board of Trinity College decided to separate the chairs of anatomy and surgery, in accordance with their policy of placing more emphasis on the teaching of surgery within the Medical School. Smith was appointed to the chair of surgery and at the same time he took up duties at Sir Patrick Dun's Hospital. He was very popular with the students and he had a clear and incisive style as a teacher. He read very widely and being a linguist he was conversant with Continental surgery. He was particularly interested in orthopaedics and he is said to have been the first to give an extended description of the reflexions of the capsule of the hip joint. According to Cameron:

> Smith was one of the most distinguished anatomists and surgeons which Ireland has produced, and as a teacher he has rarely been surpassed.... So enthusiastic was he as a teacher that he latterly almost completely abandoned practice, in order that he might devote more time to study, and to instruction of his classes. He was an accomplished linguist, and he kept himself thoroughly posted up in the medical literature of France and Germany.[4]

TREATISE ON NEUROMA

In 1847 Smith published another book entitled *Treatise on the Pathology, Diagnosis and Treatment of Neuroma*. The work described the pathological changes in several cases of neurofibromatosis, and it was illustrated with magnificent plates. The book anticipated the work of Friedrich von Recklinghausen of Strasbourg on the same subject by thirty-three years. Von Recklinghausen was to add to Smith's description by recognising that the fibromata arose from the terminal sheaths of cutaneous nerves.

William Stokes was a great admirer of Smith's contribution to Irish medicine and he dedicated his famous book *Diseases of the Heart and the Aorta* to Smith:

> In the composition of this work, on contending with difficulties inseparable from an attempt to combine the results of many years of labour, I have always been consoled by the thought that in dedicating it to you, I should be enabled to bear testimony not alone to the value of your contributions to Medical Science, but also to the signal benefits which your teaching and example have conferred upon the School of Surgery in this country.[5]

MEETING OF THE BRITISH MEDICAL ASSOCIATION

The British Medical Association met in Dublin for the first time in the second week of August 1867, providing a major opportunity for the Irish school of medicine to display its achievements. The meeting was held in Trinity College and William Stokes, Robert Smith and Dominic Corrigan gave the keynote addresses. Stokes was elected president of the association and he took the chair at a meeting in the Examination Hall. Apart from distinguished visitors from overseas, most of the leading doctors in Irish medicine were present in the audience, including Corrigan, Smith, Stokes, Adams, Collis, Cruise, Mapother, Haughton, Kennedy, Churchill and Porter. During his presidential address Stokes stressed the importance of moving away from the traditional empiricism of therapeutics: 'What is wanting', he said, 'is to have applied to therapeutics the same method of investigation which is used in other scientific enquiries.'[6] Corrigan spoke on the importance of setting adequate standards in medicine. Smith chose the practical subject of slipped epiphysis for his address, but at the beginning he spoke briefly about the history of Trinity College and its achievements. The lecture was praised very highly in an editorial in the *British Medical Journal.*

THE ONSET OF ILL-HEALTH

Smith was a fellow of the Royal Medical and Chirurgical Society of London and an honorary member of the Medical Society of Paris. He continued to edit the proceedings of the Pathological Society until his health began to deteriorate in 1873. On 20 September, the *British Medical Journal* printed the following notice under the heading 'Dr Robert W Smith of Dublin':

> We regret to state that this gentleman, whose reputation as a surgeon is well known, has been suffering for some weeks past from hepatic disease, complicated with ascites, and that he still continues in an extremely unsatisfactory condition. He has been tapped for the dropsical symptom, but suffers considerably from severe pain, which requires opiates in large quantities to procure rest.[7]

He died on 28 October 1873 at his residence, 63 Eccles Street. The editor of the *Dublin Journal of Medical Science* placed the following note under the Reports of the Dublin Pathological Society which had been submitted to him by Smith:

> As we write, the mournful tidings reach us that ROBERT WILLIAM SMITH has this day passed away. Of this loss to Surgical and Pathological Science it would be impossible to estimate the magnitude. The splendid Museum of the Richmond Hospital, the researches on Fractures and Dislocations, the classical monograph on 'Neuroma', and his labours as Secretary of the Dublin Pathological Society from its foundation to the present, are, indeed for him an imperishable record of industry and talent.[8]

18 *Introduction of intravenous saline therapy*

One of the doctors who first witnessed the effects of intravenous saline on critically ill dehydrated patients suffering from cholera wrote to *The Lancet* on 26 May 1832:

> Verily, Sir, this is an astonishing method of medication, and I predict will lead to wonderful changes and improvements in the practice of medicine.[1]

The new and revolutionary therapeutic approach was first suggested by William Brooke O'Shaughnessy, who was born in Limerick in 1809. His father was Daniel O'Shaughnessy and his mother's maiden name was Boswell. O'Shaughnessy studied medicine at Edinburgh where he attended the classes of Robert Knox who at the time was being supplied with cadavers by the notorious Burke and Hare. O'Shaughnessy graduated MD in 1829, and soon after qualification he began to take a particular interest in chemistry and toxicology. A year later he moved from Edinburgh to London.

ASIATIC CHOLERA

In the autumn of 1831 an epidemic of Asiatic cholera erupted in England. According to Robert Graves the epidemic began in India in 1817, in an area known as Jessore, about 100 miles north-east of Calcutta, and from there it spread gradually along the trade routes around the world. It first appeared in Sunderland in October 1831 which, as Graves pointed out, was directly opposite and commercially connected with Hamburg. Although the disease did not cause as many deaths as in other countries, no one knew how to cope with the outbreak. The authorities refused to accept the arguments of men like Graves that the disease was contagious, and the treatments recommended by the doctors usually aggravated the condition they were meant to improve. Treatments advocated include cayenne pepper, calomel, castor oil, emetics, rectal installation of mutton tea, turpentine enemas and bleeding. The physicians regularly complained about the difficulty of blood-letting in patients with collapsed veins. All these treatments were empirical, having no scientific basis and some, such as blood letting, were very harmful.

Shortly after the cholera epidemic began, O'Shaughnessy decided to use his knowledge of chemistry to try and find a method of treating the condition. He presented a detailed paper to the Westminister Medical Society recommending the intravenous injection of potassium chlorate. He argued that the cyanosis so obvious in the patient with 'blue cholera' could be remedied by the use of this toxic oxidising agent. He supported his argument with the details of two experiments on asphyxiated dogs. During his presentation he cast some doubt on the chemical data which he had obtained from German sources, and this may have motivated him to travel to Sunderland to carry out his own investigations. In an age when death from infectious diseases was common, O'Shaughnessy was shocked by the suffering which he witnessed when he arrived in the cholera-stricken area. He described a girl in one house stretched in front of the fireplace, with just a blanket covering her:

> The colour of her countenance was that of lead — a silver blue, ghastly tint; her eyes were sunk deep into the sockets, as though they had been driven in an inch behind their natural position; her mouth was squared; her features flattened; her eyelids black; her fingers shrunk, bent, and

inky in their hue. All pulse was gone at the wrist, and a tenacious sweat moistened her bosom. In short, Sir, that face and form I can never forget, were I to live beyond the period of man's natural age.[2]

FAMOUS LETTER TO *THE LANCET*

O'Shaughnessy acquired specimens of blood, urine and faeces from afflicted patients and he soon became totally engrossed in the work of analysis. His courage was remarkable as there was naturally considerable fear of infection among doctors at the time. On 29 December 1831 he wrote the following letter to *The Lancet* summarising his results; it was one of the shortest and yet most significant letters ever written to the journal:

Sir — Having been enabled to complete the experimental inquiries on which I have for some time back been engaged in Newcastle-upon-Tyne, I beg you will have the kindness to give insertion to the annexed outlines of the results I have obtained:

1. The blood drawn in the worst cases of the cholera is unchanged in its anatomical or globular structure.

2. It has lost a large proportion of its water, 1000 parts of cholera serum having but the average of 860 parts of water.

3. It has lost also a great proportion of its NEUTRAL saline ingredients.

4. Of the free alkali contained in healthy serum, not a particle is present in some cholera cases, and barely a trace in others.

5. Urea exists in the cases where suppression of urine had been a marked symptom.

6. All the salts deficient in the blood, especially the carbonate of soda, are present in large quantities in the peculiar white dejected matters....[3]

FIRST SALINE INFUSION

In this remarkable letter O'Shaughnessy established that the copious diarrhoea of cholera leads to dehydration, electrolyte depletion, acidosis and nitrogen retention. On 7 January 1832 he presented his findings to the Central Board of Health in London and he published them in a brilliant monograph. The book demonstrates his astonishing grasp of acid-base physiology. He wrote about the functions of carbon dioxide, oxygen and 'the colouring matter of the blood' before going on to describe his original observations on the chemical pathology of cholera. It was clear to O'Shaughnessy that treatment must depend on intravenous replacement of the deficient salt and water.

In the same year his suggestion was put to the test by Doctors Thomas Latta and Robert Lewins of Leith in Scotland. Latta gave intravenous fluids to seventeen patients, eight of whom survived. He sent a report on his work to the Central Board of Health and this was published in *The Lancet* on 2 June 1832. In this report he gave a graphic description of the beneficial effects of the first infusion of intravenous saline ever administered:

> She had apparently reached the last moment of her earthly existence, and now nothing could injure her — indeed so entirely was she reduced that I feared I would not be able to get my apparatus ready ere she expired. Having inserted a tube into the basilic vein, cautiously — anxiously, I watched the effects; ounce after ounce was injected but no visible change was produced. Still persevering, I thought she began to breathe less laboriously, soon the sharpened features, and sunken eye, and fallen jaw, pale and cold, bearing the manifest impress of death's signet, began to glow with returning animation; the pulse, which had long ceased, returned to the wrist; at first small and quick, by degrees it became more and more distinct, fuller, slower and firmer, and in the short space of half an hour, when six pints had been injected, she expressed in a firm voice that she was free from all uneasiness....[4]

O'Shaughnessy was very gratified by the apparent success of intravenous fluids and he wrote to *The Lancet*:

> The results of the practice described by Drs Latta and Lewins exceed my most sanguine anticipations. When we consider that no practitioner

would dare to try so novel an experiment, except in cases beyond hope of relief by any ordinary mode of treatment, and consequently desperate to the last degree, even a solitary instance of recovery affords matter for congratulation.[5]

An editorial in the same issue of *The Lancet* compared the new intravenous saline therapy to 'the workings of a miraculous and supernatural agent'.[6] However, there were also critics, particularly non-medical writers, who argued that the treatment hastened death. This impression was probably produced by the fact that intravenous fluids were only given to patients who were moribund, and were often not given again when new bouts of diarrhoea and vomiting led to further dehydration. When the epidemic subsided, interest in the new therapy waned, and at the same time the two main protagonists of the technique left the field. Thomas Latta died in 1833 and O'Shaughnessy left England to join the East India Company. The treatment was not used again until sixty years later, when it was introduced by Cantani in Naples. An exception was the work of Charles Fagge, who in 1874 used O'Shaughnessy's observations to advocate the use of saline in the treatment of diabetic coma.

Apart from its significance in treating dehydration, O'Shaughnessy's approach demonstrated the importance of basing therapy on sound scientific principles rather than on mere empiricism, as was universal practice at the time. Astrup, the great modern acid-base physiologist, has referred to the work of O'Shaughnessy and Latta as:

The first description of an intravenous treatment, based on the first published measurement of an acid-base status of blood. It is the most dramatic one I know of in the history of medical acid-base chemistry — actually in the whole history of medicine — when the use of simple instruments led to a correct understanding of the clinical biochemistry of a disease and to a life saving therapy.[7]

CAREER IN INDIA

In August 1833 O'Shaughnessy was appointed assistant surgeon in the Bengal Medical Service. He continued his chemical researches in India and he presented a paper to the Medical and Physical Society of Calcutta in July 1834. He did not confine his interest to chemistry however, and three years later he published a paper on electromagnetism. He served for some time as physician to Sir Charles Metcalfe at Agra. He was promoted to the rank of surgeon in 1848 and surgeon major in 1861. He was also professor of chemistry at the Medical College, Calcutta.

O'Shaughnessy wrote many books on different aspects of medicine, including a *Manual of Chemistry, The Bengal Dispensatory* and *The Bengal Pharmacopoeia*. His *Manual of Chemistry,* published in 1841, gave one of the earliest comprehensive accounts of biochemistry, and contained analyses of blood, urine, faeces, milk, pus, physiological secretions in different organs of the body, as well as analyses of the composition of different tissues such as tendons, teeth and brain. The book clearly demonstrated his vast knowledge of biochemistry. O'Shaughnessy was elected a fellow of the Royal Society in March 1843.

THE INTRODUCTION OF CANNABIS TO WESTERN MEDICINE

During his early years in India O'Shaughnessy began to explore the potential therapeutic effects of Indian hemp or cannabis. He carried out experiments using mice, rabbits and rats, and he also gave cannabis to some of his patients. The results were dramatic and he published his first observations in 1842 in the *Transactions of the Medical and Psychiatric Society of California*. Cannabis was unknown as a drug in Europe and North America at that time, and O'Shaughnessy's results generated considerable interest. Within a few years it was being used as a medication to treat a wide range of conditions by many of the leading doctors in Ireland and Britain, including Robert Graves and Sir Philip Crampton in Dublin. William Wilde drew attention to O'Shaughnessy's work on cannabis in the second edition of his book *Narrative of a Voyage to Madeira, Teneriffe and Along the Shores of the Mediterranean*, which was published in 1844.

In 1845 the physician and chemist Michael Donovan began his paper 'On the physical and medicinal qualities of Indian hemp' in the *Dublin Journal of Medical Science* with the following eulogy:

If the history of the Materia Medica were to be divided into epochs, each determined by the discovery of some remedy of transcendent power, the period of the introduction of Indian hemp into medicine would be entitled to the distinction of a new era.... The public and the Profession owe a deep debt of gratitude to Professor O'Shaughnessy.[8]

He went on to describe the clinical experiences of a number of Irish physicians and surgeons who had used the drug, and he detailed his own experiences when he took the medication for pain. However, he began by quoting excerpts from O'Shaughnessy's paper which gave details of patients whose rheumatism had been relieved by the use of cannabis:

The fourth case of trial was an old muscular Cooly, a rheumatic malingerer, and to him half a grain of hemp resin was given in a little spirit. The first day's report will suffice for all: In two hours the old gentleman became talkative and musical, told several stories, and sang songs to a circle of highly delighted auditors; ate the dinners of two persons subscribed for him in the ward; sought also for other luxuries we can scarcely venture to allude to, and finally fell soundly asleep,....[8]

Several other medical authors in Europe and North America began to report favourable results with cannabis, and it was soon being used widely. However, the doses used were generally quite low and it is thought that the improvements observed were often due to placebo effect. The enthusiasm for cannabis lasted for many years and it was not until more specific therapies became available earlier this century that its use fell into disrepute. It was finally deleted from the British Pharmacopoeia in 1932.

DIRECTOR-GENERAL OF TELEGRAPHS

O'Shaughnessy did not confine his interests to medicine. In fact, during his lifetime he became famous not so much for his medical contributions, but as the man who first introduced the telegraph to India. He had published a pamphlet in 1839 giving the results of experiments with the telegraph, but he received little official encouragement until 1847. He was then employed to lay down an experimental telegraph line between Calcutta and Kedjeree, at the mouth of the Hooghly River, and to report on the result. This experiment was a success, and in 1852 he was instructed to commence the immediate construction of telegraphs connecting the major cities.

He was appointed Director-General of Telegraphs of India and he was sent to England to collect men and materials. His energy is demonstrated by the fact that by February 1855 the telegraph extended 3050 miles, connecting Calcutta directly with Agra, Bombay and Madras. O'Shaughnessy achieved this despite many difficulties such as the lack of trained workmen, the absence of bridges across wide rivers, and the absence of roads through dense jungles. In the same year he returned to England to receive a knighthood from Queen Victoria.

O'Shaughnessy was married three times. In 1861, on retiring to England, he changed his name by royal licence to William O'Shaughnessy Brooke. He died at Southsea on 10 January 1889, in his eightieth year. In 1973, when summing up O'Shaughnessy's accomplishments, Professor Brian McNicholl wrote: 'This remarkable Irishman who showed a largely unprepared world how to base rational treatment on valid scientific observation and analysis one hundred and forty one years ago, surely deserves a high place amongst the pioneers of medicine.'[9]

ROBERT BENTLEY TODD
1809–1860

19 *A great clinical neurologist*

Robert Bentley Todd made fundamental contributions to neurology in the first half of the nineteenth century. He was also a founder of a medical school and a major teaching hospital in London, and he was in the vanguard of reforms in medical practice. He was born in Dublin in 1809, the son of Charles Hawkes Todd, professor of anatomy in the Royal College of Surgeons in Ireland. He entered Trinity College in 1825 to study law, but he was advised to switch to medicine a year later when his father died unexpectedly, leaving a large family with slender means. He obtained an Arts degree in 1829 from Trinity College and a medical diploma two years later from the Royal College of Surgeons. Todd was influenced greatly during his student years by Robert Graves: 'From him I first imbibed a taste for physiological inquiry; and, under his guidance and direction, my first studies upon that subject were pursued.'[1] After qualifying he moved to London where he joined the Aldersgate School in 1831 as lecturer in anatomy and physiology. He also became physician to the Western Dispensary and the Royal Infirmary for Children. He attended lectures at Oxford in 1832, where he was granted a medical degree a year later.

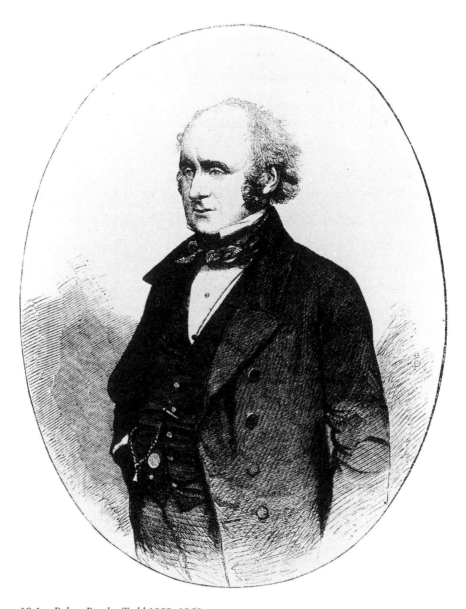

19.1   Robert Bentley Todd 1809–1860

CO-FOUNDER OF WESTMINSTER HOSPITAL MEDICAL SCHOOL

In 1834 Todd joined with three others to found a new medical school on a site in Great Smith Street, London, which they had bought for just over two thousand pounds. This school eventually became attached to Westminster Hospital, making Todd one of the founders of the Westminster Hospital Medical School. He taught in the new school for only two years, before accepting the chair of physiology and morbid anatomy in the recently established medical faculty at King's College. He was twenty-seven at the time of this appointment. Todd described himself as an anatomical physician, thus emphasising that the practice of medicine depended upon the study of anatomy just as much as did the practice of surgery.

FOUNDER OF KING'S COLLEGE HOSPITAL

At the time of Todd's appointment, King's College Medical School did not have a teaching hospital and he decided to devote his energies to rectifying this major deficiency. He established a link with Charing Cross Hospital which had recently been rebuilt and enlarged. It soon became obvious, however, that Charing Cross could not provide teaching facilities for King's College students as well as its own students. Todd argued the case for a new hospital which would serve the needs of the terrible London slums which lay to the north of the Strand and which would also serve as a teaching hospital for King's College. He leased an old workhouse in Portugal Street, just to the rear of the Royal College of Surgeons. This became the first King's College Hospital and patients were admitted in January 1840. The hospital soon became overcrowded and there was a great demand for its services. Todd urged the council of the Medical School to buy land adjacent to the hospital. The new King's College Hospital was built on this site and it was opened in 1854.

AUTHOR AND TEACHER

Todd was a very popular teacher. With his friend and former student William Bowman he emphasised the importance of the microscope in diagnosis. In 1838 he visited hospitals in Belgium and Holland with Bowman and the two men wrote a book together in 1843 entitled *The Physiological Anatomy and the Physiology of Man.* It was a standard textbook for many years and it has been recognised as one of the first physiological works in which an important place is given to histology. Todd was one of the first doctors to insist that accurate diagnosis should always precede treatment. His pupil and disciple Lionel Smith Beale developed Todd's views on this subject.

The first part of Todd's famous *Cyclopaedia of Anatomy and Physiology* was published in 1835. It was followed by four further parts which were published over the next twenty-four years. These volumes, of over six thousand pages, contained contributions from the leading doctors of the time, and it has been said that the cyclopaedia 'did more to encourage and advance the study of physiology and comparative and microscopic anatomy than any book ever published'.[2] Todd was elected a fellow of the Royal Society in 1838.

PIONEER NEUROLOGIST

Todd made several original contributions to medicine. Using the microscope, he was the first to describe hypertrophic cirrhosis of the liver. Francis Kiernan, another Irish doctor working in London, was the first to describe many of the histological features of the normal liver. Todd also wrote on valvular conditions of the heart, and there was a palatable concoction in the French Pharmacopoeia for many years known as 'Potion de Todd', which consisted of a mixture of brandy, cinnamon and sugar.

However, Todd is remembered primarily for his work in neurology. During his Harveian oration in 1934, James Collier described Todd as 'by far the greatest clinical neurologist Britain had produced until the time of Hughlings Jackson'.[3] Todd described the sensory element in sphincter control and he also wrote on peripheral neuritis, being almost certainly influenced by the earlier work of Robert Graves on this subject. He published a book on the nervous system in 1845 entitled *Anatomy of the Brain, Spinal Cord and Ganglions*, and another entitled *Physiology of the Nervous System* in 1847. In the Lumleian Lectures in 1849 he described postictal paralysis, which is still known as Todd's paralysis:

A paralytic state remains sometimes after the epileptic convulsion. This is more particularly the case when the convulsion has affected only one side or one limb: that limb or limbs will remain paralytic for some hours, or even days, after the cessation of the paroxysm, but it will ultimately perfectly recover.[4]

It was Todd who first introduced the term 'afferent nerve' to neurology:

In the motor nerve the nervous force ordinarily travels from the centre to the periphery, in the sensitive nerve it travels from periphery to the centre. The former is therefore efferent, with reference to the centre...the latter is afferent.[5]

One of his greatest contributions was his description of tabes dorsalis or locomotor ataxia, in which he approached the classification of spinal diseases which until then were all described indiscriminately under paraplegia. Todd was the first to speculate on the functions of the posterior columns of the spinal cord, and many of his views were later found to be correct by the experiments of Charles Brown-Sequard.

CHAMPION OF REFORM

Nursing standards were universally poor during the first half of the nineteenth century. Nurses were untrained, they were paid very little and their status was low. For instance, a senior nurse in King's College Hospital applied for the post of assistant cook in 1843, as she wanted promotion! Todd was most unhappy with the low nursing standards and he decided to campaign for improvements. In 1848 he organised a public meeting with the help of some influential friends. At this meeting it was decided to form an institution of religious sisters to recruit and train nurses. The sisters would live under religious discipline but they would not be bound by vows. The new movement became known as the Sisterhood of Saint John the Evangelist, and it still flourishes under the name of the Sisterhood of St John the Divine. It was the first Church of England nursing sisterhood and the first Anglican religious community to receive episcopal sanction. The nurses of this new community took charge of the wards of King's College Hospital in 1856, and the following year they established a nurses' training school. This school anticipated the nursing school established by Florence Nightingale at St Thomas's Hospital by four years.

Todd also made a great impact on the reform of medical education. He campaigned for residential facilities for medical students and he was also responsible for instituting the offices of medical dean and medical tutor. All these developments helped to organise student life and teaching, which until then had been quite chaotic. Todd introduced three open scholarships to the King's College Medical School. Two of these were subscribed by the medical professors and one by friends of the college. These scholarships were the first of their kind in the United Kingdom and probably in the world. When Todd joined the school in 1836 it had the reputation of being the worst medical school in London. When he left seventeen years later, it was thriving, and student numbers had risen considerably. Soon groups of students were coming from all over the world to study the medical and nursing reforms which Todd had introduced.

RESIGNATION

Todd resigned from the medical school in 1853 because of his inability to cope with the conflicting demands of his large practice and his teaching duties. He had also developed a significant alcohol problem, which may have contributed to his decision. As a young man Todd had seen Robert Graves rebel against the bleeding, purging and starvation remedies popular at that time for the treatment of fever. Graves advocated nourishment for these patients and alcohol was used as part of the dietary regime. Todd became an enthusiastic advocate of this approach, and more particularly of the use of alcohol. The case-notes of King's College Hospital show that he often ordered a pint and a half of brandy for his patients, in addition to wine and porter! Todd showed his faith in the remedy by taking large quantities himself, and this almost certainly was the cause of his death from a torrential gastric haemorrhage in his own consulting room on 30 January 1860. A statue of Todd by Noble was erected in the great hall of King's College Hospital after his death.

20 *Fundamental steps towards oxygen therapy*

Thomas Andrews, one of Ireland's most outstanding scientists, made the fundamental observations and experiments which ultimately led to the liquefaction of gases, previously thought to be non-condensable. Oxygen therapy is just one of the developments which ultimately grew from his basic work. He was born at 3 Donegall Square, Belfast, in 1813, the son of a linen merchant, and he attended the Belfast Academical Institution. He worked for a short period in his father's office but he was more interested in science and so he left to study chemistry in Glasgow at the age of fifteen. After his first college session and while still only fifteen he wrote a scientific paper 'On the action of the blowpipe on flame'.

He continued his education in Paris, where he obtained a place in the chemistry laboratory of Professor Dumas in the Royal College of France. He was delighted with his good fortune in obtaining this position:

If chemistry will be ever of any service to me scientifically, I am on the road both to acquire it well and to see the great men here who pursue it.... I never was in better health and spirits than at present — indeed, I must acknowledge to you that I was a little fagged and wearied in travelling.... I must confess, I prefer the fumes of the laboratory to the air of the mountains.[1]

163

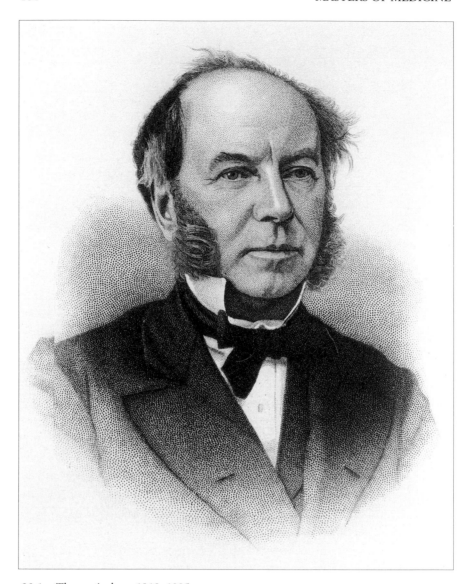

20.1   Thomas Andrews 1813–1885

He also attended clinics in the Hôpital de la Pitié. A sudden illness
forced him to leave Paris and return to Ireland, where he began his
studies in Trinity College, winning prizes in both classics and science.
He also attended lectures at the Meath and Richmond Hospitals, as well

as finding time to go to the lectures of the famous mathematician William Rowan Hamilton in Trinity College.

Andrews published a paper on 'Chemical researches on the blood of cholera patients' in the *Philosophical Magazine and Journal of Science* in 1832. In this paper he described his analysis of blood taken from six victims of cholera in Belfast. He challenged the findings of William Brooke O'Shaughnessy as he found no deficit in saline content: 'The only difference between the blood of cholera and of health consists in a deficiency of water in the serum, and a consequent excess of albumen.'[2] In the discussion of his findings he remarked, 'I cannot therefore avoid concluding that the experiments of Dr O'Shaughnessy are inexact.'[3]

It is clear from a letter which he wrote to his mother in 1833 that Andrews was a conscientious student:

> I am greatly absorbed in my hospital and medical studies; — indeed I begin to feel an enthusiasm similar to what I used to have for chemistry; the diseases I see, the treatment, everything connected with them is the general object of my waking thoughts; — and such a state of mind is one of the happiest.
>
> Dr Graves has a peculiar talent of investing every object he touches on with a deep and stirring interest; and for this alone I shall ever be indebted to him. I breakfast before seven o'clock, and, of course, by candle light; my hospital occupies me from eight till eleven or twelve. Some days I have a lecture from eleven till twelve — then during the day I either read or dissect till three — another lecture till four: the rest of the evening is devoted to reading.[4]

Andrews qualified MD at Edinburgh in 1835. His thesis for the final examination was entitled 'On the circulation and the properties of the blood'. He returned to Dublin where he was offered professorships of chemistry in two of the private medical schools, one in the Richmond School of Medicine where Corrigan and Adams taught, the other in the Park Street School where Graves and Stokes were on the staff. However, he had decided to pursue his career in his native city:

> Again I have kicked away the ball of fortune and preferred the humbler attractions of Dame Prudence to her more glittering rival. In plain language, I have declined the situation in the Park Street, and you may expect me in Belfast in a few days....

I have made a very beautiful discovery in toxicology. When I told Dr Stokes of a consequence of it in a very simple case which every one imagines he understands, he seemed greatly surprised. 'Is it new to you,' I asked him. 'Yes,' he replied, 'and to every one else: don't mention it to any one till you publish it.'[5]

CAREER IN BELFAST

Andrews developed a clinical practice in Belfast and he also accepted the post of professor of chemistry in the newly formed medical faculty in the Belfast Academical Institution. He was only twenty-two when he was appointed to this post in Belfast's first medical school. He joined the staff of Belfast General Hospital as physician in 1838. Despite these heavy commitments he found time for the research which made him one of the foremost physical chemists of his day. His early work concentrated on the heat generated in chemical reactions involving combination with oxygen, and on the same phenomenon during reactions between acids and bases. The value of the research was quickly recognised and Andrews developed friendships with some of the leading scientists in Europe, including Michael Faraday, James Apjohn and Robert Bunsen.

Largely through the efforts and prestige of its professorial staff the medical school was a success, and within a short period of its foundation there were over eighty students on the books. When consideration was being given to Belfast and Armagh as possible locations for the proposed Queen's College, the existence of the medical school was one of the factors which gave the advantage to Belfast. Andrews was a particularly popular teacher and he drew large crowds to his lectures, mostly due to his penchant for setting up chemical apparatus and carrying out experiments in front of his students. The institution had a liberal approach to education and young working men were encouraged to 'improve' themselves by attending part-time. It was common for those who were otherwise engaged in various trades or businesses in the city to attend Andrews' lectures for an hour or two each day.

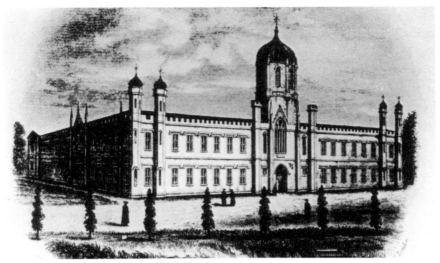

20.2　Queen's College, Belfast

VICE-PRESIDENT OF QUEEN'S COLLEGE BELFAST

In 1845 Andrews was appointed to the vice-presidency of the new Queen's College in Belfast. The presidents and vice-presidents of the Queen's Colleges at Belfast, Cork and Galway were appointed four years before the institutions were opened so that the government could have their support and advice in bringing the scheme to fruition. Andrews worked closely with Robert Kane, president of Queen's College Cork, and it was mainly due to their commitment and foresight that the new colleges developed, despite considerable opposition. During the same period the country was in the grip of the Great Famine and Andrews, despite his many commitments, was indefatigable in both raising funds for relief and caring for the poor.

Andrews' increasing involvement in the new college led to friction between him and the medical faculty of the Belfast Academical Institute, as the future of the latter was under threat by the development of a medical school in Queen's College. Andrews was also frequently away giving invited lectures as a consequence of his growing stature as a scientist. After an acrimonious correspondence, his resignation from the institute was accepted in 1848, and this was followed by a row over the ownership of chemistry equipment, much of which Andrews had bought himself. The following year the medical faculty of the institute closed, as the government grant was withdrawn on the opening of Queen's College. Some of the professors were given gratuities of £250, and others like Andrews, who was given the chair of chemistry, received appointments in the new college.

In 1849 the Queen's Colleges enrolled their first students. Andrews was a very able administrator, being approachable and direct, and having a genuine interest in all kinds of people and in their problems. Although deeply religious himself, he was broad-minded and tolerant on the subject of religion. One of his early achievements was the introduction of a chair of Celtic languages, as he believed very strongly that the ancient language of Ireland should be represented on the staff of all the new Queen's Colleges.

Pooley Henry was the first president of Queen's College Belfast, and although he was quite different in personality and background to his vice-president, both men worked closely in a partnership that lasted until their resignations in 1879. Under their regime, which was marked by 'firmness, stability and caution', the college acquired a character of its own and it developed slowly but steadily. Henry was a Presbyterian minister and Andrews a member of the Church of Ireland, and they both believed strongly in non-sectarian education. Henry delegated much of the day-to-day responsibilities of running the new college to Andrews, who was allowed to take the initiative in academic matters. Andrews carried some of the values of the Academical Institution with him into the new college. He encouraged the opening of the college facilities to the less advantaged members of society, and as early as 1851 he had introduced an evening course of lectures in chemistry for working men. He did not stand aloof from the controversial issues of his time. He wrote pamphlets on two very contentious issues, the organisation of Irish university education and the dis-establishment of the Church of Ireland. The historians T W Moody and J C Beckett described these works as towering 'above the mass of contemporary polemic for the range and depth of their learning, their scholarly precision, their independence of judgement, and their freedom from bitterness'.[6]

ORIGINAL OBSERVATIONS ON GASES

Andrews spent whatever spare time was available to him each week in his private laboratory. 'Here he delighted to receive his scientific friends, and to engage eagerly in conversation with them, while his hands were busy with the steady, deliberate construction or adjustment of apparatus for his next research.'[7] He was an excellent French and German scholar and he kept up to date with the most recent advances in science on the Continent. In 1856 he read a paper to the Royal Society in which he detailed his classic researches on the nature of ozone. In this work he proved that 'ozone from whatever source derived, is one and the same body, having identical properties and the same constitution, and is not a compound body, but oxygen in an altered or allotropic condition'.[8]

Most people of genius would be happy to retire after making a discovery of this magnitude, but Andrews persisted with his research and he was rewarded with an even bigger discovery. He found during experiments using high pressure chambers that below a critical temperature all gases can be liquefied. Conversely, no gas can be liquefied if the temperature is above the critical point for that gas, no matter how high the pressure applied. His work led him to conclude that the 'gaseous and the liquid states are only distinct stages of the same condition of matter, and are capable of passing into one another by a process of continuous change.'[9] Speaking to the Royal Dublin Society he told his audience: 'We may yet live to see, or at least we may feel some confidence that those who come after us will see, such bodies as oxygen and hydrogen in the liquid, perhaps even in the solid state.'[10]

His confidence in the significance of his work was well placed, as witnessed by the oxygen tanks now used to supply oxygen in hospitals all over the world. Andrews provided all the necessary suggestions for the adaption of his apparatus so that the 'non condensable' gases could be liquefied. He had to leave the implementation of the practical implications of his work to others, although he did carry out some further research on the subject which he reported to the Royal Society in 1876. Louis-Paul Cailletet in Burgundy and Raoul-Pierre Pictet in Geneva both liquefied oxygen within days of each other in 1877, their work following as 'a natural and almost immediate consequence of that of Andrews'.[11]

Andrews was made a fellow of the Royal Society in 1849 and he was also awarded a gold medal by the society. He declined a knighthood in 1880, a year after his retirement. Between 1849 and his death in 1885 he lived at Lennoxvale, Malone Road, which is now the residence of the vice-chancellor of The Queen's University.

WILLIAM WILDE
1815–1876

21 *Illustrious surgeon, scientist and writer*

Wwilliam Wilde, one of most brilliant members of the Irish school of medicine, was one of the first ear surgeons and he wrote the first significant clinical textbook on the subject. He was the son of a general practitioner, Dr Thomas Wilde, and he was born in County Roscommon in 1815. He received his early education, like Oliver Goldsmith, at Elphin, County Roscommon. He began his medical studies in Dublin when he became apprenticed to Abraham Colles at Dr Steevens' Hospital. Apart from being a good teaching hospital, Dr Steevens' also had literary associations as Jonathan Swift was one of the hospital's original trustees and Stella was a benefactor. Wilde also studied at the Park Street Medical School. Here he came under the influence of Robert Graves and William Stokes.

Soon after Wilde's arrival in Dublin, Asiatic cholera began to spread throughout the country. Wilde was advised to stay with relatives near Conna in Connacht so that he would not contract the disease. However, when the epidemic spread to the west of Ireland, Wilde willingly involved himself in a situation of great danger. The owner of a lodging house in Kilmaine, near Conna, fell victim to the disease and no one would go near him. Wilde took up residence with the patient and nursed him. Despite Wilde's efforts the patient died and the young student had to bury him, as the villagers would not help beyond supplying the coffin.

JOURNEY TO THE MIDDLE EAST

Wilde spent four years at Dr Steevens' Hospital before moving to the Rotunda to study midwifery. There he became clinical clerk to Evory Kennedy. Whilst a student at the Rotunda, Wilde became very ill with fever, which was probably typhus, and it was thought that his condition was hopeless. Graves was sent for and he prescribed a glass of strong ale to be taken every hour. The student recovered and the following morning Graves found him sleeping comfortably. Subsequently Graves asked Wilde to travel as a medical attendant with one of his patients who was embarking on a health-seeking cruise to Greece, Egypt and Palestine. It has been suggested that Wilde accepted because the change of climate would benefit his health. But there was another factor which may have dictated the expediency of the prolonged absence abroad. A young woman had discovered that she was pregnant and William Wilde was the father. In September 1837 Wilde sailed off to begin a series of adventures which would last for over eight months, and which he later described in fascinating detail in his first book *The Narrative of a Voyage to Madeira, Teneriffe and along the shores of the Mediterranean.*

On his return to Dublin Wilde did not marry but arrangements were made for the care and maintenance of the child who was given the name Henry Wilson. The name was almost certainly derived from 'William's son', as this would be in accordance with common practice at the time in such situations. Henry Wilson was given a good education by his father and he eventually became an eye surgeon.

Wilde collected a considerable amount of scientific material on his journey to the Middle East and as a consequence he was invited to read papers to such bodies as the Royal Irish Academy and the British Association. He also became a popular lecturer at the Royal Dublin Society. According to Wilde's biographer T G Wilson, 'For a young medical man of twenty-four, his knowledge of the botany and zoology of his day was astounding. Had his career been in Natural Science, it is certain that he would have made major contributions to the subject.'[1]

His essay on the mechanism of suckling in whales contained original observations which were subsequently confirmed by others. In 1839 Wilde was admitted by the president, Sir William Rowan Hamilton, as a member of the Royal Irish Academy.

STUDIES ABROAD

Wilde was horrified by the number of people he saw in Egypt who had lost their sight due to trachoma, and this almost certainly awakened in him an interest in ophthalmology. As a result he began to study eye surgery at Moorefield's Hospital in London. He became a friend of Sir James Clarke, the court physician, who introduced him to London society. He soon made a name for himself in London, as his son Oscar would do later in the century. He also formed a lasting friendship with Robert Todd who, like him, had been a pupil of Graves.

After his time in London Wilde decided to visit some of the famous clinics on the Continent, starting with the Allgemeines Krankenhaus in Vienna. There he came under the influence of the great Czech pathologist, Carl Rokitansky. On leaving Vienna Wilde travelled at a leisurely pace through Germany, spending some time in Dresden and Heidelberg and studying surgery under Johann Friedrich Dieffenbach in Berlin, who at that time was making major contributions to the development of plastic surgery. Wilde carried with him letters of introduction from Maria Edgeworth, which he found gave him ready access to the leading figures and societies in the intellectual life of Berlin.

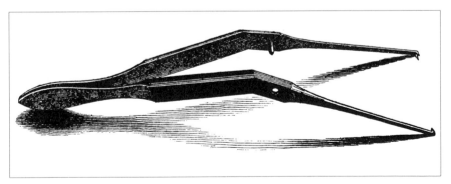

21.1   Wilde's ear forceps. Reproduced from his book Practical Observations on Aural Surgery *(1853).*

Wilde's primary objective in going to Vienna was to gain experience in eye and ear surgery. Rosas and Jager were the two leading ophthalmic surgeons there and Wilde gained considerable expertise by studying their methodology. In contrast he found that aural surgery was very neglected; it was not until later in the century that Vienna developed its reputation in this field. Several other aspiring Irish ENT surgeons followed in Wilde's footsteps to Vienna, among them remarkable men such as Sir Robert Woods, Oliver St John Gogarty and James Bowring Horgan. Gogarty (1878–1957) subsequently became famous for his literary rather than his surgical prowess. Horgan (1883–1955) achieved eponymous fame for his description of a surgical approach to the ethmoid sinuses, and Woods (1865–1938), although he specialised in ENT surgery, made fundamental contributions to the understanding of the biophysics of cardiac function.

WILDE'S EYE AND EAR HOSPITAL

On returning to Dublin from Austria, Wilde set up practice as an eye and ear specialist at his home in 15 Westland Row, and he established his own Eye and Ear Hospital at the rear of Molesworth Street. This was the first hospital in Ireland and Great Britain in which aural surgery was taught. The hospital was an immediate success and soon Wilde had to search for a bigger building. He purchased the former general hospital of St Mark's in St Mark's Street, off Great Brunswick Street, and in 1844 he reopened it as an Ophthalmic Hospital and Dispensary for Diseases of the Eye and Ear. He invited Robert Graves to become consultant physician and Sir Philip Crampton to become consultant surgeon to his hospital. William Stokes would also join the staff later.

Wilde lectured at his old medical school, the Park Street School of Medicine, on diseases of the eye and ear, and when the medical school closed in 1848 he bought the building. He paid £1100 for it and he spent another £200 on alterations. He adapted the building, which became the new St Mark's Hospital, to accommodate twenty public patients, and there were also three private rooms, an operating theatre, an out-patients department, living quarters for a house surgeon, and a lecture room. This hospital is still standing and it now houses the genetics department of Trinity College. Many students, undergraduates and postgraduates, came to the hospital from abroad, particularly from England and America. Wilde examined the cases at the out-patients in front of the students, while a 'shorthand writer' made notes. He then examined the students on the cases they had seen and gave a short tutorial. After the out-patients he did a teaching ward-round which ended with a session in the lecture room, where he elaborated in more detail on the treatment of the cases seen. Students were encouraged to study the pathological drawings and specimens from Wilde's large collection in the hospital and they were also allowed to watch him operate. Wilde had no illusions about the quality of the teaching at St Mark's: 'I have reason to believe that the instruction in this institution is the most efficient of its class afforded by any institution in the Kingdom.'[2]

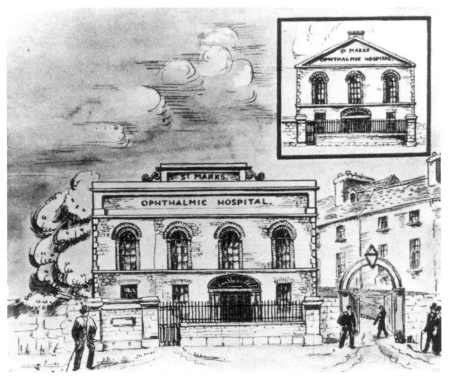

21.2   St Mark's Ophthalmic Hospital. This building still stands at the back gate of Trinity College and it now houses the genetics department of the university. In 1897 St Mark's Hospital amalgamated with the National Eye and Ear Infirmary to form the Royal Victoria Eye and Ear Hospital, which is situated in Adelaide Road. (Courtesy of the Board of the Victoria Eye and Ear Hospital)

Wilde was very dedicated to his hospital and visited it several times each day and often at night. He developed a very good reputation as an eye and ear surgeon and his practice grew rapidly. In 1862 he handed over the management of the hospital to a Board of Trustees for the use and advantage of the afflicted poor of Ireland. In doing this, he joined the distinguished ranks of founders of Dublin voluntary hospitals, such as Richard Steevens, Mary Mercer, Jonathan Swift, Sir Patrick Dun and Bartholomew Mosse.

INNOVATIONS AND PUBLICATIONS

Wilde established himself as one of the great ear specialists of his time and he helped to place the subject on a scientific footing. He introduced many new instruments, including the first dressing forceps and an aural snare known as Wilde's Snare. One of the operative approaches he devised for mastoiditis became known as Wilde's Incision. He also established the role of the middle ear in the aetiology of aural infections.

In 1853 he published his textbook *Practical Observations on Aural Surgery and the Nature and Treatment of Diseases of the Ear.* This was the first textbook of importance on the subject and it is now regarded as a classic in its field. It is based largely on bedside observations and investigations. In the preface he wrote:

> I have laboured, and I trust not in vain, to expose error and establish truth; to lay down just principles for an accurate diagnosis of Diseases of the Ear; to rescue their treatment from empiricism and found it upon the well-established laws of modern pathology, practical surgery and reasonable therapeutics.[3]

An American edition of the book was brought out by Addinel Hewson, who had been a pupil of Wilde's in Dublin. It was translated into German and it remained a standard textbook for many years. Wilde also wrote a book describing his experiences on the Continent, entitled *Austria. Its Literary, Scientific and Medical Institutions,* which was published in 1843. It has recently been republished in a German translation. He became editor of the *Dublin Quarterly Journal of Medical Science* in 1845 and held the post until 1850.

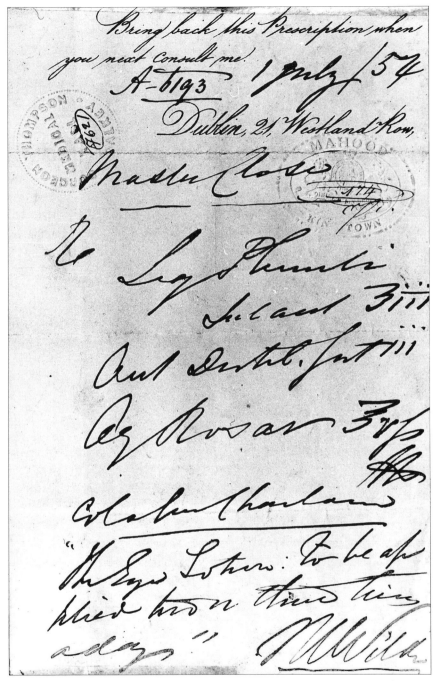

21.3 *A prescription for an eye lotion signed by William Wilde in 1854. (Courtesy of RCPI)*

PIONEER OF DEMOGRAPHIC STUDIES

Wilde was appointed medical adviser and compiler of the tables of the causes of death in the census of 1841, and assistant commissioner for the 1851, 1861 and 1871 censuses. In these he collected and collated social and biological data which was not being collected in any other country at the time. Sir Peter Froggatt has described Wilde's work on the 1851 census as 'one of the greatest demographic studies ever conducted'.[4] This study became a standard work of reference on the Great Famine which devastated Ireland between 1845 and 1849. It was probably his experience on the 1841 census that prompted the Victoria Assurance Company to recruit him as their medical referee.

MAN OF MANY INTERESTS

Wilde's mother and sister lived with him at 15 Westland Row. In 1848, after the death of his mother, he moved along the street to number 21. Three years later he married Jane Francesca Elgee, a poetess, who wrote under the name of Speranza for *The Nation*. They had three children: William, who became a barrister and later a journalist with the *Daily Telegraph*, Oscar the famous poet and playwright, and a girl named Isola who died in childhood.

Wilde had many interests outside medicine. He did important work on natural history, ethnology, topography and related subjects. He was a noted archaeologist and antiquary and he compiled the great *Catalogue of Antiquities* in the Royal Irish Academy. He used the experience which he had gained through several years of fieldwork in the Boyne Valley to write his book *The Beauties of the Boyne and Blackwater*, editions of which are still appearing. He also wrote a book on the life of Jonathan Swift. His biography of Bartholomew Mosse, which was published in the *Dublin Quarterly Journal of Medical Science*, rescued the founder of the Rotunda Hospital from years of neglect. He also wrote a memoir of Sir Thomas Molyneux which was published as a serial in the *Dublin University Magazine*. Molyneux, who was educated at Leiden, was the first Irish medical baronet and he published on many aspects of natural history and medicine. His most famous medical contribution was a treatise on the influenza epidemic of 1693, in which he monitored the

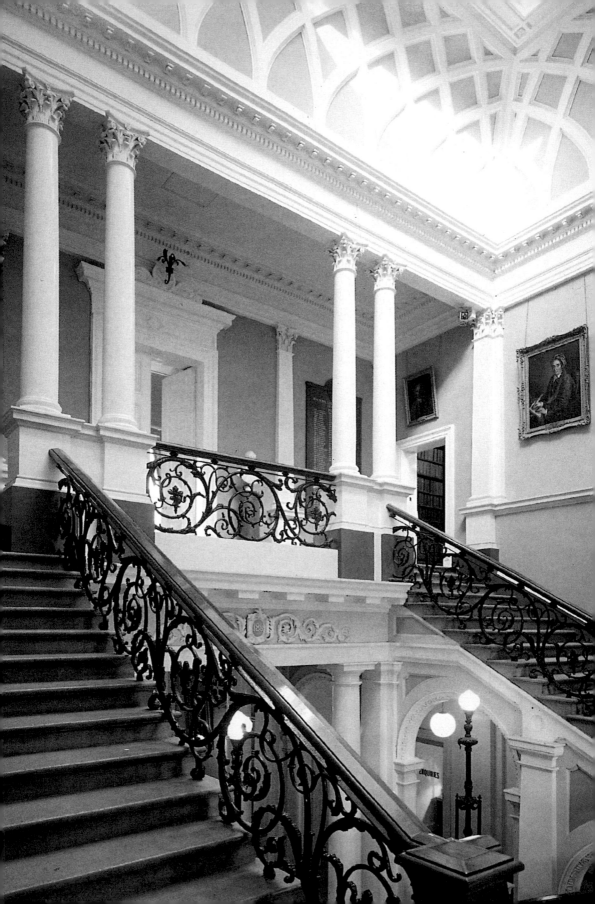

Pl 1 (Previous page)   The upper staircase leading to Dun's Library in the Royal College of Physicians of Ireland, Kildare Street, Dublin. (Courtesy of RCPI)

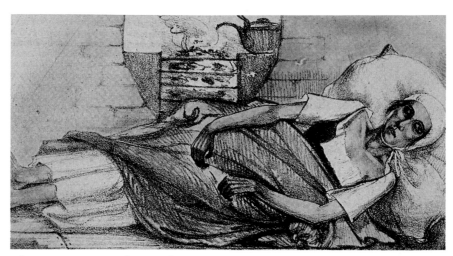

Pl 2   A contemporary drawing of a victim of the cholera epidemic in Sunderland, from The Lancet, *18 February 1832.*

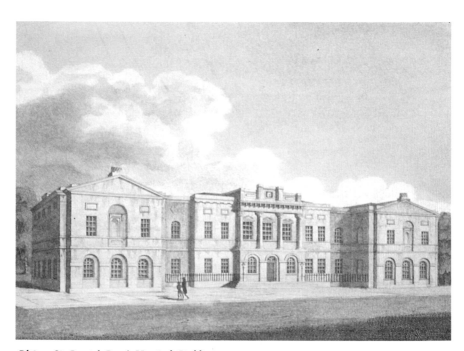

Pl 3   Sir Patrick Dun's Hospital, Dublin.

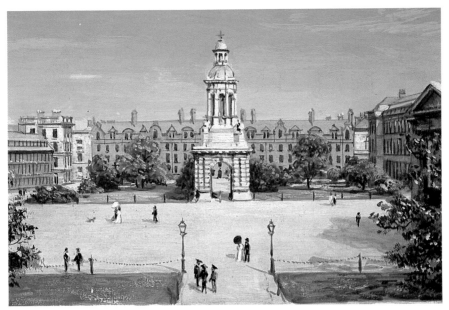

Pl 4   Watercolour of Trinity College Dublin c 1920 by Thomas Nisbet.

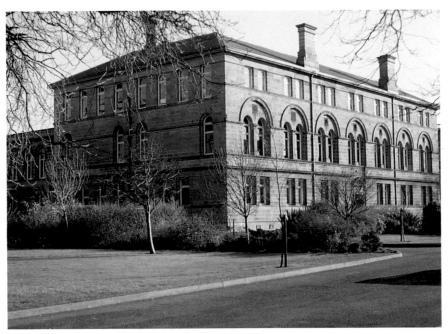

Pl 5   The medical school building at Trinity College Dublin, which largely replaced Macartney's school towards the end of the nineteenth century.

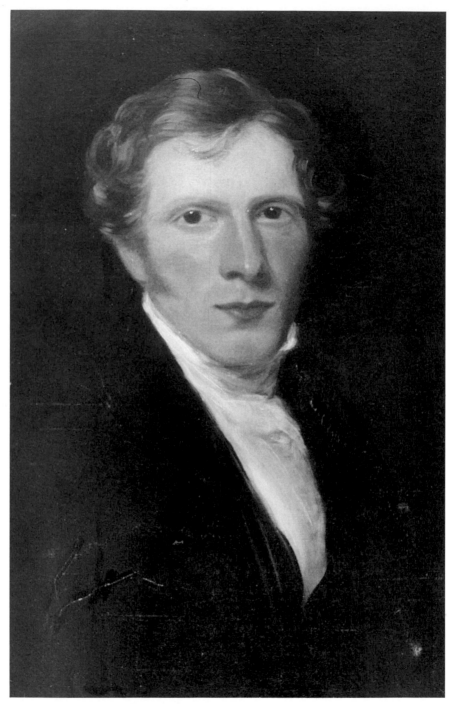

Pl 6   John Houston 1802–1845 (Courtesy of RCSI)

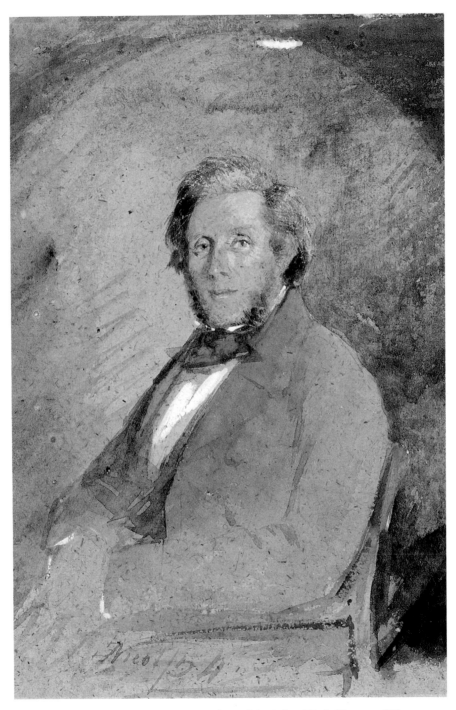

Pl 7   Watercolour of William Wilde (1815–1876) by Erskine Nicol. (Courtesy of The National Gallery of Ireland)

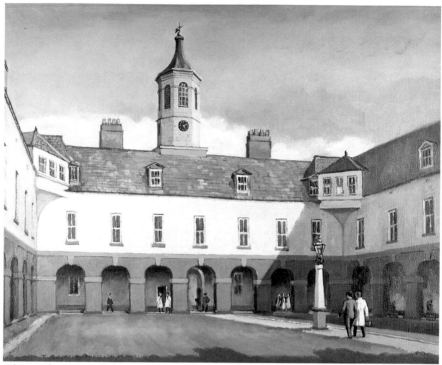

Pl 8   The courtyard of Dr Steevens' Hospital, Dublin, by T G Wilson. Photograph by David Davidson. (Courtesy of RCSI)

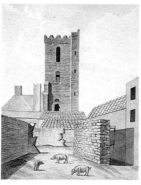

Pl 9   St John's Tower drawn by Gabriel Beranger in 1780. It was the only remaining part of the hospital and priory of St John the Baptist which had stood on the site now occupied by the Augustinian Church in Thomas Street, Dublin. (From Beranger's Views of Ireland, *RIA, 1991.)*

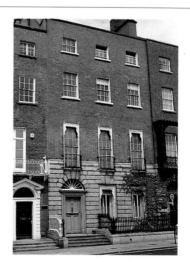

Pl 10   Number 5 Merrion Square, Dublin, formerly the home of William Stokes.

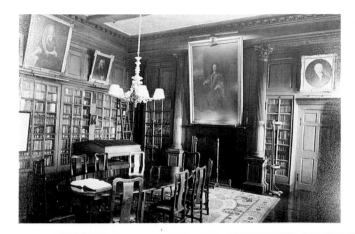

Pl 11 The Worth Library at Dr Steevens' Hospital, Dublin.

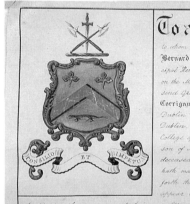

Pl 12 Grant of Arms to Dominic Corrigan from the Ulster King of Arms of All Ireland in 1860. (Courtesy of RCPI)

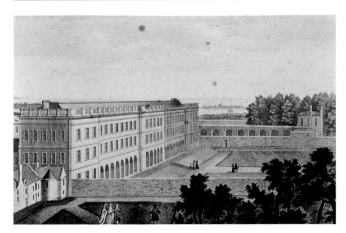

Pl 13 The Library of Trinity College Dublin in 1753, with the Anatomy House, the first medical building in the university, on the right. (Courtesy of TCD)

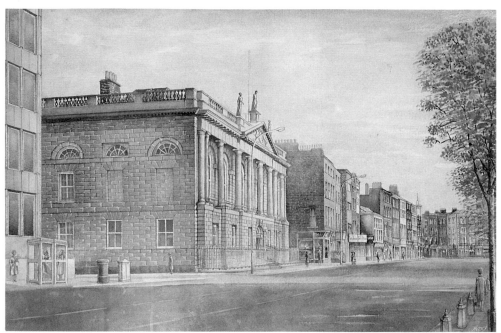

Pl 14   The Royal College of Surgeons in Ireland by Patrick Heney. (Courtesy of RCSI)

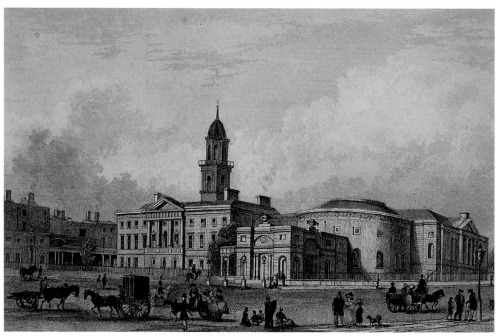

Pl 15   The Rotunda Hospital, Dublin, by W H Bartlett.

progress of the epidemic by estimating the volume of coughing at church on Sundays! Sir Peter Froggatt has suggested that Wilde may have been influenced by Molyneux as Wilde describes him as a very able physician with 'a well-deserved reputation in general literature, natural history, and antiquities'.[5]

Wilde's entry in the *Medical Directory for Ireland* in 1852 is the largest and most varied. It mentions, among many other accomplishments, that Wilde was a member of several medical, literary and scientific societies, including societies in Athens, Vienna, Berlin, Stockholm and Paris.

The Wilde's moved to 1 Merrion Square in 1855 and here they entertained on a grand scale. Their house became a meeting place for the country's artistic and literary élite. The medical historian Charles Cameron was a regular guest and he later recalled:

> There were two well-known 'diners out' at that time who, like myself, were always invited to the Wilde's dinner parties, namely, the Rev. Charles Tisdall, DD, and Dr Thomas Beatty, an obstetrician in large practice. Beatty was the only medical man who had been president of both the Royal College of Physicians and the Royal College of Surgeons. The reverend and medical doctors had excellent voices. Their habit was to meet in Wilde's study and then to ascend the stairs very slowly, singing a duet.[6]

LEGAL BATTLE

Wilde was knighted in 1864 for his census work. However, his career suffered a severe setback when a young woman named Mary Travers, with whom he had unwisely formed a relationship, set out to ruin him. She had become very demanding and Wilde decided to end the relationship. Infuriated, she sought revenge by circulating a rumour that she had been assaulted sexually by Wilde during a consultation. Lady Wilde condemned Mary Travers' activities in no uncertain terms in a letter to her father, Robert Travers, who was lecturer in medical jurisprudence at Trinity College. Mary saw the letter and she brought a civil action for libel against Lady Wilde and her husband. The jury found for Mary Travers but awarded her only one farthing damages. Wilde was left with the expenses of the case, which were quite considerable.

FINAL ACHIEVEMENTS

After the trial Wilde spent more and more time at his country home, Moytura, which he built in 1865 on the banks of Lough Corrib, and he wrote a book on the history and antiquities of the area. He received several honours, including the Order of the North Star of Sweden in 1862. Two years later he received the degree of MD *honoris causa* from Trinity College.

Wilde died on 19 April 1876 after a long illness. Lady Wilde described his last weeks in a letter which she wrote shortly after his death:

> His health was failing in the winter — no actual complaint — except bronchial attack, and we hoped for spring — but spring brought no strength. He faded away gently before our eyes — still trying to work, almost to the last, going down to attend professional duties. Then he became weaker, and for the last six weeks never left his bed. He himself still hoping and planning as usual for his loved Moytura, but still he grew weaker day by day, no pain, thank God, no suffering....[7]

For three years following Wilde's death, the annual report of St Mark's Hospital was framed in black. He left three uncompleted manuscripts behind him. One was planned to be a major history of Irish medicine, but this was never completed. The others, a manuscript on Irish folklore and a Life of the eighteenth-century painter and architect Gabriel Beranger, were completed by his wife and subsequently published. According to Peter Harbison in his introduction to the beautiful edition of *Beranger's Views of Ireland,* published by the Royal Irish Academy in 1991, the painter 'would have been largely consigned to oblivion had his cause not been championed in the 1870s by Sir William Wilde'.[8]

SAMUEL HAUGHTON
1821–1897

22 Champion of mathematics and medicine

When Samuel Haughton began his medical studies he was already a well-known mathematician and geologist. He used his scientific training to carry out fundamental research on joint and muscle function in animals and man. Haughton came from an old Quaker family, and even though both his parents had withdrawn from the Community of Friends, he spent his childhood in Quaker surroundings. He was born in Carlow on 21 December 1821 and he received his early education in a large school supervised by the rector of the parish. Here Haughton came under the influence of a teacher who had a profound interest in nature. Master and pupil went on several field trips together to explore the topography of the local countryside. This stimulated Haughton's interest in botany and geology.

STUDENT OF DISTINCTION

At the age of seventeen Haughton entered Trinity College where he immediately distinguished himself as a student and won the Lloyd Exhibition in mathematics in 1842. His brilliance was recognised by his election to a fellowship in 1844, shortly after his graduation, making

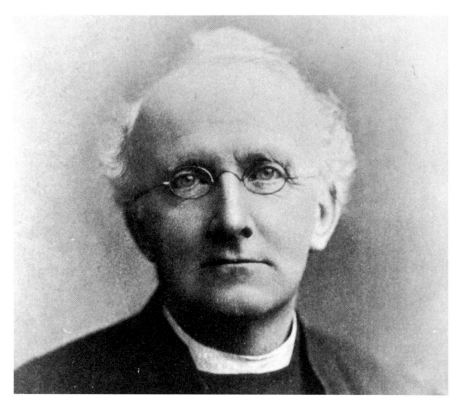

22.1   Samuel Haughton 1821–1897 (Courtesy of RCPI)

him the youngest graduate ever to be elected fellow. He then had to comply with the college regulation that all fellows should take Holy Orders.

At this time Haughton came under the influence of the remarkable Trinity mathematician James MacCullagh, with whom he shared a house in the college. It was probably due to his influence that Haughton's early work was in the discipline of physical science. When he was only twenty-six years old he was awarded the Cunningham Medal by the Royal Irish Academy for his paper 'Equilibrium and motion of solid and fluid bodies'. He became a leader in applied mathematics, working on problems such as the modelling of the earth and its inner structure, and calculations on the depth of the sea. In 1851 he was appointed professor of geology and seven years later he was elected a fellow of the Royal Society.

HAUGHTON GRADUATES IN MEDICINE

As a child Haughton had been interested in medicine and had considered devoting his life to work as a medical missionary in China. Now as a young geologist his interest in medicine was re-awakened. He had come to the conclusion that he could not interpret the many fossil remains in geology without a knowledge of comparative anatomy. He decided to remedy this gap in his knowledge by entering the medical school at Trinity College at the age of thirty-eight. Haughton carried out his dissections and laboratory work as enthusiastically as his young colleagues and he attended ward rounds and lectures until his graduation in medicine in 1862. During this time he continued to fulfil the duties associated with his chair of geology and he also published at least twelve geological papers.

REGISTRAR OF THE FACULTY OF MEDICINE

During his undergraduate years Haughton began to realise that the medical school needed reform. He used his influence with the senior members of Trinity College to obtain the post of registrar of the faculty. Once appointed, Haughton set about re-organising the teaching within the faculty. With this in mind he established a medical committee with William Stokes in the chair and he himself acted as secretary. Several reforms were introduced which greatly improved the efficiency of the medical school.

WORK ON ANIMAL MECHANICS

As a result of his work in the anatomy department, Haughton became extremely interested in the mechanical principles of muscular action. Following his graduation he continued to do research on the subject. It was his practice to spend two hours in the dissection room every day working on the comparative anatomy of the muscular system of vertebrates. He published a number of papers on the subject and his ideas took final shape in his book *Principles of Animal Mechanics* which was published in 1873, after nearly a decade of research. The work was a comprehensive study of the physiology of a wide range of animals and it pioneered the use of mathematics to analyse physiological functions such as the movements of the limbs and muscle contraction. Haughton was solely responsible for the development of the oppositionist theory of animal mechanics. In the preface of his book he set out his principle of 'least action in nature':

> I have met with numerous instances in the muscular mechanism of vertebrate animals of the application of the principle of least action in Nature; by which I mean that the work to be done is effected by means of the existing arrangement of the muscles, bones, and joints with a less expenditure of force than would be possible under any other arrangement; so that any alteration would be a positive disadvantage to the animal.[1]

The principle of least action was introduced into physics originally by the French mathematician and astronomer Pierre Moreaude Maupertius (1698–1759). Haughton used this principle in his research to demonstrate that the bone-muscle arrangements were such as to require the least expenditure of energy for the performance of limb movements. He argued that changes in this optimal system would bring no advantage to the animals, no matter how gradually these changes took place. He presented this as an unanswerable theoretical contradiction to Darwin's theory of slow evolution through progressive perfection of a species. N D McMillan has pointed out that at the time Darwin and his supporters such as Huxley could not answer the fundamental questions raised by Haughton's research, however 'recent formulations of evolutionary theory have emphasised the discontinuous revolutionary change of species as opposed to the slow evolutionary change proposed by Darwin'.[2]

Haughton used opportunities in the clinical setting to perform ingenious experiments which allowed him to measure circulation time, the mechanical work of the heart and blood pressure. His conclusions compare favourably with the results obtained using modern technology. This is all the more remarkable when one considers the circumstances of some of his experiments!

On the 18th of March, 1863, a large fibro-cellular tumour was removed by Mr M H Colles, in the operating theatre of the Meath Hospital, from the left groin of a middle-aged, large-sized man; in the course of the operation the external epigastric artery, which appeared enlarged to feed the tumour, was divided, and before it could be ligatured, strong jets of blood from it were thrown in various directions about the room. I noticed, as the poor fellow moved about on the operating table, that jets of blood fell short, or enjoyed a long range, according to the angle of elevation of the orifice of the bleeding artery, and that there was a certain maximum range on the floor of the theatre, which was not exceeded.

I saw immediately that I had before my eyes the solution of the problem that had puzzled me; as by measuring the co-ordinates of the maximum range, I could calculate the velocity with which the blood left the artery.[3]

Haughton's approach of using mathematical principles to elucidate biological mechanisms was used to great effect in this century by another Irish anatomist Michael Aloysius MacConaill (1902–1987). Perhaps the last of the great Irish medical polymaths, MacConaill helped to lay the foundations of modern biomechanics through his work at University College Cork on the structure and functional anatomy of joints.

HAUGHTON'S DROP

In 1866 Haughton published a paper entitled 'On Hanging' in the *Philosophical Magazine*. It was common practice at that time, particularly in England and Scotland, to allow the condemned man to fall just three or four feet and then to watch his agonies while he died slowly from cerebral anoxia. Haughton argued for a longer drop for humane purposes and he used his mathematical and anatomical knowledge to support his case:

Instead of the 'short drop' generally used, we ought to employ the 'long drop', which causes instantaneous death. It has been ascertained by me that the shock of a ton dropped through one foot is just sufficient to fracture the anterior articulating surfaces of the second vertebra at their contact with the atlas; and that this fracture allows the shock to fall upon the medulla oblongata so as to produce instantaneous death. As the result of some consideration bestowed upon this subject, I would recommend the adoption of the following rule:

Rule 1. 'Divide the weight of the patient in pounds into 2240, and the quotient will give the length of the long drop in feet.' For example, a criminal weighing 160 lbs should be allowed 14 feet drop.[4]

Haughton's medical background is apparent in this passage as he refers to the condemned man as a 'patient'! His formula was adopted generally and it became known as Haughton's 'Drop'. This gave him a certain notoriety, especially among the 'fresher' medical students. The medical author Johnston Abraham, who was a student at Trinity College, remembered when Samuel Haughton was first pointed out to him:

One day a benevolent-looking old gentleman of about seventy wandered into the dissecting-room looking for the Professor; and, as he passed, a third-year man working opposite me murmured;
'That's Sammy Haughton. Invented "the drop", you know.'
I gazed at the old man, fascinated. He looked so gentle. It seemed incongruous. The other man read my thoughts.
'Yes. It does seem an odd thing for a clergyman to have thought of, even though he was a doctor. But it really is much more merciful. The old method was terribly brutal.'[5]

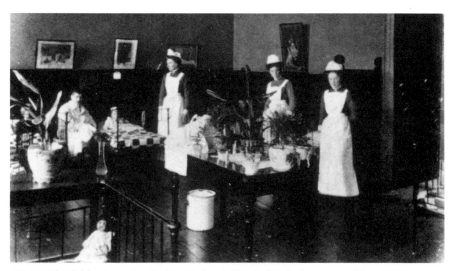

22.2   The children's ward at Sir Patrick Dun's Hospital at the beginning of this century. (Courtesy of RCSI)

GOVERNOR OF SIR PATRICK DUN'S HOSPITAL

Haughton served for thirty-four years as a governor of Sir Patrick Dun's Hospital. During this time he campaigned relentlessly for better hospital facilities for the sick poor. During the epidemic of cholera in 1866 there was a major crisis in the Dublin hospitals. The disease was spreading rapidly and there was an acute shortage of nurses. Haughton called for volunteers from amongst the students and he organised them into a nursing staff which did duty until the epidemic had passed. In organising the rotas, he drew no distinction between himself and the students, and he took his turn at nursing along with the rest. This direct contact with the sick and panic-stricken poor had a major impact on him and led him to stress the value of bedside work in student training. He founded medals for the encouragement of clinical work in Sir Patrick Dun's Hospital and the last act of his life was to make these awards more substantial and more permanent.

INVOLVEMENT WITH THE ZOOLOGICAL SOCIETY

Haughton's involvement in the Zoological Society formed a major part of his life. In 1860 he became a member of its council and in 1864 he was elected its honorary secretary. He served in this post for twenty-one years and he relinquished it to take up the duties of president. The Zoological Society at that time had, as it still does today, major financial problems. Haughton tackled these problems with great energy and managed to keep the society viable. He enjoyed relating how the bank, on one occasion, had threatened to close the society's account and he had met the difficulty by offering to deposit a ferocious Bengal tiger as security for the debt.

He performed autopsy examinations on animals which died in the Zoological Gardens and from time to time he presented his findings to the Dublin Pathological Society. In February 1864 he presented the post-mortem findings on a seal who had died after he was attacked by some boys with 'brick bats' two weeks previously. In February 1878 he described an autopsy which had been carried out on a lioness. The animal died from tuberculosis but Haughton pointed out that the commonest cause of death amongst the large carnivora at the zoo was pneumonia and that he based his observations on the fact that he had dissected 'upwards of a hundred large cats, lions, tigers, leopards, pumas and jaguars...'[6] In the same presentation he mentioned that it was commonly believed, largely on the authority of Robert Graves, that the high mortality amongst the monkeys was due to tuberculosis. However, Haughton diagnosed scurvy after he had dissected several monkeys: 'I found purpuric spots in the kidneys, pericardium, and heart, which proved that the cause of death was internal purpuric scurvy. I attributed this to their bread and milk diet, and accordingly we stopped it, and gave them fruit and fish and from that moment the mortality stopped.'[6]

At that time it was the custom for members of the council to meet in the Zoological Gardens for breakfast, before proceeding to business. These 'zoo breakfasts' were a distinctive feature of the social life in Dublin and at these meetings Haughton appeared at his very best. Surrounded by friends of long standing such as Dominic Corrigan, he gave full scope to his playful nature. The restaurant building at Dublin Zoo was erected in his memory by public subscription and it is still known as Haughton House.

Haughton had a multiplicity of interests and he was an authority on many subjects apart from medicine. His contributions to physical science were principally in the areas of elasticity (continuum mechanics), the theory of light and solar radiation and the tides. His work on the tides was originally undertaken with the purpose of making the navigation of the Irish Sea and English Channel safer. He became a recognised international authority on tides and a consultant on the subject to arctic explorers. He also used his knowledge of tides to throw light on a number of other subjects, such as the incidence of shipwrecks and the sequence of events at the Battle of Clontarf. He wrote around two hundred and seventy papers on different aspects of science and he was author or editor of over thirty books. He received many honours, including the DCL of Oxford, the LLD of Cambridge and of Edinburgh, and an MD from Boulogne. He died in 1897, leaving behind him a remarkable record of achievement.

ARTHUR LEARED
1822–1879

23 Inventor of the bi-aural stethoscope

René Laënnec introduced auscultation as a diagnostic aid in the early years of the nineteenth century. The stethoscopes used for many years were simple tubular devices through which the doctor listened with one ear. Credit for the introduction of the first bi-aural stethoscope goes to Arthur Leared, medical scientist, traveller and writer. Leared, the son of a merchant and a native of Wexford, was born in 1822. He was educated at Trinity College where he obtained the MB degree in 1847, having become a licentiate of the Royal College of Surgeons the previous year. After qualifying he spent six months in the Meath Hospital where he worked with his professors, William Stokes and Robert Graves, before taking up the post of medical officer at Oulart dispensary in County Wexford.

WIDE-RANGING INTERESTS

Leared went to India in 1851, but poor health forced him to return a year later to work as a physician in London. He became a member of the London College of Physicians in 1854 and a fellow in 1871. During the Crimean War he was appointed physician to the British Civil

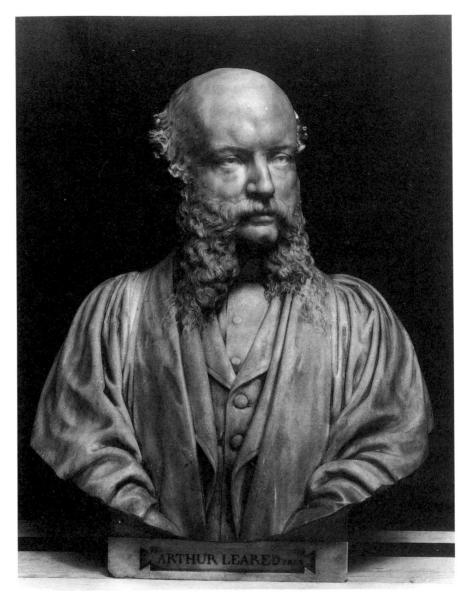

23.1   Arthur Leared 1822–1879 (National Portrait Gallery, no 11130. Courtesy of RCP, London)

Hospital at Smyrna, and he left to take up this post in 1855. Leared enjoyed travelling and after the war he visited the Holy Land. On his return to London he was appointed to the Great Northern Hospital and to the Royal Infirmary for Diseases of the Chest at Brompton. He also became lecturer on the practice of medicine at the Grosvenor Place School of Medicine.

Leared was a member of several societies, including the Royal Irish Academy, the Royal Geographical Society and the Icelandic Literary Society. He contributed several papers to medical literature, on topics as diverse as the blood, tuberculosis, the gastrointestinal tract and cardiology. His most remarkable achievement was his invention of the bi-aural stethoscope which, according to his obituary in the *Medical Times and Gazette* was 'one great proof of his medical skill and his interest in chest infections'.[1] Leared was a man of culture, and because of his interests outside medicine he had a large circle of literary, scientific and artistic friends.

THE BI-AURAL STETHOSCOPE

The instrument was constructed using gutta-percha tubes and was exhibited by Leared at the Great Exhibition which was held in London in 1851. This exhibition was formally opened by Queen Victoria on 1 May 1851 and it ran for 140 days. Over six million visitors flocked to see the exhibits on view in the Crystal Palace, which was specially designed by Paxton for the event.

Leared's stethoscope was displayed with the other medical instruments in the section entitled 'Philosophical, Musical, Horological and Surgical Instruments'. As Leared walked around the area where his stethoscope was exhibited he would have seen some rather intriguing exhibits. For instance, Madame Caplin, inventor and patentee, was demonstrating hygienic corsets and chest expanders. There was also 'a medical walking stick containing an enema-syringe, a catheter, a test-tube, a test-paper, a pair of forceps, a number of wax matches and a pill box'.[2] The medical profession was beginning to appreciate the importance of the microscope and several different varieties were exhibited. A French firm displayed a small dentist's mirror with a long handle. It attracted little attention but it was subsequently bought by Manuel Garcia for six francs in September 1854 and with it he made the first laryngoscope.

It would appear that Leared failed to take appropriate steps to realise the commercial potential of his double stethoscope. Within a few years similar stethoscopes were being manufactured in America and shipped across the Atlantic. When Leared returned to London from the Crimean War in 1856 he wrote to the editor of *The Lancet* refuting a statement that a Dr Camman of New York and a Dr Marsh of Cincinnati had invented the instrument before him:

> To prove priority of invention is often a troublesome, and sometimes an unpleasant, task; but, in the present instance, the difficulty at least is not great.... I have now before me the copy of a description sent with my instrument to the Executive Committee of the Exhibition, dated January 28th, 1851; and I may add that I had a double instrument constructed in 1850, if not earlier. Now, I think the above date is conclusive that it was impossible for me to copy from the American instrument, while from the position in which mine was placed, it is not only possible, but highly probable, that the idea of the instrument was pirated, and the patent for it obtained on the other side of the Atlantic within the year. This, however, I can declare, that I never heard or read anything which gave me the least clue to the invention....
>
> I must apologise for intruding thus largely on your space, but I was anxious to explain the matter fully now that, as a foreign importation, the double stethoscope has a fair chance of being tested.[3]

Camman's design was first illustrated in the *New York Medical Times* in January 1855. Leared is now acknowledged as the inventor of the first bi-aural stethoscope in Garrison and Morton's *A Medical Bibliography*. He was granted an MD by Trinity College in 1860 for a dissertation on 'The sounds caused by the circulation of the blood', which he published the following year, and he was also admitted MD *ad eundem* at Oxford in 1861.

CONTRIBUTIONS TO GASTROENTEROLOGY

Four years after Leared described his stethoscope, he read a paper to the physiological section of the Medical Society of London, in the course of which he made another fundamental contribution to medical knowledge. Through an ingenious combination of clinical observation and scientific experiment he established that pancreatic juice 'decomposes fat into its proximate elements'.[4] In proposing this he was challenging the teaching of leading physiologists of the time. Leared published his paper 'On the pancreatic juice in relation to the digestion of fat' in the *Medical Times and Gazette* in 1854: 'My inference, therefore, is, that besides the conversion of starch into sugar, one of the true offices of this secretion is the separation of fatty bodies into their immediate principles.'[4] In 1860 he published a book entitled *The Causes and Treatment of Imperfect Digestion*, which established his reputation as a medical writer and which reached a seventh edition twenty-two years later. During his life he was known chiefly for his writings on gastrointestinal problems.

FOREIGN TRAVELS

Between 1862 and 1874 Leared visited Iceland on four occasions and he became so proficient in the language that he published a book in Icelandic, *Fatal Cystic Disease of Iceland*. In 1870 he visited America and in 1872 he went to Morocco. His book *Marocco and the Moors* was published in 1876. In the preface he claimed that one of his reasons for writing the book was to draw attention to 'the incomparable climates to be found in Marocco for persons suffering from affections of the chest'.[5] The second edition, which appeared in 1891, was edited by the famous traveller Sir Richard F Burton, who described Leared as 'A learned physician, a skilled practitioner, an observer of no common powers, and a genial, liberal, travelled man....'[6]

Morocco was very unsettled at the time and not safe for Europeans. Leared's curiosity and desire for discovery placed him at risk on several occasions, even when he and his friends donned disguises. In spite of turban, beard, sunburn and flowing Moorish robes they were readily recognised as Europeans wherever they ventured. At times they were surrounded by a hostile mob shouting curses: 'Many of these would not bear translation, one of the mildest being, "May God burn your father, Christian dog!" The Moors consider it the greatest insult to curse the parents of those they hate.'[7]

On one occasion Leared led his intrepid group to a large open space where the markets and festivities were usually held:

Proceeding farther into the square, we observed a snake-charmer and a man with monkeys, the place being noted for these exhibitions. I requested the former to begin his performance, and the man at once pulled out two hideous reptiles from a basket and began to flourish them about his head. A crowd of roughs, men and boys, rapidly collected. We kept aloof as much as possible, nevertheless the mob showed signs of hostility and began to jeer...we all thought it prudent to beat a retreat as fast as spurs could induce our animals to move.[8]

The fact that Leared was a doctor was sometimes an advantage to him in his explorations, although he often found the demands it placed upon him exhausting. At many of the places where he stayed he was immediately mobbed by large groups of Moors demanding medical attention. Occasionally he was also expected to cure the relatives of local dignitaries:

At every stopping-place there were no end of patients, and when stationary for some days, one's practice increased immensely. Some were fever-stricken, others loathsome from skin diseases: the lame, the blind, the deaf, the childless, and the lean — for the last two were conditions for which remedies were eagerly sought — all thronged round our tent.[9]

Leared returned to Morocco in 1877 as physician to the ambassador of Portugal, who was travelling to congratulate the sultan of Morocco on his accession. Leared's wife accompanied him on this journey. The sultan gave Leared a free pass and so he was able to visit the cities of Morocco, Fez and Mequinez. He explored many of the more remote parts of the country on this occasion and he succeeded in identifying the site of the famous ancient Roman town at Volubilis. He published an account of this remarkable achievement in 1878 and it was subsequently appended to the edition of *Marocco and the Moors* which was published in 1891.

Leared read a paper on Morocco to the geographical section of the British Association in Dublin in 1878. He expanded his lecture into another book entitled *A Visit to the Court of Morocco*, which was published in 1879. Around the same time he secured some land north of Tangier with the intention of building a sanatorium for tuberculous patients, as he believed the climate was more suitable than that of southern Europe.

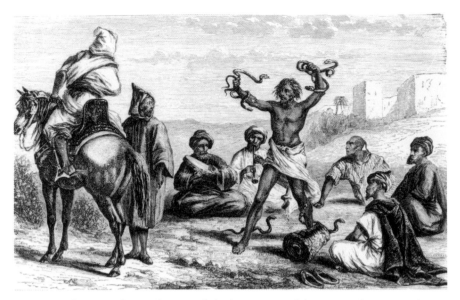

23.2   An illustration from Arthur Leared's book Marocco and the Moors, *showing a snake charmer. Leared and his group had to leave this scene quickly when a hostile crowd gathered around them. (Courtesy of TCD)*

Leared travelled to Morocco for the last time in the summer of 1879. He made the visit in connection with his proposal to build a sanatorium, but he became ill in Tangier and decided to return to London. He broke his journey at Lisbon, where his condition deteriorated. Typhoid fever was diagnosed when he arrived in London. He appeared to improve at first but then he deteriorated again and died on 16 October 1879.

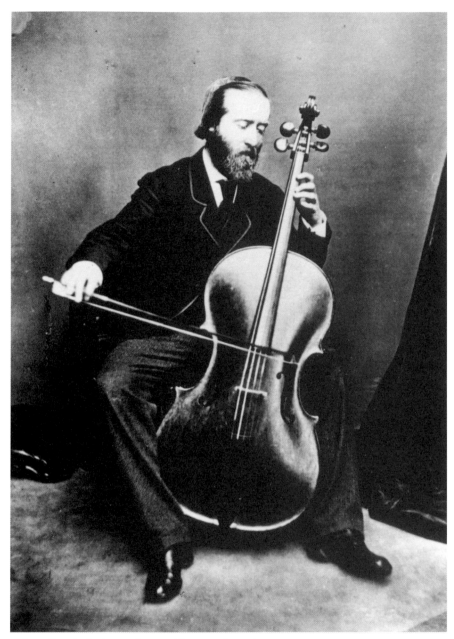

24.1   Francis Cruise 1834–1912 (Courtesy of RCPI)

FRANCIS CRUISE
1834–1912

24 An early endoscopist

Francis Cruise designed the first effective endoscope. He was born in Mountjoy Square in Dublin on 3 December 1834. He was the son of a Dublin solicitor and he received his early education at Belvedere College and Clongowes Wood College. Cruise studied medicine at Trinity College and he gained clinical experience under Corrigan, Adams and Smith at the Richmond Hospital. He also helped Robert McDonnell with his research and this was a valuable experience for him. It was McDonnell who carried out the first blood transfusion in Ireland in 1865. Corrigan had a major influence on Cruise during his undergraduate days and Cruise found his teacher's lectures very stimulating as the material was always presented in a lucid manner. Corrigan was fifty-two at the time and at the height of his professional practice. Cruise later recalled the first day he approached his teacher:

I can never forget the first day I spoke to Corrigan in the grounds of the Hardwicke Hospital. Of commanding figure, very like Daniel O'Connell, his face beamed with kindness, and his manner, if a trifle brusque, was most fascinating. I put a question to him about a patient we had just seen in the hospital ward, and the painstaking manner in which he explained all I asked established a confidence never after shaken or forgotten. Of his subsequent kindness to me I could never speak without emotion. If I had been a favourite son he could not have been more partial, and, as I later found, more devoted.'[1]

Corrigan selected Cruise to be his resident clinical clerk. They attended meetings of the Dublin Pathological Society together and Cruise prepared the specimens under Corrigan's direction. The friendship which developed between teacher and student was remarkable and was to last a lifetime. Years later, when Corrigan was dying, Cruise slept in an adjoining room in readiness for any emergency.

After his graduation in 1858 Cruise was in poor health so he accepted an invitation to visit the United States with a famous traveller, Count Henry Russell. There, in the backwoods, he became an expert rifle shot. On returning to Dublin he became a licentiate of the Royal College of Physicians of Ireland in 1859 and a member of the Royal College of Surgeons of England the following year. In 1861 he was granted an MD by Trinity College for a thesis on abnormal development of the female genital organs. He was made a fellow of the Irish College of Physicians in 1864. Cruise was attracted initially to surgery but later he turned to medicine. In 1858 he lectured on anatomy and physiology in the Carmichael School, which was attached to the Richmond Hospital, and from 1864 he lectured in medicine. He was appointed junior physician at the Mater Hospital when it first opened in 1861.

THE DEVELOPMENT OF ENDOSCOPY

Cruise wrote on many medical subjects but his most famous contribution was his account of the cystoscope, which was published in 1865. The cystoscope was first introduced by John Fisher in Boston in 1827. In 1853 Antonin Jean Desormeaux of the Hôpital Necker in Paris developed Fisher's instrument and he became known as the 'father of cystoscopy'. However this instrument had severe limitations because of the poor illumination. Cruise addressed this problem and he improved the lighting by using the thin edge of the flat flame of a paraffin lamp in which camphor had been dissolved. Light from the flame passed through an adjustable aperture. It was then reflected from a specially positioned silver mirror which was perforated by a small hole through which the observer could view the inside of the bladder by means of an eye lens. His endoscope tubes included designs for both direct and right-angle vision. Cruise intended that his instrument should be used not only in the bladder but in other organs, and there were attachments for examining the rectum, uterus, auditory meatus, nasal fossae, pharynx and larynx. These attachments were made to his specifications by Dublin craftsmen. He also thought that his instrument could be adapted for investigation of the oesophagus. 'There is no portion of the human body', he wrote, 'into which a straight tube can be introduced in which it will not be found of service'. [2]

Cruise demonstrated his instrument for the first time on 15 March 1865, at a meeting of the Medical Society of the College of Physicians in Dublin. The instrument generated considerable interest and received favourable comments in some of the London medical journals, including *The Lancet* and the *British Medical Journal*. The report in *The Lancet* was written by the journal's correspondent, who had been present at the meeting:

> Dr Cruise's endoscope is a modification of Desormeaux's, and possesses the great advantage over it of an illuminating apparatus so brilliant, and admitting of such easy and perfect adjustment, that little or no previous training is required to enable the practitioner to obtain a satisfactory view of deep cavities which heretofore have been generally looked upon as quite inaccessible to sight, such as the bladder, urethra, remote portions of the rectum, &c.
>
> We have now at our command an instrument which will enable us to extend and correct our ideas respecting the nature of ailments about which formerly we were very much in the dark.... I think it only a simple act of justice to this gentleman to notice his labours and improvements, to compliment him on the very favourable reception his communication met with, and to give him the credit of priority in following up in this city the study of the long-neglected endoscope, of having so modified it as to give us a really valuable instrument, and of demonstrating for the first time in Dublin its unquestionable value as an aid in diagnosis and treatment. [3]

Cruise wrote a detailed paper 'The utility of the endoscope as an aid in the diagnosis and treatment of disease' which appeared in the *Dublin*

Quarterly Journal of Medical Science in 1865. In this paper he stated that he had long dreamt of becoming a proficient endoscopist, even as a student. He first tried the instrument described by Desormeaux but gave it up in despair because of the poor illumination. Some years later he returned to the subject when a modification of the lighting source of the instrument occurred to him. When he built his instrument he found that the new arrangement worked far better than the older design. However he proceeded cautiously:

> Rendered distrustful of success by repeated failures, for months I worked in silence and in private, until I became familiar with its use and manipulation. Then, for the first time, I exhibited it to others. Early in March I showed it to Dr Fleming, of the Richmond Hospital, and demonstrated to him and Professor R W Smith an organic stricture of the urethra. Subsequently, by the kind invitation of medical friends, I examined a variety of cases at many of the Dublin hospitals, and also in private. I am quite satisfied that it is an unquestionable success, and I feel justified in stating that I believe the field of its practical utility is almost illimitable. I venture even to hope that in the course of time it may work as complete a revolution of our knowledge of many obscure diseases as the stethoscope has wrought in the diagnosis of infections of the lungs and heart.[2]

Cruise went on to give a detailed description of the instrument and he described his experiences in examining the urethra, the rectum, the uterus, the nose and the ear with the endoscope. He used the instrument primarily to investigate diseases of the urethra and bladder, and was the first to describe the upward extension along the course of the urethra of the disease process in gonorrhoea. His paper in the *Dublin Quarterly Journal of Medical Science* is a masterly account of clinical investigation, but he finished it with the description of an experiment designed to convince the most sceptical of his readers!

> However, on this day (April 4) my friend and colleague, Dr Robert M'Donnell, submitted my instrument to a test upon the dead body, which I think may fairly be considered an 'experimentum crucis', and, in illustration of its capacity, I record the trial, for the veracity of which Dr M'Donnell is as responsible as I am myself:— He first prepared a subject by opening the bladder and introducing into it three substances of a

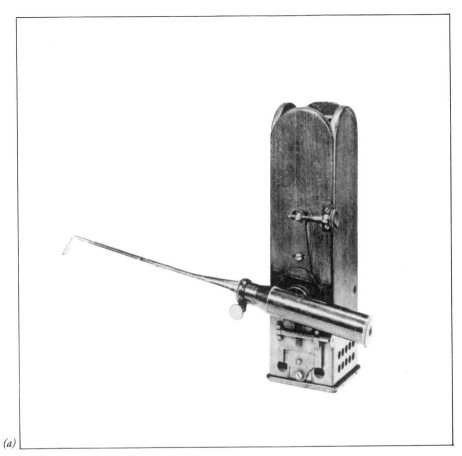

(a)

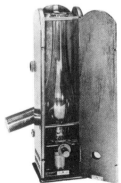

(b)

24.2   (a) The cystoscope designed by Francis Cruise
       (b) The illumination system of the endoscope

nature the most unlikely to be thought of and respecting which I was in total ignorance. He then brought me to the body, and challenged me to tell with my endoscope what the articles in the bladder were. In a few minutes I was able to do so, and to demonstrate them to him. The articles were — a brass screw with a milled head, a short Minié bullet, and a mass of plaster of Paris.[2]

Cruise's endoscope was introduced to the London Lock Hospital by Christopher Heath, and from there its use spread to several parts of England. The endoscope was exhibited at the Dublin meeting of the British Medical Association in 1867. William Stokes praised the instrument as a very significant development in an address delivered before the Medical Society of the College of Physicians in Ireland in 1866:

> Originally described by Desormeaux, it was reserved for Dr Cruise to make the idea practically applicable; and so much has he made the instrument his own that, while Paris can claim to be the best place for the stethoscope, Vienna for the laryngoscope and Berlin the ophthalmoscope, Dublin is entitled to the honour if not of the discovery, at least of the application of endoscopy.[4]

Ernest Mark in his history of cystoscopy has pointed out that Cruise kept the practice of endoscopy alive until his instrument was superseded by one developed in 1877 by the German Max Nitze. Nitze developed an endoscope with incandescent lighting using an electrically heated platinum loop.

THE USE OF HYPNOSIS

In his later years Cruise became interested in psychiatry and in particular in the application of hypnosis to medicine. In 1890, when he was fifty-six years old, he travelled to Nancy in France to study hypnosis under Henri Bernheim, the professor of medicine. Later Cruise went to Paris and studied at La Charité and at La Salpêtrière. When he returned to Dublin he began to use hypnosis as a form of treatment. One of his students recalled Cruise using hypnosis in an attempt to relieve pain:

'On one occasion I saw him making a trial of the method in the case of a female patient: having placed a small coloured glass globe on a table and told her to keep looking steadily at it he, after some minutes, very slowly and solemnly uttered the words: "you will have no more pain".'[5]

OTHER INTERESTS

On St Luke's Day in 1881 Cruise was elected president of the Royal College of Physicians. He was a member of the senate of the University of Dublin and of the Royal University of Ireland. He was also a member of the Royal Irish Academy. Cruise had many interests outside medicine. He was a gifted cellist and he also composed for the instrument. He founded his own instrumental club and he was a governor of the Royal Irish Academy of Music. He lived at 93 Merrion Square.

Cruise was a classical scholar of some standing. He translated the *Imitatio Christi* (Imitation of Christ) into English in 1887 and he also wrote a biography of Thomas à Kempis of which he said: 'To me it was a labour of love to pursue this study, to snatch half-hours from the turmoil of a wearisome life to turn over dusty volumes and trace out as best I could his saintly career.'[6] Cruise mastered the art of photography so that he could take photographs as he journeyed through Holland seeking information about places which had associations with the life of the German monk. In the preface of his biography he wrote: 'Probably very few can be as conscious as I am of the many faults and deficiencies of the book, but the life of a physician in active practice is, to say the least, not favourable to literary work, as the only leisure he can command is made up of the spare half-hours he steals while on very anxious rounds.'[7]

For these works he was honoured in 1905 by Pope Pius X, who conferred on him the Grand Cross of St Gregory the Great, and a street in Kempen was named after him. His library, containing many books relating to Thomas à Kempis, has been preserved by the Jesuit community in Gardiner Street. Cruise wrote a short biography of Sir Dominic Corrigan in 1912, which was included in a book entitled *Twelve Catholic Men of Science*, edited by the medical polymath Sir Bertram Windle, president of Queen's College Cork. The biography was also published separately as a pamphlet by the Catholic Truth Society.

Cruise's contribution to medicine was recognised in 1896 when he was knighted, and five years later he was appointed honorary physician to Edward VII.

Cruise did not forget the expertise that he had gained with the rifle whilst in the backwoods of America as a young man. He used to demonstrate his skill at meetings of the Medical Club in the Dublin Mountains. One admiring colleague wrote: 'The distance from which he can shatter the neck of a champagne bottle without breaking its body is surprising, especially when it is considered that the shooting at Bohernabreena commences after the champagne bottles have been emptied.'[8]

As he grew older he was greatly respected by the people of Dublin for his personal goodness. The novelist and doctor John H Pollock recalled standing as a boy under a gas lamp at the junction of Clare Street and Merrion Square on a windy autumn night waiting for a small brougham to pass:

> There is a candle burning within, steadily, which serves to illuminate the occupant: a shrunken, aged man, with a white beard, his head bent low over an open book, absorbed by his reading in this doubtful illumination. The carriage turns to the right, approaching a house on the southern side of the Square: Sir Francis Cruise, whom the wits nick-named Kempis Cruise, knowing his life-long addiction to The Imitation of Christ as a subject of study. Looking up his appointment book against tomorrow? Writing prescriptions, perhaps? Or, it may be, prudently considering his fees, to be presently sent out? I do not choose to think so. Rather is he reading in the insignificant volume of his choice; the twenty-third chapter, paragraphs 1 and 2: 'Very quickly must thou be gone from hence; see then how matters stand with thee. A man is here today, and tomorrow he is vanished. And when he is taken away from the sight, he is also quickly out of mind'.[9]

Francis Cruise died on 26 February 1912 and he was buried at Glasnevin Cemetery. His nephew, the Lord Abbot of Downside, read the graveside prayers, and the coffin was lowered to the chanting of 'Benedictus' by the clergy and students of Holy Cross College, Clonliffe, to which Cruise had been physician for forty years.

EDWARD HALLARAN BENNETT
1837–1907

25 Original observations on fractures

Edward Hallaran Bennett, whose name is remembered in Bennett's Fracture, was born at Charlotte Quay, Cork, on 9 April 1837. He was the fifth son of Robert Bennett, barrister and recorder of Cork. Bennett received his early education at Hamblin's School in the South Mall, Cork, and later at the Academic Institute in Harcourt Street, Dublin. Although Bennett's father was a barrister, there was a strong medical tradition in the family. He was a close relative of the anatomist James Richard Bennett who was a student at the College of Surgeons before going to Paris in 1822. There he studied under Dupuytren and Laënnec before becoming a very successful teacher himself at the Hôpital de la Pitié. Edward Hallaran Bennett's grandfathers were both doctors: James Bennett was a physician in Cork and his mother's father, William Saunders Hallaran, was a distinguished Cork physician and a pioneer in psychiatry. He published two works on mental illness, one in 1810 and the second in 1818.

UNIVERSITY ANATOMIST

Edward Hallaran Bennett became a student at Trinity College in 1854 and he attended clinics at the Meath, Dr Steevens', the Richmond and Sir Patrick Dun's Hospitals. Robert Smith was his professor of surgery and under his guidance Bennett developed a lasting interest in bone pathology. When he qualified in 1859 he was appointed demonstrator in anatomy in Trinity College. In 1863 he became a fellow of the Royal College of Surgeons and the following year he was awarded the degree of MD by Trinity College. In the same year he became university anatomist at Trinity, a post which he held for nine years. He now embarked on the difficult task of obtaining a position in one of the Dublin hospitals. Bennett's diary, covering the years 1864 to 1871, has recently come to light and it provides a fascinating new insight into the lives of those great men who dominated the medical life of the country at the time. It gives an intimate and 'behind-the-scenes' picture of that golden age in Irish medicine, something which was not given in the obituaries or eulogistic biographies that until now have been the sources of our information.

SURGEON AT SIR PATRICK DUN'S HOSPITAL

Bennett recorded in his diary that early in 1864 he began negotiations with James Apjohn with a view to buying the latter's practice in Sir Patrick Dun's Hospital. He spent most of January speaking to other members of the staff to ensure their support. However these negotiations came to nothing and he consoled himself by spending the best part of a week at the end of the month skating in different parts of Dublin. In October of the same year he began renewed negotiations with Samuel Haughton and with the professors of the medical school about a place in Sir Patrick Dun's. The professors agreed to support his candidature provided that he made appropriate arrangements with the medical and surgical staff of the hospital. Robert Smith also supported his application in writing and Bennett was appointed in October 1864.

AN UNUSUAL INTEREST

Professional advancement was not the only thing which occupied Bennett's mind at this stage, as he also embarked on the rather unusual

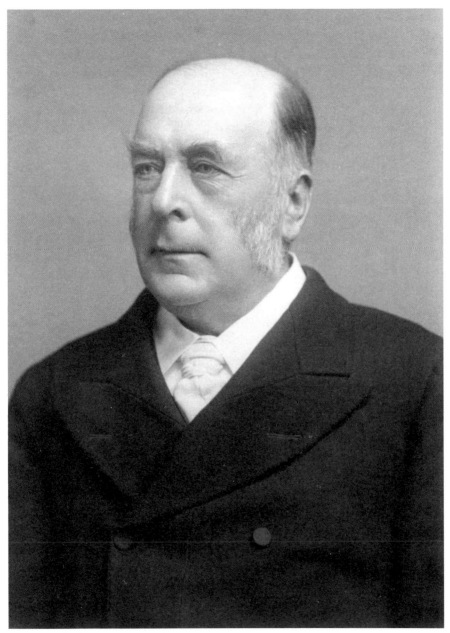

25.1   Edward Hallaran Bennett 1837–1907

project of breeding snakes. The absence of reptiles in Ireland was, according to legend, due to the fact that St Patrick had banished them from the country. Dr Guithers, an eccentric fellow of Trinity College, had brought frogspawn from England in 1696 and bred frogs successfully in a ditch in the college grounds. Soon there was a healthy population of frogs in Trinity, and according to a report in the *New Philosophical Journal* in 1735 'these prolific colonists sent out their croaking detachments through the adjacent country, whose progeny spread from field to field throughout the whole kingdom'.[1] There was no report of a similar successful experiment with snakes until Bennett reported his observations to the National History Society of Dublin in 1866. Four years previously he had purchased some snakes in Covent Garden Market in London, not with the object of introducing them permanently into Ireland, but:

> .... in order that I might watch their habits for a time, and finally dissect them whenever they should fall a victim to the prayers of St Patrick. I purchased three, and brought them over to Dublin; and, as I was going for sometime to the county of Cork, took them with me there.... I watched their habits and mode of feeding, &c., for some time; but, as I feared, one morning I found, on visiting the case, that some one had let them out.[2]

The snakes, which were about three feet long, escaped into a closely planted area of about twenty acres surrounded by a high wall. During the following two years Bennett was informed whenever they were sighted. Then in June 1865 they were seen again, and two young snakes, each about four inches long, were observed with them!

THE SEARCH FOR A NEW APPOINTMENT

In January 1868 Bennett set his mind to more serious business when he began a campaign to get himself appointed to another hospital because the emphasis in Sir Patrick Dun's Hospital was on medical rather than on surgical practice. He said that he got a 'hint' to hold himself free for the Richmond Hospital to succeed Robert Adams. Bennett approached Robert Adams' brother but he failed to get a response. He also

negotiated with Robert Smith on the possibility of succeeding him at
the Richmond. In the middle of all this, Bennett was brought before the
Board of Trinity College in connection with problems within the School
of Physic. He told the Board that he and other members of the staff
were unhappy about the efforts which the registrar of the faculty,
Samuel Haughton, was making to transfer all power to himself. He said
that Haughton's conduct 'was not that of a gentleman'.[3]

In July Bennett opened negotiations with Robert Adams again and
the latter agreed to resign following consultation with Sir Dominic
Corrigan. The negotiations lost their momentum during August as most
of the parties involved were in Oxford at a medical meeting. It was a
very hot summer and Bennett would have gone abroad but he stayed at
home to hold himself in readiness as he knew 'that Mr Adams had some
notion of resigning but could not make up his mind'. The new
academic year began and Bennett was soon absorbed in teaching his
students. On 23 December 1868 he noted in his diary that 'all talk of a
change of a hospital is at an end for the present, Mr Adams seems better
this season than ever'. [3] Adams was seventy-five at this time.

ROMANCE AND CONTROVERSY

In April 1870 Bennett, who by now was very frustrated, recorded some
rather frank sentiments about Robert Smith in his diary: 'R W Smith
says he will resign before next session. If he does so much the better in
one way, he does us no good and is always abusing the place. So I am
myself — I work he does not.'[3]

Bennett had fallen in love with a girl named Frances Connolly
Norman and had proposed to her. She said she would give him an
answer at the end of the year. All this placed him under increasing
pressure and he wanted to establish a more secure financial base. He was
also anxious to get a definite answer to his proposal. He wrote in his
diary in early September: 'in a short month I will be hard at work at a
new session and cannot get the time then to make love — I have had
my hands in blood enough for the last four days....'[3] This rather
gruesome remark referred to operations he had been involved in with
the surgeon Richard Butcher on harelips. Within a few days of writing
this note, Bennett had a letter from Frances inviting him to visit her

parents, thus signalling that she was about to accept his offer of marriage. His joy in receiving this letter was short lived as he had new worries within a few days. On 10 September he made the following note in his diary about a child who was admitted with a foreign body lodged in his airway: 'I had desperate work today in Dun's with the child — had to dilate the opening in the trachea — touched but could not get out the body.'³ Bennett was eventually forced to open the child's larynx. The child recovered but the matter did not end there, as rumours began to circulate among his colleagues that Bennett had mishandled the case. The whole episode was very unpleasant for Bennett, but he emerged from it eventually with his reputation untarnished.

In October 1870 Bennett acquired a house at 26 Lower Fitzwilliam Street and he was married on 20 December at Chapelizod Church.

A RESPECTED FIGURE

In 1873 Robert Smith died and Bennett was appointed professor of surgery. Like Smith, Bennett became secretary of the Pathological Society of Dublin, and in 1880 he became its president. He was one of the principal promoters of the amalgamation of medical societies in Dublin, which resulted in the formation of the Royal Academy of Medicine in 1892. He was elected president of this academy in 1897. He was also a member of the Royal Irish Academy and the Zoological Society. Bennett has been described as a model of honour and uprightness. He was straightforward to the point of bluntness, and he was particularly intolerant of pretence. He was known in Sir Patrick Dun's as 'the Boss'.

Bennett was one of the early exponents of antiseptic surgery in Dublin, as is apparent from the following lines describing him in a poem written by a student in 1876:

But see, what other figure comes in view!
Broad-faced, broad-chested, and broad-bottomed too.
Around him shines a mist of odorous spray,
By which his patients scent him miles away.⁴

BENNETT'S FRACTURE

Bennett was particularly interested in bone pathology and he published several papers on fractures. At a meeting of the Pathological Society of Dublin on Saturday 12 November 1881 in the School of Physic, he described the fracture dislocation of the first metacarpal bone, now known as Bennett's Fracture. He presented several specimens of fractures of the metacarpal bones and he commented that the first metacarpal bone appeared to be involved more often than its fellows. He went on to observe:

> Of greater interest is the fact that in each of the five examples of fracture of the metacarpal bone of the thumb, allowing for shades of difference such as must always exist, the type and character of the fracture is the same — a form and type of fracture not hitherto described in these bones;.... The fracture passes obliquely (a b in woodcut) through the base of the bone, detaching the greater part of the articular facette with that piece of the bone supporting it, which projects into the palm.... Seeing the value of the movements of the thumb, no injury of it is to be lightly regarded, and this fracture, though it unites readily by bone and with almost inappreciable deformity, renders the thumb for many months lame and useless.[5]

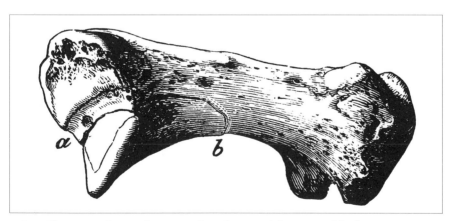

25.2   *Illustration of Bennett's Fracture, from the original description of the fracture.*

Bennett was the third Dublin surgeon in the nineteenth century to describe a fracture in the forearm, the others being Colles and Smith. These three men made major contributions to the development of orthopaedic surgery. The high standards which they achieved in this subject have been maintained in the twentieth century by the work of Irish surgeons such as Arnold K Henry (1886–1962), author of *Extensile Exposure,* a classic work on surgical approaches in limb surgery, and James M Sheehan who has gained international recognition for his development of the Sheehan Knee, now used all over the world in knee-replacement surgery.

LAST YEARS

In 1882 Bennett chose 'The physiology of plastic surgery' as the subject of his presidential address to the Biological Association in Trinity College. In 1904 he resigned from active work because of failing health, and Edward Henry Taylor was appointed lecturer in his place. Two years later, Bennett resigned his chair and Taylor was appointed professor of surgery to succeed him.

Bennett died on 21 June 1907 at his residence in Dublin. The same year, the Bennett Medal was founded. This bronze medal is given to the winner of the postgraduate award in surgery in the Faculty of Health Sciences of Trinity College. There is a portrait of Bennett on one side and on the other side there is a representation of a fractured first metacarpal bone.

26 *Pioneers in cardiac research*

HENRY NEWELL MARTIN

Henry Newell Martin's work on the isolated mammalian heart was a major stimulus to research on the physiology of cardiac function. The cardiologist Jeremy Swan brought the benefits of the knowledge which accrued from this research to the bedsides of seriously ill patients in this century.

Speaking at Denver, Colorado, in 1900, the famous English physiologist Michael Foster said, 'So if I have done nothing more, at all events I sent Henry Newell Martin to America.'[1] Henry Newell Martin was born in Newry, County Down, in 1848, the eldest of twelve children. Martin received most of his early education at home from his father who was a schoolmaster. At the age of fifteen he matriculated at University College London and began his studies in its medical faculty. At the same time he became an apprentice to an Irish doctor, James McDonagh, at Hampstead Road, and in return for his board he dispensed all the doctor's medicines. He attended the lectures of Michael Foster at University College and Foster was so impressed by his ability that he appointed him as his demonstrator.

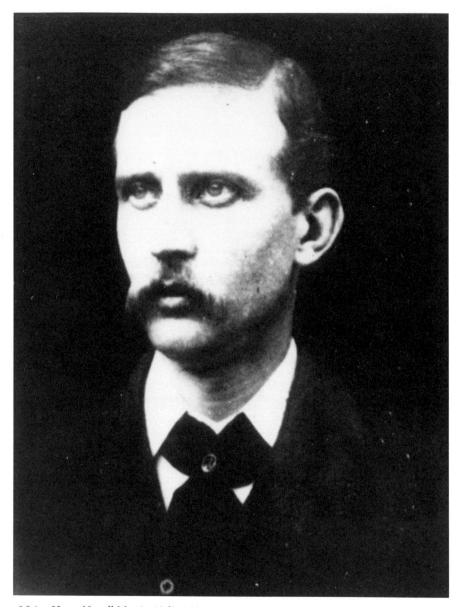

26.1   Henry Newell Martin 1848–1893

SCHOLARSHIP TO CAMBRIDGE

In October 1870 Martin went to Christ College Cambridge on a scholarship. At around the same time Foster moved to Cambridge as prelector of physiology at Trinity College, and he was delighted that his pupil could continue as his assistant. Martin had a very distinguished undergraduate career at Cambridge and after graduating with a B Sc, he proceeded to the degree of D Sc in physiology. He also took the MB degree in London. He worked for a time with Thomas Henry Huxley at the Royal College of Science in London, and the two collaborated on a book entitled *Practical Biology* which was published in 1876. Meanwhile Martin was made fellow of his college in Cambridge in 1874 and it appeared that he would have a brilliant career ahead of him in academic physiology in England. However, in 1876, on the recommendation of Huxley and Foster, Martin was invited to become the first occupant of the chair of biology and physiology in the newly established Johns Hopkins University in Baltimore.

PROFESSOR AT JOHNS HOPKINS UNIVERSITY

Johns Hopkins was a wealthy Quaker merchant who had bequeathed seven million dollars, which was to be divided equally to found a university and to establish a hospital. The plans for the university materialised first. It was established with a nucleus of six distinguished professors, which included Newell Martin. These professors were very carefully selected, as Daniel Coit Gilman, who spearheaded the development of the university, believed in spending more money on men and their tools than on buildings. The hospital was under construction for nearly twelve years, receiving its first patients in 1889, and the medical school was opened four years later.

Martin stayed there for seventeen years and made several fundamental contributions to physiology. He was a very popular teacher with both his undergraduate and postgraduate students. In 1879 he married Hetty Cary, the widow of General Pegram, a Confederate officer. She was a very beautiful and remarkable woman. After their marriage Martin established the custom of inviting his pupils to a weekly informal conference at his home, and his wife acted as hostess. One of his pupils,

Henry Sewall, has left us his impressions of his first meeting with Martin:

> ...called on Professor Martin at his rooms and my spirits were lightened when I saw a young man, he was then twenty-eight and looked younger, who treated me at once something like a companion. He was scarcely of medium height, of slight but well developed frame. His head was rather small, the eyes blue and wide open, nose thin and fine, complexion fair and mustache blond. His dress was always strikingly neat without being foppish.... Martin accepted me as his assistant in the biological laboratory at a stipend of 250 dollars for the first six months. Not for many months did I suspect that this was at first a private and not a University appointment.[2]

MARTIN'S HEART-LUNG PREPARATION

At that time little was known about the physiology of the mammalian heart as it was not technically possible to isolate it in the same way as one could isolate a frog's heart for study. It was therefore a major step forward when Martin developed his heart-lung preparation:

> It occurred to me that the essential difference probably lay in the coronary circulation; in the frog, as is well known, there are no coronary arteries or veins, the thin auricles and spongy ventricle being nourished by the blood flowing through the cardiac chambers, but in the mammal the thick-walled heart has a special circulatory system of its own and needs a steady flow through its vessels, and cannot be nourished (as appears to have been forgotten) by merely keeping up a stream through auricles and ventricles.[3]

Henry Sewall recalled the occasion when Martin first tested his ideas by experiment:

> I very well remember one morning, I think it was in the fall of 1880, Martin said to me, in effect, 'I could not sleep last night and the thought came to me that the problem of isolating the Mammalian heart might be solved by getting a return circulation through the coronary vessels.' The idea seemed reasonable and at the close of the day's work we

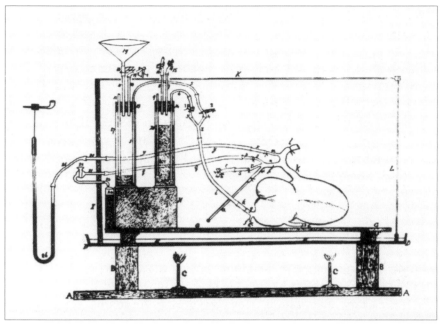

26.2   Martin's isolated mammalian heart, from the original paper.

anaesthetised a dog, prepared him for artificial respiration and then Professor Martin opened the chest and ligatured one by one the venae cavae and the aorta in such a way as to leave sufficient amount of blood in the heart itself. The heart continued to beat in a normal manner, the circuit made by the blood being from the right side, through the lungs to the left side and back through the coronary vessels in the heart wall to the right auricle again. Thus heart and lungs were completely isolated from the rest of the body and could be studied unaffected by the interference of factors foreign to itself....[2]

Martin, with the help of his students Frank Donaldson and William Henry Howell, spent the next three years developing the heart-lung preparation. Howell would eventually succeed him at Johns Hopkins University in 1893. Martin's achievement in isolating the mammalian heart has been described by L T Morton as 'one of the greatest, single contributions ever to come from an American physiological laboratory'.[4] Using his heart-lung preparation, Martin went on to make several original observations on the mammalian heart, and he was among the first to study the effect of temperature changes upon the isolated heart. The significance of his work was acknowledged when it was selected as the subject for the Croonian Lecture of the Royal Society of London in 1883. Martin was elected a fellow of the society in the same year.

Martin was the first to place a cannula in a coronary artery of a living dog's heart and to measure the blood pressure and pulse wave in the coronary system. He also did original research on the respiratory system, and his work with E M Hartwell, which he carried out shortly after going to Johns Hopkins University, settled the controversy regarding the function of the intercostal muscles.

PERSONAL TRAGEDY AND EARLY DEATH

During his years in the Johns Hopkins University, Martin was involved in the plans to establish its famous medical school and he took part in the preliminary organisation. However, during the second decade of his time there, things began to go wrong for him. He was extremely sensitive to any kind of criticism and he may also have had a tendency to depression. On one occasion Sewall, who attributed some of Martin's problems to agnosticism, was shocked to hear him say 'I am thirty years old today and am ready to quit; have had enough'.[2]

Whatever the reasons, it soon became clear that although the laboratory as a whole was prospering, Martin's own 'verve and inspiration were dying out'.[5] His wife became seriously ill in the late 1880s, probably from tuberculosis. She was twelve years older than him and she had helped him with the writing of his popular textbook *The Human Body*. By the end of 1891 it became obvious to his colleagues that Martin himself was very unwell. He had developed a serious problem with alcohol. Although he made some progress under the care of his colleague William Osler and the leading American neurologist Weir Mitchell, his wife's death in 1892 led him to resume drinking and his physical condition deteriorated once again. He resigned his post in 1893 when he was only forty-five years old, and his chair was filled in May of that year by his pupil William Howell.

The new medical school at Johns Hopkins opened in October 1893. That same month Martin died from a haemorrhage while he was striving to recover his health in the dales of Yorkshire.

HAROLD J C SWAN

Ernest Starling and other physiologists built upon the work of Henry Newell Martin so that in the early years of this century the physiology of the heart and circulation was gradually elucidated. According to Henry Sewall, many of the advances in cardiac pathology made in the early years of this century followed 'along the path first cleared by Martin'.[3] However, it took several years before the principles underlining the basic functions of the cardio-pulmonary system were applied to clinical practice. The development of cardiac catheterisation in 1938 by André Cournand accelerated interest in the pathophysiology of the cardio-pulmonary system in patients with heart disease. Monitoring devices for measuring oxygen saturation in different parts of the cardiovascular system also became available. However, it was the work of Jeremy Swan and William Ganz which made cardio-pulmonary physiological measurements possible in a wide variety of clinical situations. The ability to obtain critical physiological information in a temporarily changing disease state with safety, revolutionised clinical investigation in the 1970s. The haemodynamics of anaesthesia, myocardial ischaemia and infarction, pulmonary disorders, sepsis, and other conditions, were rapidly appreciated and logical therapies evaluated. As a result, the routine management of patients in critical or potentially critical situations changed dramatically.

Jeremy Swan was born in 1922 in Sligo, the son of a general practitioner who practised in the town from approximately 1920 to the time of his death in 1948. He was christened Harold James Charles Swan but his mother called him Jeremy as a fond name and he is known by this name. His parents' marriage was not a success. His mother, Marcella Kelly, who was also a doctor, practised medicine in England from approximately 1938 until her retirement in 1968. His father had a busy practice in Sligo and Swan remembers visiting some of the great houses, such as Lissadell, Hazelwood, and Markree Castle, with him on calls. He has memories of meeting W B Yeats when his father treated the poet during an illness.

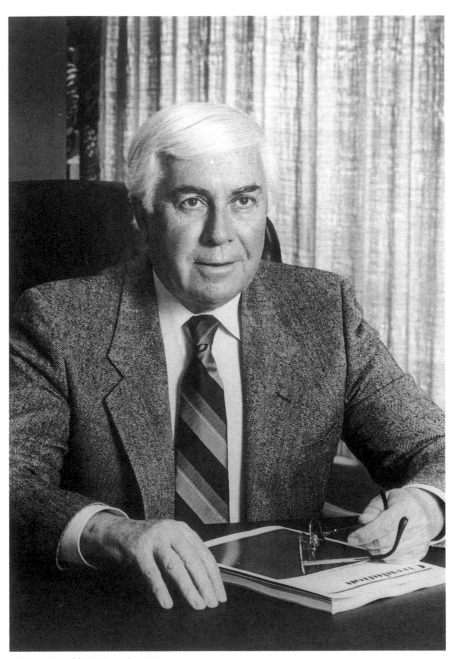

26.3   *Harold J C Swan* b 1922

THE EARLY YEARS

Swan was educated initially at Glenstal Abbey in Limerick and subsequently at St Vincent's College, Castleknock, Dublin. His years at Castleknock had a strong moulding influence on him and he learnt that 'one must work hard if goals are to be achieved in life'.[6] The biographer and medical historian J B Lyons was also a student at Castleknock at that time and he recalls that Swan stood out among his peers 'as a gentle and refined youth'.[7] He studied medicine at St Thomas's Hospital, London, between the years 1939 and 1945. In his early years as a medical student he developed a near-fatal meningococcaemia. He survived only because his mother made the diagnosis within six hours of the onset of symptoms and he was given large doses of intramuscular sulphapyridine as he lapsed into coma. After qualifying he served as casualty officer and later as house physician at St Thomas's Hospital.

He became a member of the Royal College of Physicians of London in 1946 and in the same year he entered the Royal Air Force medical service. He was placed in charge of the medical division of one of their hospitals in Habaniyia in Central Iraq. After the war he became assistant to the distinguished physiologist Henry Barcroft at St Thomas's Hospital. In 1949 he published the first paper on the effects of noradrenaline, which had just been discovered, on blood flow in human muscle and skin. He was also co-author with Henry Barcroft of Volume I of the monographs of the Physiological Society, *Sympathetic Control of Human Blood Vessels,* which was published in 1953.

WORK AT THE MAYO CLINIC

After obtaining his PhD in 1951, Swan joined the Department of Physiology at the Mayo Clinic where he worked with Earl Howard Wood, who pioneered the development of much of the technology of cardiac catheterisation laboratories. Swan soon made his mark at the Mayo Clinic and he began to receive many attractive offers in the United States. Between 1954 and 1955 he studied physical chemistry, electrical measurements and biostatistics at the University of Minnesota. In 1955 he was appointed consultant physician to the Mayo Clinic, and a year later he was also appointed assistant professor of physiology.

Further promotion followed in 1959 when he became director of the cardiology laboratory. In the same year he went to Stockholm to become familiar with the new discipline of cardiac angiography, and when he returned to Rochester he established a diagnostic catheterisation and angiographic laboratory. He began to work closely with John W Kirklin, a pioneer in cardiac surgery, and this experience allowed him to develop a perception of the practical requirements of physiological measurement in the clinical setting.

MAJOR 'BREAKTHROUGH' IN LOS ANGELES

In 1965 Swan was appointed professor of medicine at the University of California in Los Angeles (UCLA), and also director of cardiology at the Cedars/Sinai Medical Centre. Here he began the task of building a research team which would eventually become internationally famous. The concept of coronary care units had just been developed by Dr Hughes Day at the Bethany Hospital in Kansas City. It soon became apparent to the physicians who were running these new coronary care units that some patients admitted in an apparently stable condition subsequently died because of cardiogenic shock and pump failure. Because of his background in cardiac catheterisation, Swan realised that a greater understanding of the problems associated with acute myocardial infarction could be obtained if it were possible to use catheterisation at an early stage. However, it became obvious that this was impractical because of the severity of the cardiac arrhythmias which were induced by the procedure. Then Swan read a paper in *The Lancet* by Ronald Bradley, who had been a student at St Thomas's Hospital when Swan was a lecturer in physiology there in 1950. In his paper Bradley described how he had measured pressures in the pulmonary artery using extremely fine plastic tubing, without a significant incidence of arrhythmias.

Swan tried Bradley's approach but it proved extremely difficult to advance the catheter from the peripheral veins particularly in critically ill patients with low cardiac outputs. It was a major problem which had to be overcome if further progress was to be made in the management of myocardial infarction. The breakthrough came in an unexpected fashion:

In the fall of 1967 I had occasion to take my (then young) children to the beach in Santa Monica. On the previous evening I had spent a frustrating hour with an extraordinarily pleasant but elderly lady in an unsuccessful attempt to place one of Bradley's catheters. It was a hot Saturday and the sailboats on the water were becalmed. However, approximately half a mile off shore, I noted a boat with a large spinnaker well set and moving through the water at a reasonable velocity. The idea then came to put a sail or a parachute on the end of a highly flexible catheter and thereby increase the frequency of passage of the device to the pulmonary artery. I felt convinced that this approach would allow for rapid and safe placement of a flotation catheter without the use of fluoroscopy and 'solve' the problem of arrhythmias.[8]

Swan had been appointed a consultant to Edwards Laboratories, a small manufacturing company whose products included the Starr-Edwards heart valve and the Fogerty embolectomy catheter. He discussed his ideas with the company. They had facilities for the extrusion of catheters of different sizes and the ability to alter stiffness based on the chemical and curing characteristics of the materials. It was decided to construct a double-lumen extruded catheter, with one lumen available to inflate a flotation balloon in order to test the concept initially. As a consequence five catheters with flotation balloons were manufactured.

William Ganz, a graduate of Charles University, Prague, was working with Swan at this time. Swan recalls that Ganz was in the laboratory when the first catheters arrived, so they tried one on an experimental animal. The technique proved such an immediate success that they could not believe their results:

Repeat visualisation revealed that the catheter had migrated in one heartbeat through the right heart and was recording the wedge pressure in a distal pulmonary artery. Deflation of the balloon allowed its prompt return to the superior vena cava. Several repeat inflations of the balloon confirmed the near instantaneous progression into the pulmonary artery and into the (low pressure) wedge position.[8]

The concept was a success and Swan and Ganz began working on the further development of the device. Swan introduced the new technique to the cardiac catheterisation laboratories and to the coronary care unit where it was equally successful. Soon catheters were being borrowed by the staff of other departments to monitor the treatment of very ill, non-cardiac patients. Swan's breakthrough meant that clinical decision-making regarding the critically ill patient could now be based on an understanding of the fundamental physiological processes involved and the factors which might modify them. The use of the Swan-Ganz catheter became widespread and within a decade it was estimated that as many as two million catheters were being marketed annually.

Swan and his colleagues first published the results of their work in a paper in the *New England Journal of Medicine* in 1970, and this paper became one of the most frequently cited references of the decade.

AN INFLUENTIAL FIGURE

Swan has influenced numerous trainees and colleagues by his caring approach to patients. Even though he is recognised as one of the masters of modern technology, his medicine has remained very 'patient centred'. He has been described as 'the perfect blend of scientific cardiologist and compassionate physician'.[9] In 1985 he was awarded a mastership in the American College of Physicians. This is a very prestigious honour as only eight masters are elected each year in the United States.

Swan is one of the leading figures in American cardiology and is a former president of the American College of Cardiology. He has maintained links with Ireland and is a member of the American Irish fund. He has received many international awards, including the James B Herrick Award of the American Heart Association in 1985. He felt particularly honoured in 1990 when asked to deliver the Stokes Lecture to the Irish Cardiac Society. These honours are well deserved, as Swan's work has led to a total change in the understanding of the pathophysiology, diagnosis and treatment of ischaemic heart disease and other disturbances of cardio-pulmonary function.

27 First to describe the cytochrome system

Charles Alexander MacMunn published the first description of the respiratory pigment now known as cytochrome, which plays a fundamental role in the respiratory system of cells. It was one of the most significant discoveries ever made by an Irish doctor. Charles MacMunn was born at Seafield House, Easkey, Sligo, in 1852. His father, Dr James MacMunn, had an MD from Glasgow and he was medical assistant at Dromore West Dispensary, as well as being medical attendant to the Royal Irish Constabulary in a number of local districts. As a child MacMunn was noted for his keen interest in nature. He was educated at Trinity College Dublin where he obtained a BA with honours in 1871, an MB in 1872 and an MD in 1875.

MacMunn went to Wolverhampton in 1873 to work in his sixty-two-year-old cousin's medical practice. His cousin died shortly afterwards and MacMunn decided to settle in Wolverhampton and develop the practice. He also married the daughter of his deceased cousin. The 1881 census records that he and his wife had three sons, and they had a cook and nurse living in the house with them. MacMunn became honorary physician and the first pathologist to the South Staffordshire General Hospital, later renamed the Royal Hospital, Wolverhampton. A few

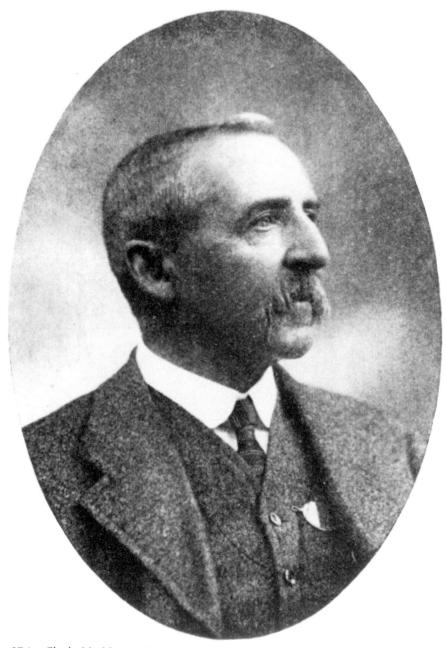

27.1   Charles MacMunn 1852–1911

years after his honorary appointment his wife died. He remarried, and his second wife was the sister of Captain Webb, the first man to swim the English Channel. MacMunn subsequently became honorary pathologist and physician to the General Hospital, Wolverhampton.

RESEARCH ENTHUSIAST

MacMunn had a keen interest in research, and as he devoted all his spare time to it he decided to set up a laboratory in the loft of his stable. He received a grant from the Birmingham Philosophical Society and from the Royal Society with which he bought equipment. Two years later he published an account of his research in a paper entitled 'Studies in medical spectroscopy' in the *Dublin Journal of Medical Science*. This paper gave an excellent overview of the subject and it also contained some original observations. In 1880 he wrote a monograph entitled 'The Spectroscope in Medicine'. He had a busy practice which allowed him very little time for research, but his wife recalled later:

> His research problems were always on his mind and during his medical rounds he had the habit of writing down his ideas on his shirt cuffs so that he could try them out at the next opportunity. When, some time later, he received a grant from the Birmingham Philosophical Society to build a small laboratory in his garden, he had a small horizontal iron pipe built into the wall, the purpose of which was to enable him to see which patients were coming up the garden path so that if he did not wish to interrupt his work, he could warn the maid to say he was out.[1]

DISCOVERY OF INTRACELLULAR PIGMENTS

Through his research he discovered that there were respiratory pigments in cells other than those in the blood. These intracellular pigments were widely distributed in the muscles, tissues and organs of vertebrate and invertebrate animals. He used the terms myohaematin and histohaematin to describe the pigment when present in muscle and tissue respectively. The pigments showed marked absorption in the visible spectrum and, most significantly, they were capable of oxidation and reduction. They were therefore respiratory pigments, similar to the haemoglobin of red blood cells. The discovery of these led MacMunn to conclude that the absorption of oxygen and the formation of carbon dioxide took place in the tissues and not in the blood, as was commonly believed until then. In December 1884 MacMunn read a preliminary communication on his discovery to a meeting of the Physiological Society in London. Two years later his first paper on cellular pigments was published in the *Philosophical Transactions*. This was followed by a paper outlining further results, which appeared in the *Journal of Physiology* in 1887. It began as follows:

> In a former paper I have shown how by the examination of the fresh organs and tissues of Vertebrates and Invertebrates by means of the microspectroscope I was led to discover the presence of the histohaematins and of myohaematin....
>
> In the present paper I can go further and show how they can be got into solution, and although as yet the pigmented portion cannot as in the case of haemoglobin be separated from the proteid constituent, yet one can definitely prove: (1) that a peculiar colouring matter is present in solution, (2) that it yields decomposition products which prove its near relationship to haemoglobin, while at the same time it fails to yield all such decomposition products, proving that it is distinct from haemoglobin or any of its decomposition products; and (3) one can form a fairly accurate idea as to the physiological role which it may play and as to its reactions.[2]

MacMunn went on to describe detailed experiments using the spectroscope, and he concluded by observing that the cellular pigments have a respiratory function and that 'they are as important as haemoglobin'.[2]

THE INFLUENCE OF WILLIAM STOKES

It is difficult to understand why MacMunn, remote from any major scientific institution, became involved in such fundamental research using the spectroscope. Who inspired the young doctor to such an extent that he devoted so much of his spare time to this work? It would appear that the credit should go to William Stokes. Stokes was still a physician at the Meath Hospital when Charles MacMunn was a student there. MacMunn was one of the brighter students and in 1872 he won the Hudson Prize for Medical Cases. Stokes was nearly seventy at the time and he was very aware that the great Irish school of medicine, of which he had been such a prominent member, was beginning to decline. He attributed much of this decline to the fact that the Dublin school had not kept abreast of scientific developments in the rest of Europe. Stokes outlined his ideas in a lecture which he delivered to the College of Physicians on 16 November 1870. When discussing the recent developments in medical science he stressed the potential of the spectroscope:

> The addition of the spectroscope to our means of research promises results, the importance of which are incalculable, and it is not improbable that by its assistance many questions relating to essential, as distinguished from local disease, may yet be elucidated, especially when its results are taken in connexion with those of organic chemistry. Its marvellous powers of qualitative analysis are shown by the researches of Mr Huggins, and Dr Millar, into the chemical composition, even of the fixed stars, while its powers, as regards the composition of the colouring matter of blood are established by the researches of Professor Stokes of Cambridge....[3]

The Professor Stokes mentioned in the lecture was George Gabriel Stokes (1819–1903) who was a cousin of William Stokes. They were both grandsons of Gabriel Stokes, who was deputy surveyor general between 1680 and 1721. George Gabriel Stokes was born in Skreen, County Sligo, in 1819, the youngest son of the rector of Skreen. He was Lucasian professor of mathematics at Cambridge and he made many contributions to the world of science, particularly in fluid mechanics. An additional remarkable contribution was his discovery in 1852 of the nature of fluorescence. He also made a very fundamental contribution to the science of biology, as he was the first to describe the function of haemoglobin in a paper which he read to the Royal Society in 1864. On the basis of his work with the spectroscope, Stokes concluded that haemoglobin existed in two states of oxygenation and that these two states accounted for the difference in colour between venous and arterial blood, and that blood changed colour by either loosing or acquiring oxygen.

William and George Gabriel Stokes corresponded with each other regularly and they exchanged ideas about the possible value of spectroscopy in medicine. In volume 51 of the *Dublin Quarterly Journal of Medical Science* William Stokes published one of the letters from his cousin on the subject of spectroscopy in clinical medicine. At the time when these two great men were exchanging ideas, MacMunn was a student of William Stokes at the Meath Hospital. He was obviously inspired by his mentor's enthusiasm for spectroscopy and this probably explains why he set about establishing a laboratory soon after beginning his practice at Wolverhampton.

MacMunn's research was attacked by the physiological chemist Felix Hoppe-Seyler in 1890, and as the latter had great influence MacMunn's work on respiratory pigments was neglected. This was a great blow to him and the disappointment, together with ill health, sapped his energy. He lost confidence in his work and as a result he discontinued his research on respiratory pigments. The importance of his work was appreciated when, in 1925, David Keilin (1887–1963) of the Molterno Institute at Cambridge realised the significance of the pigments and renamed them cytochromes A, B and C.

It is a remarkable coincidence that George Gabriel Stokes and MacMunn, who were responsible for revealing respectively the function of haemoglobin and the respiratory pigments of the cell, were born in villages just a short distance from each other in County Sligo. There is evidence from correspondence in the Stokes papers at the University Library, Cambridge, that George Gabriel Stokes advised MacMunn on the presentation of some of his experimental findings. However, the relationship between the two Sligo scientists appears to have been very formal. Two other Irish men, Joseph Barcroft (1872–1947) and Quentin Gibson (*b* 1918), made very significant contributions to respiratory physiology in this century. Barcroft, from Newry, County Down, was professor of physiology in Cambridge, where he developed a sensitive method of blood gas analysis and demonstrated that oxygenation of the blood in the lungs is accomplished by simple diffusion through the alveolar membrane. Gibson elucidated the cause of hereditary methaemoglobinanaemia at Queen's University Belfast in 1948 by correctly identifying the enzymatic defect involved.

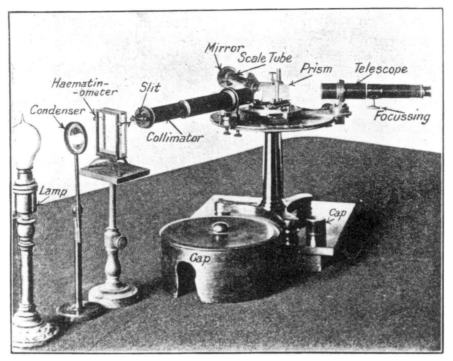

27.2   *The spectroscope used by MacMunn to carry out his experiments.*

SERVICE DURING THE BOER WAR

Charles MacMunn played an active part in the social life of
Wolverhampton. He took a great interest in the Volunteer movement
and he became a surgeon to the 3rd (Wolverhampton) Volunteer
Battalion, South Staffordshire Regiment. During the Boer War he
volunteered for service, and from 1899 to 1902 he was attached to the
special hospital staff. He was medical attendant to Field Marshal Lord
Roberts, who later appointed him staff officer on the Royal Hospitals
Commission which was set up to inquire into the administration of the
medical services during the war. There had been much disquiet in
England over the enormous number of cases of 'enteric fever'. Almroth
Wright had produced a successful vaccine by this time, but it was only
offered to the army on a voluntary basis. MacMunn got malaria whilst
in South Africa and this led to chronic ill health throughout the

remaining years of his life. During the war he was mentioned in dispatches and received the Queen's campaign medal. Subsequently he acquired the Coronation Medal of Edward VII and the Long Service Medal. He was appointed a justice of the peace for the county of Stafford in 1907, and was made a life governor of Birmingham University. MacMunn died in 1911 and he was buried with military honours, his coffin being carried on a gun carriage.

IMPORTANT CONTRIBUTION

MacMunn's work on the cytochrome system must rank as one of the most significant and fundamental discoveries made by an Irish doctor, yet curiously he has received little recognition for his achievement. His last book *Spectrum Analysis applied to Biology and Medicine* was published three years after his death. He began the work during his last illness but he died before he had an opportunity to revise the initial drafts. The work bore the following dedication: 'To one who helped me through days of toil and trouble when everything seemed hopeless, I, her husband and companion, dedicate this small tribute of affection.'[2] Ironically it was his wife who oversaw the preparation of the book for publication, with the assistance of some of MacMunn's friends. She described her task as a labour of love.

CHARLES DONOVAN
1863–1951

28 Research on tropical diseases

The Indian Medical Service was a popular career choice with young Irish doctors and a number of them found an exciting challenge in elucidating the nature of the diseases which were prevalent in the great subcontinent. Some, like Charles Donovan, made very significant discoveries. Donovan was born in Calcutta in 1863 and he received his early education in India. As a child he developed a keen interest in natural history, particularly in birds. His father, also named Charles, was an Irish civil servant in the Bengal Civil Service and he sent his son at the age of thirteen to live in Ireland. Donovan stayed with his grandfather and he attended Queen's College Cork (now University College Cork) and later Trinity College. In 1889 he qualified with an MD from the Royal University of Ireland, which was the degree-granting body for students of the Queen's Colleges at that time. Two years later he entered the Indian Medical Service. During his early years in India he was involved in active service and he was awarded the India Frontier Medal. He was stationed at Fort Dufferin in Mandalay and attached first to the 27th Madras Infantry and then to the 10th Gurkhas.

233

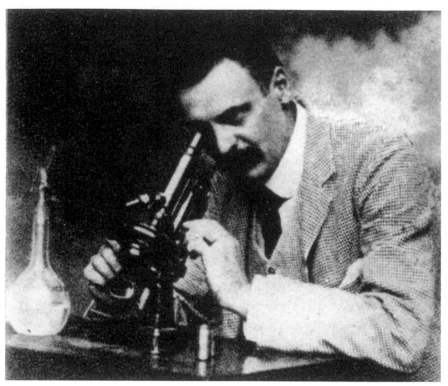

28.1   Charles Donovan 1863–1951 (From Notable Names in Medicine and Surgery *by H Bailey and W J Bishop. 1959. H K Lewis, London.)*

MEDICAL APPOINTMENTS

After two years he joined the staff of Madras Medical College where he became professor of physiology. He was also appointed physician to the general hospital in Madras. A few years later he became superintendent of the Royapettah Hospital, a position which carried with it the responsibility for the medical care of civil servants in Madras. Within a short time he had turned the Royapettah into a hospital with significant research interests.

Donovan was a tall man of athletic build, and his assistant, Captain P Krishnaswami, remembered him as a magnificent figure:

> ....with a cheerful smiling face and kindly expression, large-hearted and generous. He used to drive into the Hospital in a brougham, and after a

few minutes in the office, came punctually into the Havelock ward at 7.20 a.m., where he stayed for about 3 hours, after which he went round the other wards till 11.30 a.m. He was throughout talking to the patients or students. His bedside manners were perfect and the patients felt considerably better and encouraged when he moved systematically from one bed to another.[1]

MAJOR DISCOVERIES

Donovan's commitment to research was rewarded, as he shares with William Leishman the credit for discovering the small oval intracellular forms of the protozoan parasite which causes kala-azar, one of the major infectious diseases of India. Kala-azar is characterised by intermittent fever, darkening of the skin, anaemia, weight loss and splenic enlargement. In the last century an epidemic swept through parts of India, decimating the population. Donovan made his discovery in 1903 when examining blood taken by splenic puncture from an emaciated patient who was suffering from diarrhoea and irregular fever. Leishman, a protégé of Almroth Wright, who was working independently at the Royal Army Medical College at Netley, reported similar findings at necroscopy in the spleen of a soldier who had been invalided from an area known as Dum-Dum, about seven miles from Calcutta. He reported his observations in the *British Medical Journal* in May 1903. He speculated that the bodies he observed were trypanosomes which had degenerated after the death of the patient. Two months later Donovan reported similar necroscopy findings, but then he reported that he had also found the bodies in a splenic biopsy:

> Yesterday (June 17th) I had occasion to puncture *intra vitam* the spleen of a native boy, aged 12 years, suffering from irregular pyrexia, with no malarial parasite in his peripheral blood (careful examination of stained films on four several (*sic*) occasions), and found identical bodies in the blood from the spleen, thus removing any doubt there was as to the products being due to *post-mortem* changes.
>
> It is unwise to theorize on the insufficient grounds at present in hand. I hope to contribute something more definite on the subject after further and more prolonged study of these organisms.... There was nothing resembling trypanosomata in the peripheral blood of the boy in question.[2]

It occurred to Donovan that the patients with these intracellular bodies might be suffering from kala-azar, so he wrote to the *Indian Medical Gazette* in 1903 appealing for specimens of splenic pulp from patients with the condition. He also sent his slides and charts to Major Ronald Ross, FRS, professor of tropical medicine at the University of Liverpool. Ross published an analysis of Leishman's and Donovan's observations in the *British Medical Journal* in November 1903, and he also made the link with kala-azar:

> Lastly, as Donovan observes, his two preparations made intra vitam exclude post-mortem changes altogether, and should, therefore, contain some unaltered trypanosomes. Prima facie, then, I am strongly inclined to think that we have to do with some quite novel organism. As it has already been found in eight cases of fever and cachexia, it promises to be a common and important one. The charts of two of Donovan's cases sent by him to me certainly recall the chronic pyrexia with enlarged spleen so frequently observed in India, and are, indeed, not a little suggestive of kala-azar.[3]

In a further communication to the same journal two weeks later, Ross proposed that the bodies which they discovered should be called Leishman-Donovan bodies and the parasite should be known as Leishmania donovani. Kala-azar is endemic today in India, China, Russia, the Middle East, Egypt, Sudan, East Africa, several Mediterranean countries and parts of South and Central America.

In 1905 Donovan made another major discovery when he identified the organism responsible for granuloma inguinale or granuloma venereum. This disease is caused by Donovania granulomatosis, a micro-organism found in the cytoplasm of the white blood cells of infected patients. The disease, which became common in Britain in the 1950s following substantial West Indian immigration, presents with genital lesions and painless inguinal swelling, which later ulcerates. Donovan's discovery of the causative organisms of kala-azar and granuloma inguinale was wholly due to his own enthusiasm for research, as the work was carried out before any organised research or research institutes developed in India. He was never jealous of other workers and was always very open about his work, which he never published until he was sure of its accuracy.

A number of other Irishmen in the Indian Medical Service, such as John Wallace Megaw (1874–1958) and Robert McCarrison (1878–1960), also made fundamental contributions in the area of infectious diseases. Megaw's work on tick typhus has been recognised as 'the starting point of modern work in Asia on the rickettsial diseases'.[4] McCarrison identified the sand-fly as a vector for what was until then one of the unclassed fevers of India, and he also became an international expert on endemic goitre.

RELATIONSHIP WITH STUDENTS AND ASSISTANTS

Donovan managed to instil great enthusiasm for research in the staff of his hospital at all levels. On one occasion he led a field research expedition of the hospital staff which was witnessed by a medical locum at the hospital. The locum was very impressed by Donovan's dynamic personality and the loyalty and affection of his staff, who were all adept at making slides. Donovan had the capacity to bring out the best in people. He encouraged his Indian medical assistants and he always treated them with consideration, as Captain P Krishnaswami has recorded:

> I had the unique good fortune of being Donovan's Assistant Physician in General Hospital and later, 2nd Assistant Professor of Physiology for Research, Madras Medical College, during the years 1909 to 1916. During those days, all Professors, Physicians and Surgeons, were European I.M.S. Officers, and there was a great deal of 'sub-sternal tension' in serving them as assistants. The only exception was Col. Donovan, whose treatment of his assistants was most courteous, kind, and gentlemanly.[1]

Donovan also shared the work of his staff, often lifting patients in and out of bed. He taught his students how to prepare meals for their patients and how to perform mundane jobs such as giving enemas, as he realised that many of them would work without nursing support after graduation. He was a man of great personal integrity and he always refused to do anything which might compromise him in any way. He was noted for his sensitivity when dealing with patients, particularly those with a hopeless prognosis. Like Graves and Stokes he realised the importance of nutrition, and insisted, often against administrative resistance, that the patients on his wards should be given good diets. 'Diet is everything, and these patients have improved on diet alone. There is no use wasting money on drugs', he told his students.[1]

Many of Donovan's students became leading members of the Indian medical profession. One of them, Professor A S Mannadi Mayar, later recalled that his teacher was:

> The only Professor who entered the lecture-room with a black gown on accompanied by his assistants. He taught only the fundamentals, and that in an unforgettably impressive way, profusely illustrated by graphic diagrams, so beautifully drawn by himself. He entered the wards also in a dramatic way, attended by his assistants, nurses, and students. His remarkable bedside clinical teachings were based on physiological principles. He spent hours on microscope work and stimulated his students to do likewise and also to make full use of laboratory facilities in clinical diagnosis.[5]

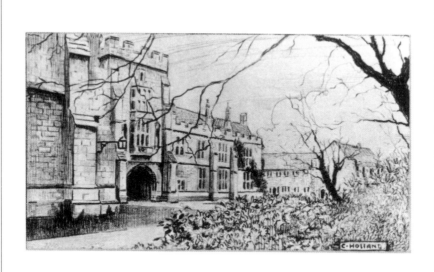

28.2   Queen's College Cork, with the medical school in the background.

He was an extremely hard worker:

> He made evening rounds of wards on many days. It could be said, that
> he was the only Physician, who did it. Sundays were observed as holidays
> by Physicians and Surgeons. Donovan, on the other hand, used to give
> lecture-demonstrations in the clinical laboratory, illustrated, by copious
> diagrams. As soon as he received his weekly B.M.J.'s he would throw
> them on the ward-table for students to look over. If there was any
> interesting article, he drew the attention of the students to the same.
> There was no day when he did not spend an hour in the Laboratory, and
> another hour in the Hospital ward, teaching students.[1]

Donovan had many interests outside medicine. He had a keen interest
in natural history and he was an expert on butterflies. He was also a
gifted artist, and one of his students recalled 'when he drew a dog or
rabbit illustrating an experiment, there was vociferous cheering from the
class'.[1]

RETIREMENT

Donovan resigned from the Indian Medical Service in 1920 when he
was fifty-seven years old. He returned to England and settled in the
village of Bourton-on-the-Water, Gloucestershire. Unfortunately his
collections of butterflies from the Nilgiris and the neighbourhood of
Madras were damaged during the voyage home. He devoted much of his
time to entomology after his retirement and in 1936 he published his
Catalogue of the Macrolepidoptera of Ireland. In this comprehensive work
he brought together the records of pioneering entomologists with those
of later observers, and he included his own work. His occasional remarks
about some of the earlier studies were said to have lent the work 'a
distinctive character'.[6]

Donovan was primarily a field lepidopterist, and with the great
experience he accrued from studying natural history in India, he made
two significant contributions to the subject. The first was his rediscovery
of the haunts of the White Prominent in County Kerry, and the second,
and more outstanding, was the discovery of the existence of Webbs
Wainscott in certain coastal bogs in County Cork.

He was a frequent visitor to the home of his sisters at Ummera House, Timoleague, County Cork. They shared his interest in natural history and they spent many hours on field trips together. A friend later recalled: 'To visit Ummera House with its walled gardens, its blue hydrangeas under shady trees and its peaceful old world atmosphere was to step back for a time into a kinder and more gracious age.'[7]

Donovan died in 1951 at the age of eighty-eight. Two years later a commemorative plaque was unveiled at a special ceremony in Madras to mark the fiftieth anniversary of his discovery of the organism responsible for kala-azar.

29 *A leader in bacteriology and immunology*

Almroth Wright pioneered the concept of the full-time, dedicated research worker in medicine, and he emphasised the importance of adequate funding to support major programmes of medical research. He devoted his own life to such research and he made fundamental contributions to bacteriology, haematology and immunology. He also developed a major research institute at St Mary's Hospital, Paddington, and it was here that Alexander Fleming discovered penicillin in 1929.

Almroth Wright was the second son of an Irish clergyman, the Reverend Charles Wright, and his Swedish wife Ebba. He was born in 1861 in the rectory of a Yorkshire village, Middleton Tyas, near Richmond, where his father was a curate. His uncle, Perceval Wright, was the professor of botany at Trinity College Dublin, and he took a great interest in his nephew. Almroth's Swedish grandfather, Nils Almroth, was professor of chemistry in the Carolinska Medico-Surgical Institute, and he was the author of several books on chemistry.

A STUDENT IN BELFAST AND DUBLIN

After a period as chaplain to English churches in Dresden and

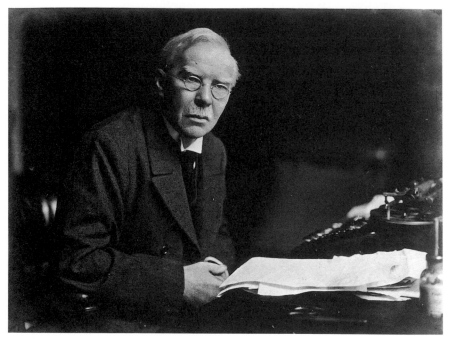

29.1   Almroth Wright 1861–1947

Boulogne, Charles Wright was appointed vicar of St Mary's Church, Belfast, in 1874, when Almroth was thirteen. Almroth attended the Belfast Academical Institution until he entered Trinity College Dublin at the age of seventeen to study arts and medicine simultaneously. He received his BA with first class honours in modern languages and literature in 1882, and he was also awarded a gold medal. He qualified in medicine a year later.

During his undergraduate years he was greatly influenced by the scientific approach of John Mallet Purser, King's professor of the Institutes of Medicine at Trinity College. Purser used his vacations on the Continent to visit leading centres in medical science, and thus to keep abreast of the latest developments.

MEDICINE OR LITERATURE?

Wright was interested in both medicine and literature and he was unsure which one he should choose as a career, so he approached Edward Dowden, his professor of literature, for advice. Dowden, quoting Charles Lamb, said: 'Literature is a good stick but a poor crutch. So if I were you I would go on with medicine. It is the finest possible introduction to life, and, if you have got the gifts to write afterwards, it will give you an invaluable background.'[1] Wright took Dowden's advice, and later in his life he used his literary ability to write on subjects related to medical science and philosophy. This ability was acknowledged by Bernard Shaw, who wrote to Wright telling him, 'You can handle a pen as well as I.'[2]

With Professor Purser's support, Wright was awarded a travelling scholarship by Trinity College. He chose to study at Leipzig, at that time one of the most advanced medical centres in the world. There Carl Ludwig was making fundamental discoveries in physiology, Julius Cohnheim was discovering the part played by white cells in the inflammatory process, and Carl Weigert was developing stains to study microbes.

EARLY EXPERIENCE

Wright moved to London in 1885 but he could not find any suitable opportunity there to develop his interests in scientific medicine. He won a scholarship to study law, but having completed a course he decided that he did not want to be a lawyer. He then competed successfully for a clerkship post in the Admiralty. This provided him with a regular income and he used his evenings to do voluntary medical research at the Brown Animal Sanatory Institute in Wandsworth Road. This was the first experimental pathology laboratory in Britain and it was established as a centre for investigating and curing 'maladies of Quadrupeds and Birds useful to man' by the bequest of an eccentric Irishman named Thomas Brown. The institute played a key role in fostering pathological research in the last century and apart from Wright several distinguished medical scientists, including Victor Horsely and Charles Sherrington, worked there.

Wright then moved to Cambridge where he began to work with the physiologist Michael Foster. He won a scholarship which enabled him to study again in Germany, and on this occasion he spent time in Marburg with Friedrich von Recklinghausen and in Strasbourg with the physiological chemist Felix Hoppe-Seyler, who was famous for his work on haemoglobin.

A SIGNIFICANT DISCOVERY

In 1889 Wright married a Cambridge graduate, Jane Wilson, whose father was a justice of the peace in County Kildare. They would have three children, two sons and a daughter. After their marriage the couple moved to Sydney for two years, where Wright worked as a demonstrator in physiology. He returned to London in 1891 and began working in the laboratories of the Colleges of Physicians and Surgeons in London. He carried out research on a variety of subjects, including diabetes, acidosis, the optical principles of the microscope, colour blindness and blood coagulation. During his work on the coagulation process Wright discovered that calcium in the blood is essential for the clotting process. This discovery had great practical importance subsequently as it enabled blood banks and laboratories to store blood simply by the addition of substances which remove calcium. Wright's position at the laboratories of the two Royal Colleges was temporary and he was seeking a more permanent post. In 1892 he applied successfully for the post of professor of pathology at the Army Medical School at Netley. His principal opposition for this post was David Bruce, who had been assistant to the previous professor and who was already well known for his discoveries in bacteriology. It was Bruce who identified the organism responsible for Malta Fever, which belongs to a group of organisms now known as Brucella. Bruce was very embittered by Wright's success as Wright was a civilian and only thirty-one at the time.

RESEARCH IN BACTERIOLOGY

At Netley Wright began to devote his time to the rapidly developing field of bacteriology. The famous Irish biophysicist John Tyndall (1820–1893), who was awarded an MD for his contributions to medicine by the University of Tübingen, stimulated considerable interest in bacteriological research in these islands. Tyndall, who was born in Carlow, carried out extensive studies on atmospheric germs and dust, and his findings 'gave the final blow to the doctrine of spontaneous generation as much if not more than Pasteur'.[3] He also discovered the process of fractional sterilisation (Tyndallisation). Pasteur made a major advance when he demonstrated to the farmers at Pouilly-le-Fort that sheep could be made immune to the lethal anthrax by inoculation with an attenuated culture. Max Grüber in Austria, Emil Pfeiffer in Germany and Fernand Widal in France had shown that when the serum of men recovering from typhoid fever was added to a culture, it caused the typhoid bacilli growing on the culture to form clumps, whereas serum from non-infected men had no such effect. Wright demonstrated that the same phenomenon occurred to the microbes of Malta Fever (brucellosis) when exposed to the serum of patients who had the condition. His research also showed that by testing the blood of patients who were suffering from undiagnosed fever, against the microbes of typhoid and Malta Fever respectively for this 'agglutination effect', it was possible to say whether one of these conditions, or neither, was responsible for the fever.

Early in 1893 Wright was visited by a Russian bacteriologist named Waldemar Haffkine, who had been working on cholera at the Pasteur Institute in Paris. His work had shown that guinea-pigs did not die after a lethal injection of the cholera organism if they had been vaccinated previously with an attenuated culture of the microbe. Armed with this information Haffkine was on his way to India to begin the first big human inoculation programme. Wright decided to tackle the problem of Malta Fever which the agglutination test had shown was a common cause of fever all round the Mediterranean coast. By experimenting with a few monkeys he showed that some degree of protection could be obtained both by living and killed vaccine. Wright put his faith in immunisation to the test by injecting himself with a killed vaccine and afterwards with a living culture. Unfortunately the vaccine did not give him adequate protection and he became very ill. The illness lasted several weeks, but Wright's commitment to immunisation remained unshaken. Even as he was recovering, his mind began to dwell on the much more challenging problem of typhoid fever, which at that time was a major cause of death.

THE CHALLENGE OF TYPHOID FEVER

Although the incidence of typhoid fever had fallen in cities with high standards of sanitation, Wright realised that these measures would not work with large armies in war, owing to the almost impossible task of dealing effectively with excreta. More than 60 per cent of the German deaths during the Franco-Prussian War were attributed to typhoid. Wright realised that typhoid fever was not just an infection of the bowel, but that death occurred when the bacilli invaded the blood stream. If the circulating blood could be made lethal for typhoid bacilli, then these patients should survive. Wright set out to discover if the inoculation of a heat-killed typhoid culture would induce antibody formation in man. To do this with accuracy he had to develop new technical methods which would allow him to standardise the potency and the duration of effect of his vaccines. Through repeated tests on his own blood and the blood of young army surgeons who volunteered for inoculation, Wright made several fundamental observations on the process of immunisation.

Shortly after the publication of Wright's first paper on typhoid in 1897, the condition broke out in a large asylum in Kent. Wright was asked to inoculate the eighty-four people, from a total staff of 202, who volunteered for vaccination. None of those who were inoculated developed typhoid whereas there were four cases in the group which had not been inoculated. Despite this favourable result, Wright encountered considerable opposition to his inoculation campaign. When the Boer War started he was reluctantly given permission by the War Office to inoculate 'such men as should voluntarily present themselves'. In the end only 14 628 men volunteered for the vaccine out of a total of 328 244. It was difficult to get accurate information from the field, but the data which accumulated favoured the inoculation programme. It is not surprising that typhoid was a major problem during the Boer War as only 4 per cent had volunteered for inoculation. Throughout the three year campaign, there were nearly 58 000 cases of typhoid fever amongst the British troops, and there were 9000 deaths.

The debate on the immunisation issue continued after the war. In 1904 Wright published his views and the results of his research in a book entitled *A Short Treatise on Anti-typhoid Inoculation*. Eventually the War Office, which was now more supportive, decided to set up a special study under Colonel William Leishman. Leishman had been trained by

Wright. The results of the four-year study, which began in 1905, were unequivocally in favour of vaccination. Wright's victory undoubtedly reduced the British death toll from typhoid during the First World War as it became policy to vaccinate all soldiers being sent abroad.

In 1906, during the long dispute over typhoid vaccination, Wright was given a knighthood. That same year he was awarded an honorary D Sc by Trinity College Dublin for his contribution to medical science. In 1913 Wright returned to Trinity to give one of the Purser Lectures, which commemorated his former professor of medicine. Two years previously Wright had been awarded one of the first two honorary fellowships of the college, an honour which gave him great pleasure.

THE MOVE TO ST MARY'S

In 1902 Wright had moved from the Army Medical Service to become pathologist and bacteriologist to St Mary's Hospital, Paddington. He was allocated two rooms and a little equipment with which to provide the hospital's pathology service and to develop his research. One of his assistants recalled going along to the laboratory one evening just after his appointment to 'spy out the land'. He found Wright:

> all alone, bunched up over the laboratory bench and carrying out in semi-darkness some tricky work with a bead of mercury and a capillary glass tube. 'I say semi-darkness' because the whole big laboratory was lit solely by the two smoky yellow flares from bunsen burners with the air cut off at their base. Only his great head and hands were lit up by the dancing flame — a most Rembrandtesque effect. When I found him, Wright was swearing heartily at the hospital parsimony which ordered that 6 p.m. was late enough for any pathologist to be using up electric current. I gave one look at this queer scene and ran into Praed Street to buy a couple of incandescent gas mantles which were then coming into use. With these screwed into the top of his two Bunsens, we soon had the laboratory lit up like any gin palace, 'Now we can work all night', was Wright's only comment.[4]

WORK ON IMMUNITY

At St Mary's Wright began to carry out a detailed study of the phenomenon of phagocytosis. He was joined in his work by Stuart Douglas who had worked with him at Netley. They soon discovered that the disposal of microbes by phagocytes was not a simple affair. The microbes had to be 'prepared' by some property of the blood before phagocytosis could take place. Wright gave the name 'opsonic' to this property, from the Greek *opsono* meaning 'I prepare victuals for'. Wright's work on opsonins started him on a long programme of research on immunity and on techniques to stimulate immunity by vaccination in order to treat as well as to prevent disease. The concepts which he advocated fell out of favour for a time after the discovery of antibiotics, but they are currently being investigated again in new approaches to the treatment of malignancy. Wright and Douglas hoped to stimulate specific circulating antibodies by their techniques, but their work is now thought to have produced its effects through stimulation of the round-cell phagocytic system and cell-mediated immunity.

Wright was very aware of the importance of funding for fundamental medical research which would be carried out by a full-time research worker. However, his views were opposed by the medical establishment in the *British Medical Journal* and *The Lancet*. Undaunted, Wright developed research programmes on several aspects of bacteriology and immunisation and he attracted many gifted young men to work with him. The most famous of these was Alexander Fleming who was to discover penicillin in Wright's department, and John Freeman who went on to explore the possibilities of immunising victims of hay fever and other allergic diseases.

THE MIDNIGHT TEA PARTIES

Wright worked with his researchers at the bench and he was the driving force behind the department. At tea time each day there was a general discussion with Wright in the chair. He usually selected a topic of conversation, and even when there were distinguished visitors present he dominated the proceedings. The topics discussed were not confined to medicine, and it was an opportunity for Wright to demonstrate his vast erudition and his prodigious memory. After this session Wright would take any distinguished visitors out to dine. Later they would all meet again in the laboratory for a 'midnight tea party' when the results of the day would be discussed and plans made for the following day's work. Some of the researchers stayed at their bench until 2 or 3 am, and they would be back there again at 9 am the following day.

THE DOCTOR'S DILEMMA

Wright found literary fame in a way which he had not anticipated. Bernard Shaw was interested in Wright's work and during the war he used to visit him in the evenings at his laboratory in St Mary's. At this time Wright was building up a very busy clinical practice by using inoculations to stimulate the immune system of patients with a wide range of conditions. During his first visit in 1905, Shaw overheard an assistant asking Wright if they should see another patient who had just come in, as their staff was already overstretched. Shaw understood their predicament and when he questioned Wright about it, Wright replied, 'Yes the time is coming when we shall have to decide whether this man or that is most worth saving.'[5] This gave Shaw the idea for his play *The Doctor's Dilemma,* which was first produced the following year at the Court Theatre. In the play Wright is caricatured in the part of Sir Colenso Ridgeon, who has to choose between saving the life of an ordinary doctor and that of a brilliant but unprincipled artist. Wright did not appreciate the play and he walked out before the end. However, there is evidence to show that Wright co-operated with Shaw during the writing of the play but he was worried that his colleagues might 'set upon me saying I got you to show them up and to puff my wares'.[6] Certainly the play did not spoil the relationship between the two men, and many years later, when Shaw and his wife were having tea at Wright's home, the latter confessed that his ideas on treatment at the time the play was written had since been shown to be wrong. Shaw replied, 'Never mind; they enabled me to write a jolly good play.'[7] Sinclair Lewis also portrayed Wright's research in his novel *Arrowsmith* which he wrote in 1925.

William Osler playfully referred to Wright as the 'Celtic siren' during a guest lecture which he gave at St Mary's Hospital in 1910, and both men 'had an amusing and friendly tilt at the dinner subsequently, when in all certainty the "Celtic siren" got the better even of Osler'.[8]

THE WAR YEARS

After the outbreak of World War I, Wright was asked to establish a research unit to study the bacteriology of wound infection and the best methods for overcoming it. Wright's unit was attached to the British Army general hospital at Boulogne. Here, in a converted casino, Wright and his co-workers studied the wounds of men who were brought straight from the battlefields of Mons, Ypres and the Marne. Most of these wounds were infected and many of the men died from septicaemia or the dreaded gas gangrene.

The first challenge was to identify the infecting organisms and their source, and this task was allocated to Fleming. He demonstrated that the men's own uniforms were a major source of infection. The team then identified two major tasks. The first was to discover why anaerobic organisms which cause gas gangrene and tetanus grew in wounds which were exposed to the air, and the second was to find out why liberal dosing with antiseptics failed to.sterilise wounds. The research demonstrated that aerobes and anaerobes were in fact symbiotic, and that anaerobic organisms would grow in porous material if aerobic organisms such as streptococci were growing in the surrounding fluid and using up the oxygen. The research also demonstrated the harmful effect of antiseptics on the white blood cells, which formed the main thrust of the patient's own defences against infection. Moreover, Wright and Fleming showed that locally applied antiseptics could not reach deeply into infected tissues where the anaerobes existed.

When Wright and his team challenged the traditional dependence on antiseptics, they called down upon themselves the wrath of the medical establishment. William Watson Cheyne was particularly vehement in his attack on Wright's work as Cheyne had worked with Lister and any criticism of antiseptic treatment was, for him, sacrilege. Because of his reaction the vast majority of surgeons did not change their approach to the treatment of wounds during the First World War. However, Wright's approach was subsequently vindicated and during the Second World War many of his ideas on wound healing were put into practice.

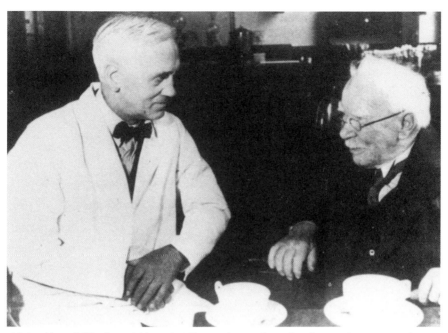

29.2   Almroth Wright and Alexander Fleming (From Alexander Fleming *by G. MacFarlane. 1984. Chatto and Windus, London.)*

During his time at Boulogne Wright continued to hold court in his laboratory, as had been his custom at St Mary's in the years before the war. Many distinguished people continued to visit his unit, including Princess Marie Louise, Sir William Osler, and his old friend Bernard Shaw. Harvey Cushing, who was also based in Boulogne during the war, visited him regularly. After the war Wright continued to develop his research department at St Mary's. He had the ability to attract the support of leading public figures and he included amongst his friends Arthur Balfour, who had been prime minister from 1902 to 1905, and Lord Iveagh, who contributed £40 000 towards the building of a new institute of pathology and research for Wright at St Mary's in 1933. Wright was elected an honorary fellow of the Royal College of Physicians of Ireland in 1932.

Although Wright was now ageing, he showed no sign of stepping down as director of the inoculation department or, as it was known later, the Institute of Pathology. He had kept both his senior assistants happy by appearing to favour each of them on occasion as his successor.

Wright did not resign from the institute until 1946, when he was eighty-five years old, and he was succeeded by the sixty-five-year-old Alexander Fleming. Some months before his death in April 1947, Wright returned to Ireland for the last time and dined at his old Alma Mater, Trinity College. He was a remarkable man and it has been said of him that he changed the whole development and application of modern medicine.

30 *Fundamental work on brain function*

G ordon Holmes was one of the great clinical neurologists of the twentieth century. He was born in Dublin on 2 February 1876 and he spent his childhood in Dellin House at Castlebellingham on the coast of County Louth. Holmes had a solitary nature, and this was reinforced by his mother's early death and the subsequent re-marriage of his father. As a child he spent much of his time exploring the countryside and consequently he developed a deep love of nature. He also worked on his father's farm during the summer months. A carpenter taught him how to make gates, wheels and carts, and later in adult life furniture-making became his hobby. He received his early education in Dundalk and he subsequently studied at Trinity College Dublin, where he was a scholar. He was taught anatomy by the famous Daniel Cunningham, whose *Manual of Practical Anatomy* was first published in 1893. During his undergraduate years Holmes loved to tramp over the Wicklow Hills and to study their flora. He graduated BA in 1897, being senior moderator and gold medallist, and the following year he qualified in medicine. He was awarded an MD in 1903.

Holmes worked for a time as resident medical officer in the Richmond Asylum, now St Brendan's Hospital. He then went to New

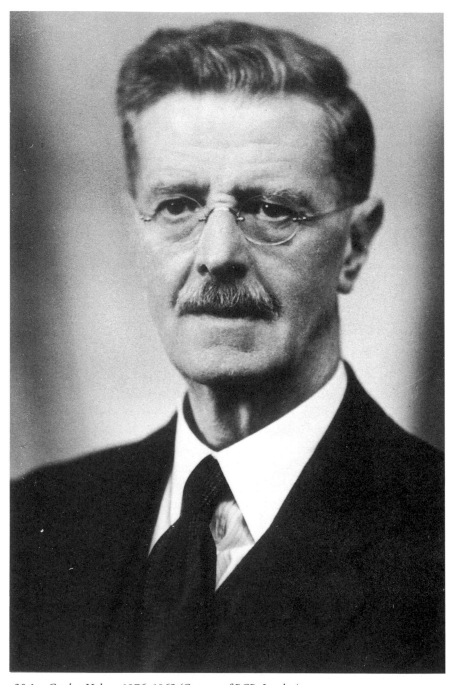

30.1   Gordon Holmes 1876–1965 (Courtesy of RCP, London)

Zealand, working his passage as a ship's surgeon. Subsequently he studied briefly in Berlin before going to the Senckenberg Institute at Frankfurt-am-Main. Here he spent two years working in neuroanatomical research under Carl Weigert and Ludwig Edinger.

QUEEN SQUARE, LONDON

Edinger was very impressed by Holmes and he advised him to pursue a career in clinical neurology. He suggested that he should apply for a vacancy at the National Hospital in Queen Square, London, and he gave him letters of introduction to William Gowers and Victor Horsley. Holmes applied for the position and he called on Gowers at his home during his dinner time. Gowers was annoyed at being disturbed and the interview took place in the hall. He told Holmes that he was not good enough and without much ceremony he showed him to the door. Fortunately Holmes evoked a completely different response when he called on Horsley. Horsley was enthusiastic about Holmes' work in Germany and he arranged for his appointment as house physician to John Hughlings Jackson at Queen Square.

Holmes became a diligent apprentice, absorbing many of Jackson's skills, and he learnt the importance of a thorough clinical examination. He took up his duties at Queen Square in 1902 and soon began to make an impression in both clinical and research areas. In recognition of the latter he was appointed director of research at Queen Square at the age of thirty. However, he did not have his membership of the Royal College of Physicians (MRCP) and it looked as if there would not be a vacancy for him on the consultant staff of the hospital. He decided to leave Queen Square and do some further travelling abroad before returning to Dublin. He met Sir Robert Scott, the antarctic explorer, and he discussed the possibility of joining his next expedition. However, before he could make any definite plans, Holmes ruptured his Achilles tendon and was forced to give up clinical work for several weeks. This gave him an opportunity to prepare for the MRCP, which he passed in 1908. A few months later a vacancy occurred on the staff of Queen Square due to the unexpected death of one of the consultants. Holmes applied for the vacancy and he was elected by a single vote. During the meeting, Jackson, who was then quite elderly and too deaf to hear the

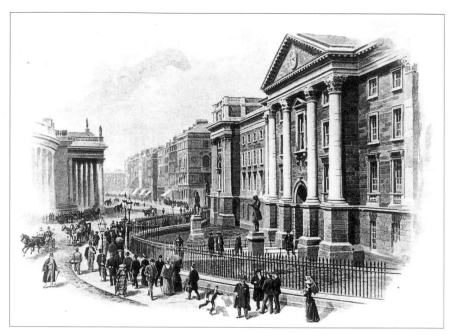

30.2   *West Front of Trinity College towards the end of the nineteenth century.*

committee's discussion about the various candidates, asked the consultant sitting next to him whom he should support. The consultant wrote 'HOLMES' on a piece of paper and Jackson cast the deciding vote. Holmes felt that he could not participate in Captain Scott's expedition because of these developments. However he did go to the quayside in 1910 to wave goodbye to the explorer as he set out on what was to be his last voyage to the South Pole.

In 1911 Holmes contributed a paper with Sir Henry Head on 'Sensory disturbances from cerebral lesions' to the journal *Brain*. This was the first systematic account of the functions of the thalamus and its relationship to the cerebral cortex, and it was the result of five years' collaborative work between the two men.

Holmes began to develop a private practice at 58 Harley Street and he was appointed consultant to Moorfields Eye Hospital and Charing Cross Hospital. He was elected a fellow of the Royal College of Physicians in 1914.

KEEN SPORTSMAN

Holmes had great physical and mental energy and he was a keen sportsman. He was a pioneer motorist and he acquired an Armstrong Sidley Special — an elegant sports car in which he competed in hill climbs. He loved to row on the Thames, and Francis Walshe later recalled how Holmes would go to Oxford with three of his residents, hire a boat and row downstream to Staines. They used to have a picnic on the way and their conversation covered many topics. Bowl-playing was another interest. One weekend Holmes and Henry Head were staying with Victor Horsley. They were joined by Ernest Starling and the four of them played bowls until lunch time. The game was resumed after lunch to test a hypothesis advanced by Head which, if correct, should improve the accuracy of the players. The four pioneers of medical science continued to play well into the night with the help of the light from the acetylene headlamps of their motor cars.

Holmes spent two months each summer at his family home in County Louth. There he worked on the farm as he had done in his childhood and he visited many friends in the locality. He also acted as coach to the village tug-of-war team, which reached the All Ireland Final one year but were beaten by the Police Team.

WAR EXPERIENCE

Holmes joined the British Army during the First World War and observed at first hand the neurological problems suffered by the soldiers on the field in Flanders. When he first applied for a commission in the Royal Army Medical Corps he was rejected on the grounds of myopia. However, he and his surgical colleague, Percy Sargent, joined the staff of a Red Cross Hospital at the front line. The officers were so impressed by their work with severely wounded soldiers that they decided to accept Holmes, and they appointed him consultant neurologist to the British armies in France. Both he and Sargent established a neurosurgical unit in Number 13 General Hospital at Boulogne. This unit, which soon became famous, won the admiration of the American neurosurgeon Harvey Cushing when he visited it on 3 May 1915.

.... After tea, Holmes and Sargent took me back to No. 13, where I saw an amazing number of head and spinal wounds, for they often receive daily convoys of 300 recently wounded. With the proper backing these two men have an unparalleled opportunity, not only to be of service to the individual wounded, but, when this is all over, to make a contribution to physiology, neurology, and surgery which will be epochal.[1]

Holmes worked long hours, dealing with the most appalling casualties. He performed post-mortems on those with brain injuries and in the evenings he worked on three major research projects. He assessed his patients under very difficult conditions and handled the primitive equipment, which included a smoke drum, efficiently enough to produce the illustrations for his paper in *Brain*. The paper assessed the effects of gunshot wounds of the cerebellum in about seventy soldiers. Much of his work was done in bitterly cold weather in an unheated room, and he had to wear a thick great coat and a rug wrapped around him, with his hands in mittens. He also did work with the distinguished ophthalmic surgeon William Lister, a nephew of Lord Joseph Lister, on the effect of occipital lobe trauma on vision. In another research project he performed cystograms on over three hundred soldiers who had sustained gunshot wounds to the spine. Holmes became consultant neurologist to the Ministry of Pensions after the war and this gave him the opportunity to make further observations on the signs of spinal injury and the symptoms of cerebellar injury.

RESEARCHER, WRITER AND EDITOR

His Montgomery Lectures in ophthalmology, which were delivered in Trinity College Dublin in June 1919, established him as a major figure in neurology. The first lecture, 'The cortical localisation of vision', is a classic in its field. The second lecture was devoted to disturbances of visual space perception, and it too contained many original observations. His work on cerebral localisation was considered a major neurological achievement and a milestone in the physiology of vision. Among the many fundamental discoveries which he made was the observation that the upper half of each retina is represented above, and the lower half below, the calcarine sulcus in the visual cortex. He also noted that the centre for macular vision lies in the most posterior part of each visual area, and that the macula does not have a bilateral representation.

Holmes published his *Introduction to Clinical Neurology* in 1946. This gave, as C S Breathnach has pointed out, 'the physiological basis for the interpretation and elucidation of neurological disorders'.[4] He was also appointed the editor of *Brain*, a post he held for seventeen years. His contribution to medicine was not restricted to neurology. In 1925 he published a paper entitled 'A case of virilism associated with a suprarenal tumour; recovery after its removal' in the *Quarterly Journal of Medicine*. This recorded the first removal of an adrenal cortical tumour. The operation was followed by the disappearance of the heterosexual symptoms, thus establishing the relationship between sexual abnormality and adrenal tumours.

HOLMES-ADIE SYNDROME

Holmes' name is remembered in the Holmes phenomenon or rebound sign seen in cerebellar disease and in the Holmes-Adie syndrome. William Adie was an Australian who had trained in Germany before joining the staff at Queen Square. In the Holmes-Adie syndrome one pupil is usually larger than the other, it reacts slowly to light or accommodation, and there is frequently an association with decreased or absent ankle jerks.

MARRIAGE AND HOME LIFE

In the early years of the war Holmes had met a young doctor named Rosalie Jobson from Scotland, who had volunteered to work in France. She was an athlete who had represented Oxford in three sports and she also played hockey at international level. She was posted home after a short period but the couple met whenever Holmes could get leave of absence. They married in early 1918 in Scotland, and soon after the war they set up house at 9 Wimpole Street. This was a large house with five floors which required a permanent staff of nine servants. Holmes now based his private practice in this house and it became a regular port of call for friends and international visitors.

Holmes was a man of strict habit and routine. Every morning he started the day with a cold bath during which he washed his hair, a habit he had started in France because of the constant exposure to lice. At breakfast he read *The Times,* and then he would walk to either Charing Cross or Queen Square Hospital. On Wednesday and Sunday morning he played golf with his wife Rosalie. His play was erratic and it did not seem to annoy him that his wife usually won. They both rowed regularly on the Thames. Holmes did not have much time for the theatre but he always read some poetry last thing at night.

PROMOTING HIGH STANDARDS

Holmes' hospital life also followed a strict routine. He expected a high standard from his staff and he did not tolerate second-rate work. However he was quick to support and encourage those whom he knew were doing their best. His ward rounds were major events of the week, and would appear to have been formidable occasions, both for the patients and the nursing and medical staff. The doors of the ward were locked and the patients encouraged by the nursing staff to lie still. They were not even allowed to read a newspaper lest the rustle should distract Holmes. Only a jug of water and a glass were allowed on the locker top. Sometimes Holmes would grasp a worried student by the lapels of his coat and gently rock him backwards and forwards as he gave him his instructions. Holmes also taught at his out-patients, and this was a major attraction for postgraduate students because, as Wilder Penfield recalled 'they knew that Holmes was a neuroanatomist and that he would, after a few simple tests, turn to the penetrating discussion of the mysteries of the structure of the brain and spinal cord, instead of repeating the text book descriptions of various syndromes'.[2]

Holmes demanded high standards and the students dreaded getting him in the clinical examination of the MRCP, even though it was generally realised that if candidates were shouted at by him they had a good chance of passing. On one occasion one of his fellow examiners became very uncomfortable when he heard Holmes shouting at a candidate. The examiner remonstrated later with Holmes, who was rather puzzled at first and then started to laugh, 'He was very good, very good and I had already given high marks when I found out he was Irish and we were having a blazing row about Dublin.'[3]

RECOGNITION AND HONOURS

Holmes was elected a fellow of the Royal Society in 1933. He received many other international distinctions and he was an honorary member of many national neurological societies. He was awarded honorary degrees by the Universities of Dublin, Durham and Edinburgh and he was knighted in 1951. Holmes, however, did not like to have his honours and achievements alluded to in public and he usually asked the chairman at meetings not to introduce him in eulogistic terms. On one occasion after an address to the Charing Cross Medical School the chairman ignored this request and began to praise Holmes to such an extent that the latter became visibly embarrassed. As the eulogy progressed, Holmes suddenly stood up and, foiling an attempt to restrain him, began to leave the podium. During the resultant confusion he fell off the stage and had to be helped to his feet.

THE LAST YEARS

During the Second World War Holmes and his wife gave their home at 9 Wimpole Street to the Americans as a service hostel and they moved to Farnham in Surrey. Gardening, Gothic architecture and the geology of Ireland were among Holmes' hobbies. He also wrote a book on the National Hospital, Queen Square. Holmes enjoyed a happy retirement with his wife and he was very distraught when she died from heart failure in 1963. He was eighty-seven at the time and he died in his sleep two years later. After his death Sir Francis Walshe said of him that he was unsurpassed as a clinical teacher, both by example and by precept, and the American neurologists Charles Aring and Derek Denny-Brown, who had both studied under him at Queen Square, acknowledged his major influence on the development of neurology in North America.

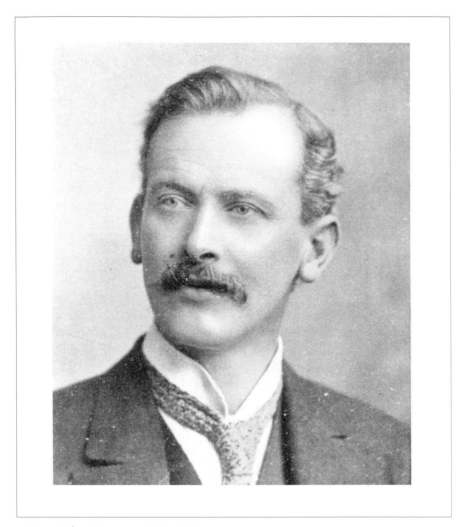

31.1   Walter C Stevenson 1877–1931

WALTER CLEGG STEVENSON
1877–1931

31 *One of the pioneers of radiotherapy*

The introduction of radiotherapy towards the end of the nineteenth century led to a revolution in the treatment of cancer, and patients with conditions which would previously have been regarded as incurable were given hope. Walter Clegg Stevenson, who was born in Calcutta in 1877, was one of the pioneers of the new therapy. His father, Walter Robert Stevenson, was a British government employee, and his mother was an Irishwoman named Elizabeth Charlotte Clegg. He was the eldest of eight children and he received his early education at St Paul's School and the High School in Dublin. Both he and his brother Frederick studied medicine in Trinity College. He qualified in 1900 and proceeded to his MD two years later. He joined the Royal Army Medical Corps as a lieutenant in 1901 and won the De Chaumont Prize at Netley during his training. He served in South Africa during the Boer War in 1901, but he resigned his commission in 1904 to work at Dr Steevens' Hospital, Dublin, as assistant surgeon and radiologist. He worked closely with Robert Lafayette Swan, one of the pioneers of modern orthopaedic surgery, and from him he imbibed a love for that branch of surgery. He soon became Swan's colleague at the Orthopaedic Hospital of Ireland in Upper Merrion Street. In 1911 he was promoted to the position of surgeon at

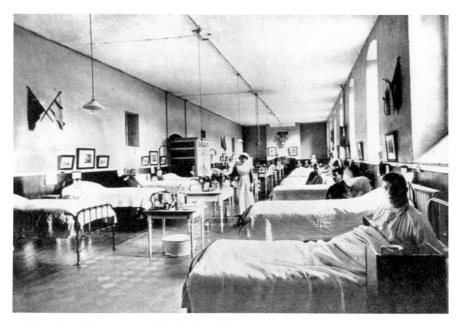

31.2   A ward in Dr Steevens' Hospital c. 1920.

Dr Steevens' Hospital, but he also continued on as radiologist until 1919, when he resigned in favour of his assistant George Pepper. Stevenson was then given the title of consulting radiologist. During the Great War he served in France with the rank of Captain. Although Stevenson was engaged in general surgical and orthopaedic practice, he is remembered today for his work on the treatment of malignant disease with radiotherapy.

THE INTRODUCTION OF X-RAYS

Wilhelm Röntgen discovered X-rays in 1895 and very soon the technique was being used in Dublin. William Steel Haughton, son of Samuel Haughton, purchased an X-ray unit in London, and within six weeks of Rontgen's discovery he was making his own X-rays in a small room in the basement of Sir Patrick Dun's Hospital. Richard Bolton McCausland, surgeon to Dr Steevens' Hospital, published the first report on the use of the 'New Photography' in an Irish hospital in May

1896. Just four months after Rontgen's discovery McCausland used X-rays or, as he described them, 'shadow graphs', to locate the position of a needle in the hand of a parlour-maid.

THE USE OF RADIUM

Interest in the whole area of radiation intensified with the discovery of radioactivity. Stevenson appreciated its potential in the treatment of cancer and he became a pioneer in the use of radium for this purpose. In 1896 the Frenchman Henri Becquerel discovered that uranium salts emitted radiation. In 1898 Marie and Pierre Curie isolated radium from pitch blende, and soon it was being used as an experimental form of treatment for different conditions. Stevenson collaborated with John Joly, FRS, who was professor of geology at Trinity College Dublin, in developing the new technique and they began their experiments in 1904. Joly made several major contributions to science. He used radioactivity to calculate the age of the earth, he invented the first commercially viable method of producing colour photographs and he solved, with Henry Dixon, one of the biggest puzzles of natural history by showing how sap in tension can be drawn up the tallest trees.

In 1910 Stevenson obtained one of his first dramatic results when he healed a rodent ulcer by exposing it to the rays emerging from a glass tube containing a few milligrams of radium which had been obtained from Berlin by Joly. Early in 1914 the Royal Dublin Society established a Radium Institute for Ireland, and Joly and Stevenson were very involved in its development. They visited the London Radium Institute and many other hospitals in England and elsewhere. The foundation funds of the Irish Radium Institute were jointly provided by the Earl of Iveagh, Sir John Purcell Griffith, and the Royal Dublin Society. The radium laboratory was based in Leinster House, the home of the Royal Dublin Society at that time.

THE DUBLIN METHOD OF RADIUM THERAPY

Of the three well-known types of radiation — alpha, beta and gamma rays — only the gamma rays are used in radium therapy. The technique of radiotherapy favoured in the early years was the insertion of one or more strong radiants centrally into the tumour. Joly realised that this centralised system was wasteful and also that it could be injurious to healthy tissues. In a communication to the Royal Dublin Society on 24 March 1914 he advocated the use of several centres of radiation:

> It is obvious that many advantages attend the use of several centres of radiation. We may omit wasteful screening. The illumination becomes more uniform. Cross-raying is favoured. The distribution of illumination is under control. In short, the methods possess all the advantages which a number of small lights possess over one central lamp when a large space has to be illuminated. In the case of the radio-active bodies, it is to be remembered that sub-division involves no loss of intrinsic efficacy.[1]

Joly and Stevenson developed this new approach by distributing the radioactive material in fine capillary glass tubes which were then inserted in thin-walled needles for application. Several of these needles coated with wax were inserted into tumours and the technique became known as the Dublin Method. They used radon, the radioactive gas emanating from radium, rather than radium itself, as the radon had a rapid disintegration rate, the radioactivity falling within a few weeks to a safe level. It was Stevenson who announced the new technique in *The Medical Press* in March 1914 in a paper entitled 'An economical method using radium for therapeutic purposes':

> It is evident that it is essential to bury the radium to obtain the greatest efficiency in its use, as otherwise more than half the Gamma rays are lost. This can be done by the use of exploring needles containing the radium or its emanation in fine capillary tubes.... The needles can be placed parallel and as close to, or as far apart from one another as is desirable, in accordance with the concentration of the radio-active material employed.[2]

The insertion of radon in sealed needles was a major step forward as it meant that it was no longer necessary to move the more dangerous and scarce radium from hospital to hospital when it was required for treatment. Now the expensive radium could be kept in a laboratory.

As Joly had expected, the use of multiple needles gave a much more even distribution of radiation throughout the tumour. The needle also acted as a filter to remove the undesirable radiation, thus giving better protection to healthy tissues. Their system was the forerunner of the modern radium needle. Joly and Stevenson were given considerable technical assistance when constructing their equipment by R J Moss, who was the registrar of the Royal Dublin Society and also public analyst.

Writing after Stevenson's death, Joly spoke of their collaboration:

> As regards the division of labour between Stevenson and the writer, those who are interested in such analyses should recognise that no amount of theory can replace in value the results of careful trial, intelligent application and thoughtful evaluation of the results. Stevenson's references to this matter are characteristic of the man; characteristic of his self-abnegation and generosity. Stevenson and the writer discussed the new technique on several occasions, and, it must suffice to say, that as regards practical details Stevenson's experience was essential to its development and final success. It is right that his name should be forever associated with it.[1]

The long hours which Stevenson spent developing the technique were in addition to those occupied by his busy surgical practice. Stevenson, like other pioneers in the field of radiation, did not fully appreciate the hazards of the new therapy. The precautions taken today to prevent unnecessary exposure were unknown then, as is apparent from the fact that Stevenson's eldest son, Joly, recalls one occasion when his father called him into his study to look for a radium needle which had fallen onto the floor.

Although radiotherapy was employed mainly to treat cancer, it was also used to treat conditions such as acute and chronic sepsis, scar formation and intractable pain from war wounds, and even a number of cases of chronic sciatica. However, over a period of time there was a growing awareness that the new therapy could also have very undesirable side effects. Stevenson finished a paper on 'The uses of radium in medicine' in 1929 by stating that, 'No account of radium is complete without a very grave note of warning to those who employ it of the risks they run of burning their fingers, starting an epithelioma in their hands or producing a fatal anaemia.'[3] His own hands were badly burnt from the radium and he actually lost the tips of some fingers.

FAMILY LIFE

In 1920 Stevenson married Hilda Davis, a nursing sister from Wales
who was working in Dublin. They lived at 60 Lower Baggot Street,
where Stevenson had his consulting rooms. They had three sons: Joly,
who was named after the physicist John Joly and who is now a
consultant in occupational medicine in Ontario; David, who practiced
as a psychiatrist in Dublin; and John, who became a tea planter in India.
Joly, who was born in 1921, has pleasant memories of his early
childhood:

> I remember that we owned an Albot automobile and later a Talbot. Both
> were open 'touring' cars with retractable cloth roof and side screens. To
> start the engine you had to hand crank. I remember when my father had
> the latest modification added to the Talbot — an internal 'self starter'
> situated on the dash board. As children we were taken on drives to places
> of interest around Dublin, including the Phoenix Park, where I have
> memories of owning a model glider operated by a catapult, which my
> father would operate. We would also drive to the Dublin mountains
> including the 'Hell Fire Club', 'Feather Bed', 'Scalp', and 'Three Mile
> Waters' a beautiful sandy beach, which I believe was in Wicklow.
>   We spent our summers in a house on the coast called Spanish Point in
> County Clare. I remember fishing for lobsters with my father while
> there. It seemed to me to be a very simple procedure, we would climb
> out on to the rocks when the tide was out and stick a long pole with a
> hook on the end under the rock, the lobster would obligingly cling onto
> the hook and be withdrawn.[4]

Sadly these idyllic holidays were ruined by tragedy, as Hilda Stevenson
was drowned when she was caught by a current while swimming with
her sister from the rocks at Spanish Point. Her husband was in Dublin
at the time of the accident and he had to drive immediately across
Ireland to bring her body back to the city. The death of his wife was a
major blow for Stevenson, leaving him to care for his three young sons.
He began to spend more time with the children, as his eldest son recalls:

> After my mother's death my father spent more time with us. I used to
> caddy for him when he played golf with his brother-in-law, Howard
> Street KC, who had been a judge in India. They played at Delgany Golf

Club. We also had more frequent visits from my aunts and they would accompany us on many drives.'[4]

However, two years after the death of their mother, tragedy struck the children for a second time when their father succumbed at the age of fifty-four to pneumonia. Joly Stevenson believes that his father's work with radioactivity undermined his resistance to infection:

> He died at home having been confined to bed for one week under the care of our family physician, Dr Winter. Following his death I attended Memorial Services where plaques were unveiled in his memory. I recall that there was one at High School Dublin; another at Dr Steevens' Hospital; St John's Ambulance Headquarters and also the Royal Dublin Society. My father had a great influence on my life which resulted in my entering the medical profession.'[4]

Professor John Joly, who had greatly influenced Stevenson's career, wrote a moving tribute to him in the *Irish Journal of Medical Science;* it finished with the admission that 'No more poignant tragedy has ever touched the present writer, who knew him and valued him from his boyhood'.[1]

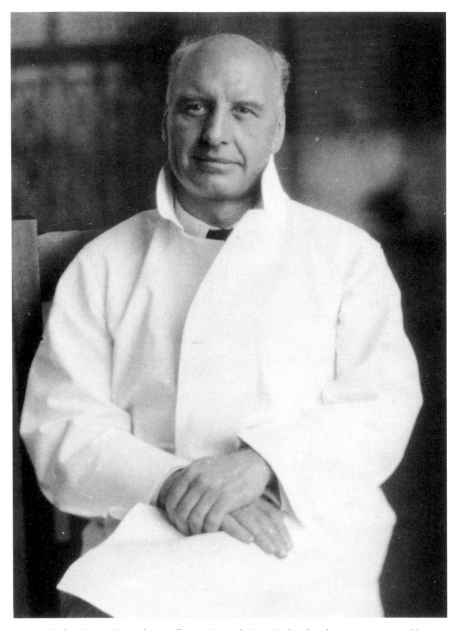

32.1   Robert Foster Kennedy at Bellevue Hospital, New York, when he was sixty years old.

32 *A leading neurologist*

Robert Foster Kennedy is one of the most famous names in American neurology. He was born in Belfast in 1884, after which the family moved to Poland where his father had accepted a post as manager of a linen factory in Czestochowa. His mother was the daughter of Robert Foster Dill, the professor of obstetrics at Queen's College Belfast. Shortly after their arrival in Poland his mother died of scarlet fever at the age of thirty-four, leaving a family of five children. Kennedy's father decided to remain in Poland but he sent his children back to Ireland. The older children went to boarding school and the younger ones went to live with relatives. Kennedy, who was still an infant, was sent to the home of his grandfather, Professor Dill, where he was cared for by the professor's two unmarried daughters, Jane and Kate.

Professor Dill appears to have been rather remote from his young grandson and he regarded caring for the child as an unwelcome responsibility in his old age. Kennedy read the newspapers for his grandfather each morning and as a reward he was allowed to read Dante's *Inferno* and the Bible on Sundays. In 1893 Dill wrote to Kennedy's older sister, who was then with her father in Poland:

Tell your father I take it for granted he will be agreeably disappointed
when he hears that I think he should now take the responsibility of
Foster's guidance and training into his own hands. Neither in point of
his health, education or conduct do I feel equal to the task — so that the
end might be such as not to satisfy his father or family.[1]

The fact that Dill wrote to his granddaughter rather than to her father
suggests that the relationship between the two men was not an easy one.
A few weeks after writing the above letter, Dill died. His daughters
moved to a smaller house in the seaside town of Bangor and they took
their nephew with them. In 1894 Kennedy was sent as a boarder to the
Royal School in Dungannon, County Tyrone, and from there he went
to study medicine at Queen's College Belfast, where he qualified in
1906. He then moved to London where he became house-physician to
Sir William Gowers at the National Hospital, Queen Square. There he
was befriended by his fellow countryman, Gordon Holmes.

TRAINING IN NEUROLOGY

Kennedy was twenty-two when he was appointed resident medical
officer at Queen Square. Here he worked with some of the greatest men
in neurology and neurosurgery at that time, including William Gowers,
Victor Horsley, and Howard Henry Tooth whose name is associated
with peroneal muscular atrophy. It was a busy post as he had to write
notes on eighty-five in-patients every morning and many letters to
doctors and relatives. His afternoons were spent with the hospital
secretary, going through applications for admission. He also had to give
the anaesthetic during some of the operations. His first three scientific
papers were written with Gordon Holmes on the subject of
syringomyelia.

Despite his busy schedule, Kennedy began to take a special interest in
patients with brain tumours. In 1908, just two years after qualifying, he
admitted a thirty-eight-year-old woman named Mary Cameron, who
was to be the first case in his classic paper on tumours of the frontal
lobe. She is mentioned in a letter which he wrote at one o'clock in the
morning to his fiancée, Isabel McCann:

I've got a very wonderful lot of cases in my beds at present. Of course I have the pick of the hospital, for I choose them myself — don't think me a callous brute. Because I'm interested in the things I see doesn't mean I forget the human side of their conditions, but do you know I have direct charge of thirteen cases of cerebral tumour!....

One of them is a Miss Cameron from Edinburgh — she is a splendid girl. I've gone over her very carefully and feel sure I know where the thing is but it will be the devil of a place to get at. The sight in the left eye has almost gone — valuable time has been wasted — she has been under the charge of a man outside who has been telling her she is suffering from 'nervous breakdown' for the last five months![2]

Mary Cameron was operated on by Sir Victor Horsley and a frontal tumour was found. However, she died shortly after the procedure.

Kennedy was very committed to his work, but he did take time off occasionally:

This afternoon Gordon Holmes and I walked up to Hyde Park and had a splendid row on the Serpentine — it has been a gorgeous afternoon — and I feel blown clean with fresh air and exercise. It's extraordinary the difference between the air in the Park and in the rest of London. Now I'm going over to examine a case, and then I'm to meet Holmes at the Society [the Royal Society of Medicine] at Hanover Square, dine with him and work all evening.[3]

THE MOVE TO NEW YORK

Despite the support of Sir William Gowers and Sir Victor Horsley, Kennedy could not find an opening in Dublin or Belfast or in any of the major centres in Scotland or England. He had now been engaged for four years to Isabel McCann, the daughter of a Belfast whiskey merchant, so he was anxious to obtain a permanent position. It would be some time before a suitable vacancy would become available in Queen Square. Consequently he accepted an offer from Pearce Bailey, co-founder with Joseph Collins and Joseph Fraenkel of the Neurological Institute in New York, to take up the post of chief of clinic. The 82-bed institute was the first of its type in America. Shortly after his arrival in New York he was also appointed as an instructor in neurology at Cornell

University on the resignation of Ramsay Hunt. 'I will have to take three afternoons out-patients and have a lot of teaching to do. The salary is small, about £80 a year, but it all helps. It's the sort of job I wanted in Dublin and it has fallen into my lap out of a clear sky!'[4]

Kennedy's reputation rests on a paper which he wrote soon after going to the United States, entitled 'Retrobulbar neuritis as an exact diagnostic sign of certain tumours and abscesses in the frontal lobes'. It was published in the *American Journal of Medical Science* in the autumn of 1911. The Foster Kennedy syndrome is described in this paper, that is, ipsilateral optic atrophy, central scotoma and anosmia, and contralateral papilloedema. It indicates the presence of a tumour or other space occupying lesion in the frontal lobe of the brain. Kennedy's reputation was rising rapidly in North America and in 1912 he was invited to give a guest lecture in Baltimore. After the lecture Harvey Cushing escorted him to the train and asked him 'to come down soon again and give them more!'.[5] In the same year Kennedy was elected a fellow of the Royal Society of Edinburgh. In 1913 he married Isabel McCann in New Hampshire.

AT THE FRONT IN WORLD WAR I

When war was declared in 1914 Kennedy volunteered to do a six-month period of service overseas. In the summer of 1915 he agreed to help an Englishman, Harold Reckitt, to convert a building in the village of Ris-Orangis near Paris into a military hospital for French soldiers. His wife joined him and worked in the 'Diet Kitchen', and after six months they returned to New York. However, in the summer of 1916 Kennedy resolved to go back to France for the rest of the war. He had hoped to join his friend Gordon Holmes at General Hospital Number 13 in Boulogne, but he was sent instead to a Field Ambulance Unit in the fighting area, as a general casualty surgeon. After ten months with this unit in Flanders he joined the Harvard Surgical Unit at Boulogne as a neurologist. This unit had been set up by Harvey Cushing in 1915. Kennedy stayed there for the rest of the war. He was mentioned in dispatches and was created a Chevalier of the Legion of Honour.

Kennedy wrote a detailed analysis of the phenomenon known as 'shell shock' and he argued that this arose from 'the antagonism on the one hand of the conscious emotions of loyalty and morale with their concomitant urge to self-sacrifice, and, on the other hand, the more or less satisfactorily repressed instincts for the conservation of individual life.'[6] He supported his theory by graphic descriptions of the horrors to which the soldiers were exposed in the trenches.

Kennedy was stationed near Holmes and both men kept in regular contact. On one occasion towards the end of the war Holmes brought interesting news:

> Today Gordon Holmes came in to tea and told me he is engaged to be married (!) to a lady doctor now working, I think, in Colchester. He seemed in great heart but I hope she's not a very sensitive soul for I think he'd be ill to live wi' — they hope to wed in the springtime.[7]

During the war years Kennedy wrote regularly to his wife. These letters were edited by his daughter, Lady Isabel Butterfield, in 1981 and they give an interesting insight into the horrors of the battlefields. The memory of men's bodies stretched out around him as far as the horizon would never leave Kennedy. His experience led him to lose faith in the idea of a personal God, and in later years he often remarked that the death of Jesus Christ no longer held any meaning for him, as each individual death in the war seemed to him as great a sacrifice.

BACK IN NEW YORK

After the war Kennedy returned to New York. During his absence his wife had stayed with her parents in Belfast. In 1919 Kennedy was appointed professor of neurology at Cornell University and he also became head of the neurological service at Bellevue Hospital. He soon had a thriving private practice and an international reputation. He was immensely sympathetic when dealing with poor patients from the lower east side of New York and he often gave them financial assistance from his own resources. His daughter, Lady Isabel Butterfield, recalls hearing of an amusing incident which took place on his ward at Bellevue around 1935:

> A Central European immigrant, a labourer who spoke no English, was

admitted to the neurological ward after a fall at work which had left him paralysed from the chest down. Taking a history was impossible because of the language barrier so my father began to go over the injured man with the infinite precision he always brought to an examination. Gradually, my father began to suspect the man was not severely paralysed, followed by the conviction that the silent man in the bed was not paralysed at all! My father then was told there was a hefty sum for accident insurance involved so he decided, after failing to get the man to talk, that he was a fraud.

My father then asked a nurse to wrap a bottle of whiskey in a towel and tubefeed it to the 'patient' in such a way that he would not know he was being given neat whiskey. The ward round then proceeded on its way when some time later there was an uproar at the far end. Turning round, my father's team of young doctors beheld the 'Central European patient' on his feet, in the hospital pyjamas, roaring drunk and roaming around, proclaiming, in a distinctly Irish accent, that it was the finest hospital he'd ever been in in his life![8]

FRIENDSHIP WITH WINSTON CHURCHILL

Winston Churchill was one of Kennedy's most famous patients. Churchill was knocked down by a car while crossing Fifth Avenue in December 1931, as a result of which he fractured two ribs as well as sustaining a severe scalp wound. Kennedy was asked to examine him from a neurological point of view and he was able to assure Churchill that no neurological damage had been done. This was the beginning of a friendship between the two men which lasted over a number of years. Before he left New York Churchill dined with Kennedy at his home in Sutton Place, and their conversation continued into the early hours of the morning. Their last conversation took place in the winter of 1941 when Churchill telephoned Kennedy at 3.00 am New York time. He asked Kennedy if he thought that the Isolationist Movement was strong enough to break up the United States if America joined the war. Kennedy replied that he considered it unlikely. Franklin D Roosevelt was also treated by Kennedy, and his daughter remembers visiting the Oval Office with her father to see the president.

HEALTH AND DOMESTIC PROBLEMS

Kennedy was affected, like many other Americans, by the New York Stock Exchange 'Crash' of 1929, when he lost approximately half his savings. He also had domestic problems and in 1938 his first marriage ended in divorce. Not long after this he suffered a massive haemorrhage from a nasal artery. The bleeding could not be stopped by conservative methods and eventually it was decided to tie off the external carotid artery on the right-hand side. Kennedy never recovered his full vitality after this episode. In 1940 he married a young medical student of Spanish extraction named Katherine Caragol y San Abria. He had two daughters by his first marriage, and a third daughter was born in 1943.

Kennedy became president of the American Neurological Society and he received many honours, including the honorary degree of D Sc from Queen's University Belfast. His health deteriorated gradually and in 1951 a diagnosis of polyarteritis nodosa was made. Early in 1952, knowing that he had only a short time left to live, he asked to be taken to his own ward in Bellevue Hospital. Although he had been attached to many of the new and more fashionable hospitals in New York, he had a special affection for Bellevue and its antiquated wards. He was always proud of his association with the hospital, which was founded in 1736 and was the first public hospital in the United States. He died soon after admission to the ward on the 7 January 1952.

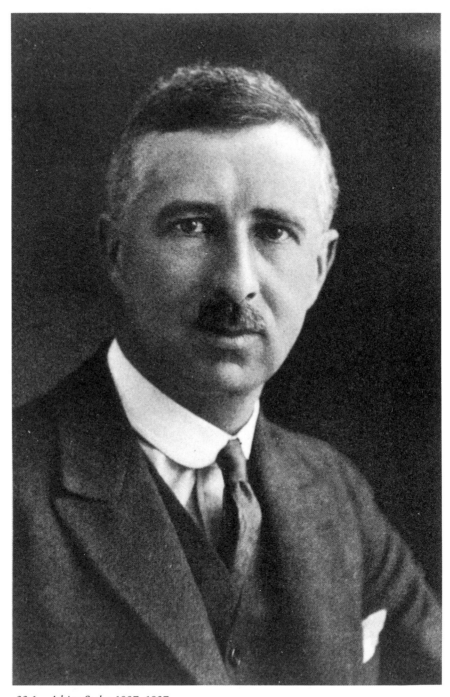

33.1   Adrian Stokes 1887–1927

ADRIAN STOKES
1887–1927

---

33 *The conquest of yellow fever*

Yellow fever, which we now know is caused by a group B arbo virus and is transmitted by the mosquito, has been recognised as one of the great plagues of the world since the first identifiable outbreak occurred in Yucatan, Mexico, in 1648. The mosquito can transmit the infection from person to person or, as in Africa, from primates to humans. Little was known about the aetiology of yellow fever at the beginning of this century and several distinguished doctors and scientists lost their lives striving to unravel the mystery. The Irish pathologist Adrian Stokes made a major contribution to the struggle to conquer the disease and he lost his life in the process. He was a grandson of the physician William Stokes, and his father, Henry John Stokes, worked in the Indian Civil Service. Adrian was born in Lausanne in Switzerland in 1887 and was educated at St Stephen's Green School in Dublin, where he won the James Robertson Medal for English Essay in 1904.

MEDICAL STUDIES

Stokes entered Trinity College in 1905 where he soon revealed his talents. He studied history for a year and obtained first class honours. He then began to study medicine and he attended the Meath Hospital:

> As an undergraduate, almost from the moment of his entering the medical school, he became a marked man, not merely for his brilliant intellectual attainments, but also for his strength of character and his capacity as a leader of men. It was recognised by all his teachers that the genius of his great predecessor William Stokes had been reborn in him.[1]

He was tall and very strong. A keen sportsman, he was in the Trinity XI, and played hockey, lawn tennis and squash. He particularly enjoyed sailing, fishing and shooting.

His undergraduate years were marked by distinction; he obtained first class honours, a senior moderatorship and the Bank's Prize. While still a student he published a paper on a 'Rare abnormality of the heart and great vessels' in the *Journal of Anatomy*. As a student he was secretary of the Dublin University Biological Association and he continued to take an interest in the proceedings of the society in later years. He graduated MB, B Ch in 1910 and was awarded an MD in 1911.

POSTGRADUATE STUDIES

Immediately after qualifying, Stokes worked as a demonstrator in anatomy. He took the fellowship of the Royal College of Surgeons in Ireland in 1912 and the membership of the Royal College of Physicians in London in 1924. He won the Travelling Prize in 1912 in Trinity, but turned it down in favour of his nearest rival, whom he thought more worthy of the distinction. His grandfather and great-grandfather had both written books on fever and now he too was interested in infection. He went to London to study bacteriology in Almroth Wright's department at St Mary's Hospital. He was awarded the Travelling Prize again in 1913 and on this occasion he decided to go to the Rockefeller Institute in New York, where he engaged in research for eight months. He returned to Dublin to take up a position as assistant to Alexander Charles O'Sullivan, the professor of pathology at Trinity College, and he occupied this post until the outbreak of World War I.

WAR SERVICE

Stokes volunteered for active service at the beginning of the war and he was sent to France. He took his old motorcycle and side-car with him to the battle front. There he was horrified by the number of men dying from tetanus and by the absence of any systematic attempt at prevention or treatment. Through persistent agitation he obtained a supply of anti-tetanic serum and he set up a mobile laboratory in his side-car. He then set off by himself, meeting ambulances and visiting the field dressing stations behind the lines. In this way he saved many lives. When typhoid fever appeared in the Guards Brigade in the early months of the war, Stokes set up an incubator on his side-car and successfully identified 'the carrier' responsible for the epidemic.

It was Stokes who first introduced the nasal catheter as a method of administering oxygen. One morning a casualty clearing station at the front was inundated with victims of a bad phosgene gas attack. It was not practical to apply the old method of administering oxygen using an individual face funnel or mask, as masks and oxygen cylinders were in short supply. Stokes conceived the idea of feeding oxygen continuously to the men through nasal catheters, four being supplied from one cylinder. The method was quickly adopted throughout the front and Stokes was again responsible for saving the lives of many soldiers. After the war the use of nasal catheters to deliver oxygen became a universal practice in all hospitals.

Stokes was the first to identify spirochaetal jaundice when it broke out in the trenches in 1916. He confirmed his clinical intuition with animal experiments and proved that the disease was identical to that first described in 1914, and more fully in March 1916, by Japanese investigators. He showed that the rats which infested the trenches were the carriers of the spirochaete, and with the aid of 'spot maps' he helped to identify which parts of the trench system were generating the majority of cases. He published joint papers with John Alfred Ryle (of Ryle's tube fame) in the *British Medical Journal* in 1916 and in *The Lancet* the following year. In these they proved that spirochaetal jaundice was caused by inflammatory changes which obstructed the small biliary ducts in the liver and that the haematuria was caused by haemorrhagic nephritis.

Stokes received several honours for his work during the war. He was awarded the DSO and the OBE by the British Government and the Belgians conferred on him the Order of the Crown.

DISTINGUISHED CAREER

In 1919 he was appointed professor of bacteriology and preventive medicine at Trinity College Dublin and assistant physician to the Royal City of Dublin and Adelaide Hospitals. He felt that clinical and laboratory medicine had grown apart and he did his utmost to remedy this situation. He published several papers, including one with Professor J W Bigger on an outbreak of dysentery in the Dublin area. He was asked to go to Lagos in 1920 with the Rockefeller Yellow Fever Commission. He was probably glad to leave Dublin at the time as he found the political upheaval which the country was undergoing distasteful.

He returned to Dublin after six months but he did not stay long as, in October 1922, he was invited to apply for the Sir William Dunn professorship of pathology at Guy's Hospital, London. He was appointed to the chair and he threw himself with enthusiasm into organising his department:

> During his four years at Guy's Stokes made a unique position for himself. Members of the staff, house officers and students constantly sought his advice and help in the manifold difficulties they encountered in the wards, and they rarely failed to profit from his wide knowledge of the literature, great experience and unbounded common sense.[1]

Stokes realised that the pathologist should not be confined to a laboratory, and he did a ward round once a week with some of his medical colleagues. He could be quite outspoken when he considered it necessary, and he fought for his subject because he believed that good experience in pathology should form an essential part of a doctor's training. He managed to expand the period devoted to pathology on the curriculum and he began to attract many students from the wards to his weekly demonstrations, much to the annoyance of some clinicians.

Stokes read widely and he encouraged his colleagues and students to do research:

Many valuable contributions to scientific literature, generally published in the hospital Reports, came from his laboratory at Guy's. Without exception, however, they appeared under the names of others, the majority being students or recently qualified men, who performed investigations suggested by him and under his direction. In spite of their protests he always deleted their acknowledgement of his encouragement and help from the manuscript. Perhaps the most important investigation of this kind was that of achalasia of the cardia (so-called cardiospasm) by one of his most promising students. In every one of the eight specimens examined inflammation or degeneration was found in Auerbach's plexus in the neighbourhood of the sphincter, thus explaining its failure to relax on the arrival of a peristaltic wave during deglutition. Other investigations dealt with the infective gastritis associated with the achlorhydria of subacute combined degeneration of the cord; acute suppurative gastritis; diffuse polyposis of the stomach; and aleukaemic leukemia.[2]

WORK ON YELLOW FEVER

In 1927 the Rockefeller Commission on Yellow Fever approached Stokes again and asked him to go to West Africa with an expedition, because of his experience with spirochoetal jaundice. It had been known for some time, largely due to the work of the Commission under the direction of Major Walter Reed, that yellow fever in South America was propagated by a domestic mosquito. The Japanese worker Hideyo Noguchi (1876–1928) had subsequently described a leptospira which he believed was responsible for the disease. This work challenged the previously held view that a virus was responsible. The Rockefeller Foundation hoped to control, if not eradicate, the infection by developing a vaccine, but first its specific cause had to be established unequivocally. This was the purpose of the expedition to West Africa.

When the expedition arrived in Africa there was an epidemic of yellow fever in a village about thirty miles from Acra. The team bought three chimps and attempted to infect them using the blood of yellow fever patients. They had no success as the African monkeys were not susceptible. They then imported some Indian rhesus monkeys, and this time Stokes recorded: 'We have infected some Indian monkeys; five out of the six inoculated with blood from yellow fever cases have died with a good pathology. We have failed to pass the strain to others; this suggests an intermediate life history.'[1] They now began to import large numbers of rhesus monkeys and the research gained increased momentum. Within a short period, they established that the disease could be transmitted from one monkey to another by mosquitoes. On 13 August Stokes wrote from Acra:

> This proves our case fairly well, and as we can get no leptospirae at all it queers that organism as the cause of yellow fever.... We still have the difficulty of not having a white man to monkey transmission and no postmortem examination on a case that has been used to infect a monkey. That will be a question of time and fortune, but I am quite confident it will be all right.[1]

Stokes was not married but he kept in regular correspondence with his relatives at home, despite the pressure of his research. He found time to write to his young nieces Aideen and Barbara Stokes about his journeys through the forest and the unusual animals he encountered there:

> I saw a lovely beast yesterday called IGUANA or something like that, he did not wait for long to talk but so far as I could see he was about your own size.... I have seen several snakes on the roads too, one really big thick one about as long as Bill and thicker than your thigh, I think he had been having a feed and was sleeping it off.[3]

Stokes worked constantly and with great determination. Monkeys were now dying regularly from the disease and he was busy performing post-mortems and preparing the tissues for examination. He worked day and night, on one occasion doing two post-mortems at 3.00 am. His team found that the serum of the monkeys was infective, even after being passed through special filters, thus supporting a viral aetiology. They also showed that 0.1cc of serum from a convalescent patient would protect monkeys against otherwise fatal doses of infected blood and against the bites of infected mosquitoes. In short, they had begun the work which would eventually produce a vaccine against the dreadful disease. Stokes also examined many mosquitoes and felt great frustration at knowing that the virus was under his eye and yet he could not see it.

Stokes had spent many hours fishing in the west of Ireland, and in a letter dated 26 August he used a fishing metaphor to describe the team's achievements up to that time:

> We are a bit full of ourselves as we have the fish hooked all right, right down in the belly, and unless we are careless and break the tackle it will only be a question of time. The time may be years, but it must come. He rose to a grey monkey in May and we hooked him fair early in July and now we can transfer it by blood or mosquitoes at will and can protect the animals by convalescent serum and so on. Of course, the gaffing of the bug will be the thing that takes time.... What we want is another strain or two isolated from human cases, and best of all, a strain isolated from a patient that comes to autopsy.[1]

SUDDEN ILLNESS

It was ironical that his own death would provide the missing link. On 15 September, about five weeks before he was due to sail home on leave, he suddenly became ill. Although he could not remember having been bitten by an insect, and both his laboratory and sleeping quarters were efficiently screened, there was no doubt about the diagnosis: he had yellow fever. His colleagues believed that he had acquired the infection in the laboratory, through abrasions on his hands when he was working with the tissues of infected monkeys. Before he was taken to the European hospital he insisted that his blood should be taken for inoculation into monkeys and that mosquitoes should be allowed to feed upon him. For the latter purpose he pushed his foot and lower leg through a long cloth sleeve into a wire cage containing about 150 mosquitoes.

Stokes realised the seriousness of his condition and he thanked his colleagues for the support he had received during the research. He asked them to do a careful autopsy after his death and he remained interested in the scientific aspects of his illness until he became comatose. There was a clinician at the base named E J Scannell, who had been with Noguchi in South America and who believed firmly in the leptospiral aetiology of yellow fever. When Stokes realised that he was dying he asked his colleague Paul Hudson to bring Scannell to see him. Hudson wrote about this meeting forty years later:

A YELLOW FEVER TRAGEDY.

DEATH OF PROFESSOR ADRIAN STOKES

WHILE INVESTIGATING THE DISEASE.

The Daily Mail regrets to announce that one of Britain's most eminent pathologists, Professor Adrian Stokes, who has been devoting six months' leave of absence from Guy's Hospital to help in conquering the scourge of yellow fever, has died from that complaint, contracted while at work, at Lagos, West Africa.

Brief cablegrams from Lagos show that he was smitten by the fever last Thursday and was taken to the European Hospital. Although the date of his death is not given, it is believed that he passed is probable he had little time for sport (in reference books his recreation is given as cricket), but although we knew little about his interest in sport we always assumed that he must have played games well when he had the time.

Here anything from 100 to 120 students passed through his hands each year. His directness never made him an enemy among them.

Professor Stokes received a commission in the R.A.M.C. in 1914, he won the D.S.O. and other decorations, and was mentioned in despatches.

∴ Yellow fever is an acute non-contagious fever usually causing a mortality of 45 to 80 per cent. in West Africa, and 25 per cent. in those parts of the American continent where it occurs. Occasionally it has appeared in Europe, the last time in Madrid in 1878. It has not occurred in England since 1865.

33.2   Report on the death of Adrian Stokes in the Daily Mail.

After casual greetings, Stokes asked Scannell to make a clinical examination and offer a diagnosis. The examination was made in complete and heavy silence. Scannell finally straightened up from the low bed, put his stethoscope in his pocket, and examined the clinical chart and record of laboratory tests. Without embarrassment, the two men exchanged long searching looks.

'Well?' asked Stokes.

'I think you have it', was the casual but sincere reply.

'You know there hasn't been any in the neighbourhood', continued Stokes, 'and you've been around the laboratory now for a fortnight, watching us work.'

Each statement was put as a question and the repeated answer was a soft 'Yes.' Scannell also agreed with Stokes's observation that he had not recently been handling the leptospira.

To the question, 'Have I been working with the virus?' the unemotional reply was, 'That's what you fellows call it.'

Somewhat upset by this apparently evasive remark, Stokes pressed on. 'Are you ready now to agree, to admit, that yellow fever is caused by a virus and not by leptospira?'

After a moment's hesitation, as though considering the choice of words, Scannell answered in a firm voice, 'I believe you fellows are right. I don't have the explanation, but I think you have yellow fever and got infected in the laboratory with what you call a virus.'

A brief silence followed. Then with a curt 'Goodbye —Scannell, Hudson,' Stokes turned his face to the wall with an air of finality. I thought I heard a faint sigh of relief and satisfaction.[4]

Stokes died on 19 September and the autopsy confirmed that his death was due to yellow fever. The mosquitoes which had fed on him were allowed to bite a monkey and it developed yellow fever as a consequence. This proved that the disease could be transmitted from man to monkey through the bite of a mosquito. Stokes was buried the day after his death at the Ikogi Cemetery, following a service conducted by the Bishop of Lagos.

Stokes's work, which was published posthumously in *The American Journal of Tropical Medicine,* established clearly that yellow fever was caused by a virus which was transmitted by a mosquito. The patients studied by Noguchi in South America were probably cases of leptospiral jaundice or Weil's disease. Within a decade of Stokes's death a vaccine of the attenuated virus, which has saved millions of lives, was developed by Max Theiler of the Rockefeller Foundation.

34 *The introduction of endotracheal intubation*

I van Whiteside Magill, who was born in Larne, County Antrim, in 1888, was one of the greatest practitioners of the art of anaesthesia. He was the son of Samuel Magill who had a drapery business in the town. He was educated at Larne Grammar School and he was awarded a gold medal for English before going on to study medicine at Queen's University, Belfast, where he graduated in 1913. He had a fine physique and was an able sportsman, boxing for his university as a heavyweight and playing rugby forward. However, his academic talents were not appreciated in the early years by his university and his MD thesis on blind nasal intubation was rejected in 1920. Twenty-five years later, the university made amends when Magill was awarded a D Sc *honoris causa*.

INTRODUCTION TO ANAESTHESIA

Magill worked as a house surgeon and then as resident medical officer at Stanley Hospital and Walton Hospital in Liverpool. When the First World War began he joined the Royal Army Medical Corps and served throughout the war as a captain. He was medical officer to the Irish

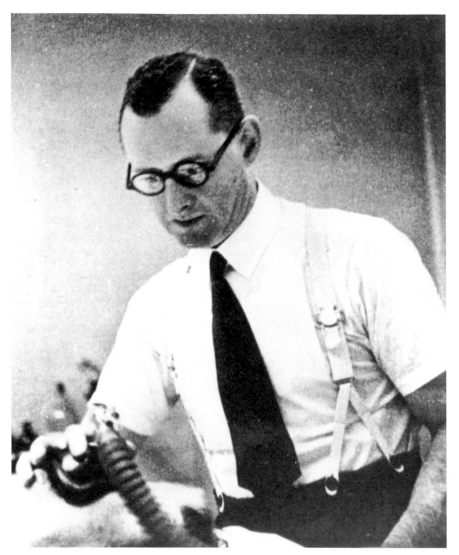

34.1   Ivan Magill anaesthetising a patient in the late 1920s.

Guards at the Battle of Loos. In 1916 he married Edith Banbridge who
was also a doctor. When hostilities ceased he was posted to Barnet War
Hospital where, among other duties, he occasionally administered
anaesthetics. Shortly after this he received a questionnaire from the
RAMC asking for his current status, in consideration of possible

demobilisation. He answered 'anaesthetist'; he said later that he was 'put up to it' by his colleagues. As a consequence he was transferred to Queen Mary's Hospital for Facial and Jaw Injuries at Sidcup in Kent. On his arrival he met Stanley Rowbotham, who was similarly posted, and so began an historic relationship as both men would make major contributions to anaesthesia. They worked with Harold Gillies who was to become famous as a pioneer of plastic surgery.

Gillies performed reconstructive operations on the faces and jaws of wounded soldiers, and Magill and Rowbotham were responsible for administering the anaesthetics. They were faced with a daunting task as there were 600 wounded soldiers in the hospital, all of whom needed face and jaw surgery. At that time anaesthesia was still comparatively primitive, making such surgery very difficult. Ether, chloroform, ethyl chloride and nitrous oxide were the gases used, and the first three of these were poured on a gauze-covered mask and inhaled by the patient. These methods were not practical when anaesthetising soldiers with severe facial injuries. Instead, rectal ether or intratracheal air and ether insufflated through a catheter were the rather crude and hazardous methods used. The surgeon also inhaled some of the anaesthetic during the procedure as he bent over the patient's face.

BLIND NASAL INTUBATION

Magill invented a forceps to facilitate the introduction of nasal catheters into the larynx under direct laryngoscopic vision. However, he noticed that on occasions the catheter entered the larynx without instrumentation, and so he began to practise 'blind nasal intubation'. This technique was used widely until the introduction of short-term relaxants, which simplified the process of intubation. Initially Magill and Rowbotham used the endotracheal insufflation technique when anaesthetising wounded soldiers. They used an air-pump driven by a motor which drew in air, to which ether was added drop by drop. However, as Magill discovered, there were major drawbacks to this technique:

> It was true insufflation — it blew in enough air, so that if there was any blood in the pharynx it would blow it out — and also it would blow out

the ether exhalations, which were not so very good for the surgeon....
Gillies, who was the surgeon at the time, said 'You seem to get the
anaesthetic into the patient all right — don't you think that you could
devise some method of getting it out, so I am not anaesthetised?' So
Rowbotham and I got to work on this and devised a two tube method of
anaesthesia. We insufflated through a catheter in the trachea but in
addition passed a second catheter to deal with expiration — the pharynx
could be packed and the surgeon protected from exhalations and the
spray of blood.[1]

ENDOTRACHEAL INTUBATION

Magill first used a single wide-bore tube in the trachea to administer
anaesthesia in 1920. The patient, a young woman, refused ether or
chloroform as she had had unfortunate experiences with both of them.
It was a formidable problem for Magill:

So, I began to think a lot about what we had. There was only one
anaesthetic that was available and that was nitrous oxide and oxygen. As
insufflation was no good I said the only way to do it was with a wide
bore tube and a bag. I made a rubber tube of $^3/_8$ inch bore and strong
'angle piece' and anaesthetised the patient with nitrous oxide and
oxygen. That was the origin of the wide bore tube.[1]

Magill had introduced 'to-and-fro' ventilation with a safe airway, and he
had made it possible to use nitrous oxide for a long operation. He said
later, 'I confess it came to me as a revelation.'[2]

Magill visited several rubber merchants to select suitable tubing of
graduated sizes, which were then stored in round tins to preserve the
curves. He and Rowbotham worked closely on the development and
simplification of tracheal intubation and the methodology which they
produced made a major impact on anaesthesia around the world. The
first description of the technique appeared in the *Proceedings of the Royal
Society of Medicine* in 1921. Victor McCormick, anaesthetist at Sir
Patrick Dun's Hospital, introduced Magill's technique to Dublin:

The pioneer work of Stanley Rowbotham and Doctor, now Sir Ivan
Magill in simplifying endotracheal anaesthesia and bringing it within the

reach of the rank and file of anaesthetists was an outstanding contribution to the development of a safer and easier anaesthesia for operations on the head and neck. Magill's first paper on 'Blind Nasal Intubation' was a model of clarity and brevity. Within a few days of reading it I successfully performed my first blind nasal intubation. Not long afterwards I made my first pilgrimage to meet Magill and was rewarded not only by helpful advice and demonstration, but also by the formation of a warm personal relationship....[3]

As might be expected, the new method of endotracheal anaesthesia made an enormous difference when operating on patients needing facial surgery. Sir Harold Gillies acknowledged this when he said: 'Plastic surgery was founded on the work of Magill and his tube; it would not have been possible without it.'[1]

CONTRIBUTIONS TO THORACIC AND CARDIAC SURGERY

Apart from helping the development of plastic surgery, the introduction of the technique of endotracheal intubation was a major stimulus to thoracic surgery. Magill was appointed as anaesthetist to the Brompton Hospital in London in 1923. Tuberculosis was rife at the time and there was no effective drug treatment. Surgery was very difficult in these patients as they produced copious sputum. Magill devised a suction catheter with an inflatable cuff as a bronchial blocker so that secretions could be aspirated from the lung being operated on. He also introduced the equipment necessary to make one-lung anaesthesia possible. Professor John Dundee has pointed out that Magill's pioneering work in this area made possible the development of thoracic and cardiac surgery as we know it today:

> An additional advantage was that the anaesthetist could now inflate the lungs of the patient at will. Thoracic surgery had been hindered by the problems of 'paradoxical' respiration, when, with an open chest and spontaneous ventilation, air would shunt from one lung to another rather than be exhaled, and hypoxia would develop. A balloon on the 'Magill endotracheal tube' sealed the lungs off from the atmosphere and not only was the anaesthetist well out of the surgeon's way but he could now control the patient's breathing.[4]

MAGILL'S ATTACHMENT AND OTHER INNOVATIONS

Magill improved the anaesthetic apparatus which was used at that time by inventing a re-breathing or reservoir bag, which became known as the Magill's attachment and which is now used by anaesthetists all over the world. He improved the technique of laryngoscopy by the simple innovation of putting batteries in the handle of his laryngoscope. He introduced several other improvements in anaesthetic technique, such as bobbin flow meters in 1928. Much of his equipment was portable, so he could give a safe anaesthetic in the ill-equipped small nursing homes which flourished at the time. He carried his cylinders under his overcoat, suspended from a yoke over his shoulders! In 1924 he joined the staff of the Westminster Hospital, where he worked with the surgeon Stanford Cade. Cade later recalled: 'To have Magill as one's anaesthetist put the surgeon in a "class".'[2] This class included Terence Millin, Harold Gillies and Tudor Edwards.

IMPROVING THE STATUS OF THE ANAESTHETIST

Magill worked constantly to improve the status of the anaesthetist. At the time when he was first appointed to the Brompton Hospital, physicians were appointed for life, surgeons for three years and anaesthetists for one year. He believed that anaesthesia would only advance when it became independent of surgical domination. He was to the fore in organising the Association of Anaesthetists of Great Britain and Ireland in 1932, and in the founding of the Faculty of Anaesthetists of the Royal College of Surgeons of England in 1947. He played a key role in developing anaesthesia as a specialty and was largely responsible for instituting the Diploma in Anaesthetics of the Conjoint Board of the Royal College of Surgeons of England in 1935. This was the first qualification in anaesthesia. In 1947 he wrote a chapter on anaesthesia in Terence Millin's book *Retropubic Surgery*. In the same year he gave the opening address at the inauguration of the Section of Anaesthetics of the Royal Academy of Medicine in Ireland.

Magill developed a very large private practice and his reputation was such that he was asked to anaesthetise distinguished members of society, including members of the British and other royal families. A W Edridge wrote in an editorial in *Anaesthesia* in 1987:

> Magill was a superb anaesthetist with an extraordinary deftness and an air of unhurried purpose. Nothing, one felt, could surprise him and nothing could go wrong. His hand never left the bag and years of the keenest observation had endowed him with an almost uncanny feel for the condition of a patient.[2]

He received many honours during his life, including a knighthood in 1960 and the Henry Hill Hickman medal of the Royal Society of Medicine. The anaesthetic department at Westminister Hospital is now known as the Magill Department of Anaesthetics.

MAN OF CHARACTER

Magill had a great sense of humour, which often broke the tedium of the operating theatre. On one occasion Gillies was operating on a patient with asymmetrical breasts. After a long period of suturing he stood back so that his handiwork could be admired by visitors in the theatre, only to be deflated by Magill who quipped, 'Surely the same effect could have been achieved with a thick sole on her right shoe.'[5] He was an inveterate practical joker. One of his favourite amusements was to put on a surgical gown and mask and then to introduce himself to a surgical colleague as a distinguished but infuriatingly stupid foreign visitor.

Fishing was his main form of relaxation. Both he and his wife went on regular expeditions and she sketched while he fished. It was an interest he kept up throughout his long life and he caught a five-pounder on his ninety-seventh birthday.

Magill died on 4 December 1986 and the obituary notice in *The Lancet* began with the sentence: 'Every anaesthetist in the world has been influenced by the work of Sir Ivan Magill and benefitted from his foresight.'[6]

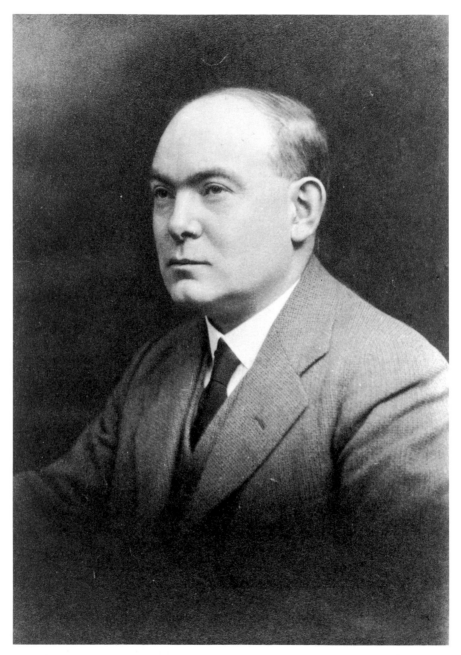

35.1   E J Conway 1894–1968

EDWARD JOSEPH CONWAY
1894–1968

35 Electrolytes and the cell

Edward Joseph Conway was a medical scientist who made a major contribution to the understanding of the physiology of the cell and its electrolytes, and his work had an important influence on the development of electrophysiology. He was born near Nenagh, County Tipperary, on 3 July 1894. His father, William Conway, was of farming stock and his mother Mary Anne, whose maiden name was McCready, came from a family of shoemakers who had been in that business for nearly two hundred years. William Conway started a drapery business in Nenagh but he retired from this after some years when his wife inherited a small legacy from a relative who had established the highly successful McCready Shoe Corporation in the United States. The family then moved to Sandymount in Dublin. However, E J Conway always retained affectionate memories of his early childhood, and many years later when he visited Nenagh for a civic reception to mark his seventieth year, he said: 'I feel that I have come home and that this very agreeable town in North Tipperary, situated as it is close to the Keeper Mountain and Lough Derg on the lordly Shannon was really a beautiful place in which to be born.'[1]

He received his early education at the Christian Brothers' School in

Nenagh, where he was noted as being very good at mathematics, and later at Blackrock College in Dublin. He was a shy and reserved boy who took his studies seriously and he was a competent pianist. He won an exhibition scholarship to University College Dublin in 1912, where he studied medicine.

INTEREST IN PHYSIOLOGY

Conway decided, while still a student, to pursue a career in the biological sciences rather than in the clinical arena. He did not believe in burdening his mind with a lot of facts which would be of no value to him later, so he did just enough study to pass his medical examinations. He was taken to task after his second medical examination for not mentioning the location of the motor area of the brain in a question on the subject. He responded by saying that he did not see any point in mentioning it as it was well known to everyone. However, he passed his examination and he then took two years out to study physiology, gaining a first class honours B Sc in 1916 and an M Sc in 1917. After graduating in 1921, he joined the staff of Professor James O'Connor, the professor of physiology at University College Dublin. He performed some teaching duties and he also became deeply involved in research, which led to a D Sc in 1927. In 1928 he obtained a grant which allowed him to carry out some research on muscle physiology and biochemistry in the laboratory of Gustav Embden in Frankfurt.

EARLY RESEARCH

In 1932 Conway became the first occupant of the chair of biochemistry and pharmacology in University College Dublin. Two years later he married Mabel Hughes from Rugby in England and they established their home in Killiney, County Dublin, where their family of four girls grew up. At UCD Conway established a very successful research laboratory, which attracted funding from sources such as the Rockefeller Foundation, the US National Institutes and Air Force, as well as the Medical Research Council of Ireland.

Conway's early research focused on renal tubular function. As he had to make several estimations of the constituents of very small volumes of fluid, he developed his own method of microanalysis. His technique was so successful that it became an integral part of the standard procedure world-wide. He devised the method originally to measure blood ammonia, but it could also be used for other estimations such as blood urea, oxygen capacity, carbon dioxide, chloride and glucose. His book on the subject *Microdiffusion and Volumetric Error*, went through five editions in thirty years.

He then undertook a review of marine geochemistry, as he had become interested in the cellular mechanisms whereby ions are transported across membranes against a concentration gradient. Macallum had advanced a theory in the 1920s which stated that vertebrate forms emerged from the ocean when the composition of sea-water and plasma were similar. It was argued that the body fluids of these early forms of modern vertebrates were isolated by membranes from their surroundings. The biochemistry of the sea then changed, but that of plasma remained static. Conway's fundamental research, using a mathematical approach, completely demolished this theory. He demonstrated that there could have been very little change in the concentration of the major ions in sea-water over the time in question, and that the sea in the early evolutionary period had three times the salinity of mammalian plasma.

ELECTROLYTE RESEARCH

In 1941 Conway made a major contribution to physiology when he demonstrated how levels of ions such as sodium and potassium are maintained at different concentrations within and without the cell. He showed how this could be accomplished if the cell membrane is selectively permeable and restraints are placed on the migration of ions, thus creating a resting or membrane potential on the cell wall. Conway postulated that the membranes were impermeable to sodium, but other workers subsequently explained the phenomenon on the basis of a metabolic pump or active transport.

Conway's work attracted the attention of the famous Irish chemist Frederick George Donnan (1870–1956). Donnan, who was the son of a Belfast merchant, was educated at the Belfast Royal Academy and

Queen's College Belfast. He worked for a time as lecturer in organic chemistry at the Royal College of Science in Dublin before moving to Liverpool, and then to University College London where he was professor of general chemistry. Donnan published his classic paper 'The theory of membrane equilibrium in the presence of a non-dialyzable electrolyte' in 1911. The Donnan theory forms part of the framework of colloid chemistry and it provides the basis for many ideas on the nature of the transport of ions and molecules across the living cell. Donnan's interest in Conway's work was therefore both flattering and stimulating for the latter. They began a remarkable correspondence which lasted throughout the years of the Second World War. Donnan was very excited by Conway's ideas on cell electrolytes and he discussed them in *Nature* in 1941 and 1942. In September 1941 Donnan wrote a very encouraging letter to Conway:

> It is *great* good luck that physiological science has found in you not only a first-rate experimenter, but also a mathematical physicist who can carry deductive mathematical reasoning right through a complex situation, and who has the imagination to *perceive intuitively* the complexity of the situation. I am glad that this has happened in a city whose streets were trod by the feet of Hamilton, McCullagh and Fitzgerald.[2]

The two men exchanged ideas and discussed complex scientific theories. There is one extant letter of Conway's which consists of several pages of abstruse mathematical formulae, broken occasionally by the odd quotation in Arabic!

Conway and his team continued to publish regularly on topics such as acid formation by the gastric mucosa, a redox pump for the biological performance of osmotic work, active transport of sodium ions and other aspects of electrolyte physiology. In 1957 he published a book in the United States entitled *The Biochemistry of Gastric Acid Secretion,* and two years later the Medical Research Council of Ireland established a Unit of Cell Metabolism under Conway's direction.

Conway tended to stay aloof from his colleagues, and many of his staff were in awe of him. However, as Maizels, his biographer, pointed out: '....those who succeeded in breaking through the barrier set by his shy and retiring nature, had a real affection for him and were honoured to have been associated with him.'[1] James Deeny, former chief medical officer in the Department of Health, remembers asking Conway for facilities which would enable him to do some research on a part-time basis. Conway willingly gave him the bench space and he was also very encouraging.

Several young men and women who worked under Conway's direction subsequently developed very successful departments of biochemistry in other colleges in Ireland, and a number achieved distinction in the clinical field. Apart from Conway's work, there have been several other major Irish contributions to biochemistry this century. Vincent Barry synthesised one of the first-line drugs for leprosy at the Medical Research Council laboratories in Trinity College. Nina Carson discovered the hereditary metabolic disorder of homocystinuria in Belfast. The work of John Scott, Donald Weir and John Dinn in Trinity College has led to a new understanding of vitamin B12 and related neuropathies.

HONOURS AND DISTINCTIONS

Conway received many honours during his life. He became a fellow of the Royal Society in 1947 and he received an honorary D Sc from Trinity College Dublin in 1952. In 1953 he was made an honorary fellow of the Royal College of Physicians of Ireland and after the conferring he delivered an address on 'Science and the physician'. In this he emphasised the historical connections between medicine and the sciences of biology, chemistry and physics, and he concluded by observing that: 'It may be said that judged from the most "practical" basis, advance in the pure sciences allied to medicine is not only fruitful but necessary, and that it is short-sighted to support or confine medical research only to the immediate objective of treating disease.'[3]

Conway was elected a member of the Academie Septentrionale in 1958, a society which was founded in 1935 to bring together the most illustrious European names in science and art. He was appointed chairman of the Dublin Institute for Advanced Studies in 1960 and in the same year he was elected a member of New York Academy of Sciences. Conway was also a member of the Pontifical Academy of Sciences. He received the Boyle Medal of the Royal Dublin Society in 1968.

INTERESTS OUTSIDE MEDICINE

Conway played a leading role in the foundation of the Graduates Association of the National University of Ireland and he was its first chairman. However, like many scientists, he was not a practical organiser. According to Maizels it was 'not unknown for him to arrange several independent lunch appointments for the same day, and then to spend time on an experiment in his laboratory, lunching on tea and a bun'.[1] He was very absent-minded and lost his glasses so often that he kept a few pairs of Woolworth's spectacles near him so that he would not lose valuable time looking for his own. He had a rather reserved nature but he could be quite forceful when defending his theories. According to Professor F G Young, he was:

> ....a doughty controversialist and the discussions that resulted from his papers on the mechanism of gastric secretion are still remembered by many, particularly for the dogged charm and wit with which Conway defended his ideas in scientific meetings. Like many Irishmen he was interested in the philosophical aspects of scientific thought and an evening by his fireside could be of memorable interest.[1]

The Irish Times published a portrait of Conway in 1953, praising him for the honour he was bringing to University College Dublin. It then went on to paint a pen picture of the scientist:

> His brows are of bronze. Meeting in the middle, they give an oddly Oriental slant to his green eyes. His slightly nasal voice is soft; his manner almost meek. At first he seems shy and vague; but if he is interested, his whole face becomes illuminated with a cherubic smile. His conversation becomes animated and seasoned with subtly humorous allusion. Then you notice for the first time his small, fastidious hands — hands as much at home in manipulating the delicate instruments of his own invention as in weaving fine phrases in the language of music.[4]

The last sentence referred to his musical skill. He had a grand piano in his house and he usually played for his guests after dinner. He was very fond of more obscure German pieces — particularly those which presented him with a technical challenge. He was also very interested in

the work of German philosophers such as Immanuel Kant and Georg
Hegel.

Conway enjoyed gardening and he took a special interest in the
cultivation of roses. He was also a keen fisherman and was particularly
expert at fly-fishing. For a number of years he and his family rented a
house in Dog's Bay in Connemara, where he would fish for salmon and
sea trout. In 1958 he built a bungalow on the shore of Lough Sheelin in
County Cavan. It was at the end of a holiday there in 1967 that he
developed a stroke from which he made only a partial recovery.
However, he was spared a very long period of incapacity as he died in
Dublin on 29 December 1968. On one occasion, at the height of his
international fame, a medical associate asked him why he did not accept
a professorship abroad and increase his income considerably. 'But I like
working here', he protested mildly, and when pressed further for a
reason he replied with an uncharacteristic display of sentiment, 'Perhaps
it's the people of Dublin.'[4]

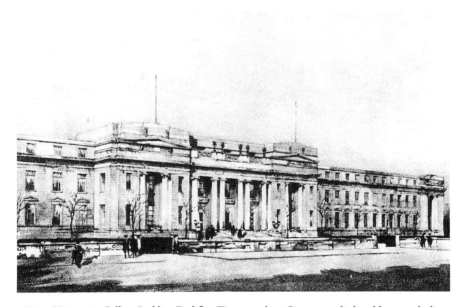

*35.2   University College Dublin, Earlsfort Terrace, where Conway studied and later worked.
The* aula maxima *is now the National Concert Hall, a development which would have interested
Conway as he was an excellent pianist. Physiology is still taught to UCD medical students in part
of the building.*

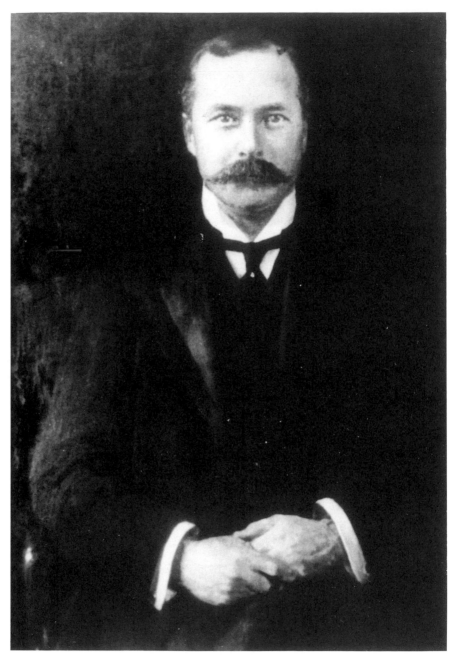

36.1   Peter Freyer 1851–1921 (Courtesy of RCSI)

36 *Irish contributions to urology*

Over the centuries Irish surgeons and physicians have made several significant contributions to the development of urology and nephrology. George Daunt invented an instrument for performing operations for bladder stone in 1750 and his work received the recognition of the Royal Academy of Surgery in Paris. Jonathan Osborne was a pioneer nephrologist who made several original observations on proteinuria and renal disease. In 1878 Sir Philip Crampton introduced a suction device to evacuate the fragments after a stone had been crushed in the bladder, anticipating the American surgeon Bigelow who perfected the technique forty years later. Sir Francis Cruise improved the cystoscope and Thomas J D Lane made a major contribution to Irish urology when he established the Meath Urological Department. Two Irish surgeons, Peter Freyer and Terence Millin, became internationally famous for their work on the surgery of the prostate gland.

PETER FREYER

Peter Freyer was born at Ballynahinch, County Galway, in 1851, and he was educated at the Erasmus Smith College, Galway, and at Queen's College Galway. He subsequently studied at Dr Steevens' Hospital, Dublin. He was awarded a BA with first class honours and a gold medal in 1872 and two years later he passed his medical degrees with similar distinctions. After graduating he did some work in Paris before joining the Indian Medical Service, where he became particularly skilled at the removal of calculi from the bladder. One patient, the Nawab of Rampur, was so grateful that he gave Freyer one lakh of rupees, which was worth approximately £6600 at that time. This led to a battle between Freyer and the Indian Medical Service, which demanded that he should return the money to the prince. He objected and won his case. In 1896 he commenced practice in Harley Street and quickly developed a very large and lucrative private practice. He was appointed surgeon to St Peter's Hospital for Stone, succeeding another Irish surgeon named Ambrose Todd.

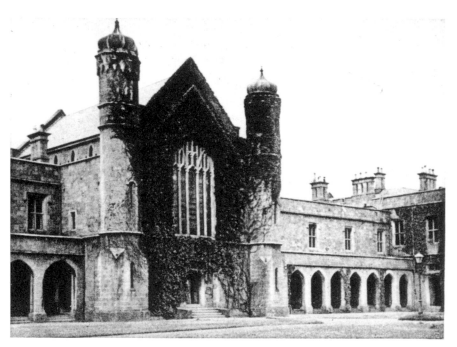

36.2   *Queen's College Galway (now University College Galway) where Freyer studied.*

A NEW OPERATION

Freyer's fame rests mainly on a paper which he published in the *British Medical Journal* in 1901. In this paper he stated:

> I have in four cases undertaken a new and, at first sight, very formidable operation for radical cure of the enlarged organ, namely total extirpation of the prostate, in one and all with entire success. These four operations have completely revolutionised my views with regard to the treatment of this painful and widespread malady, and I submit that the complete success with which they have been attended opens up a new and promising era in this field of surgery with far reaching results.[1]

Freyer was immediately attacked for his assertions by the medical press and his priority was disputed. A particularly bitter feud arose between him and Lord Moynihan, the latter claiming that the operation had been first performed by his old chief McGill in Leeds, but that he had died before having an opportunity to publish his account. Others also claimed that they had performed the operation before Freyer. He responded characteristically with the following statement:

> But if these gentlemen have, as they say, been doing my operation, they have neither recognised its significance, explained the anatomical considerations under which it would be performed, nor put it forward before the profession in such a clear and forcible form and backed by that success that commands attention and respect. This I respectfully submit I have done in my lectures; and it is under these considerations I claim it as new.[2]

Garrison and Morton have credited the American surgeon Eugene Fuller with the original description of the operation, but they also acknowledge Freyer's contribution. Certainly suprapubic prostatectomy was not generally practised before Freyer's paper in 1901, and it was his constant and forceful advocacy that secured its acceptance throughout Europe.

Freyer was the author of several successful books on different aspects of urological surgery. During his life he received many honours, including the Arnott memorial medal for original work in surgery in 1904 and a knighthood in 1917. He was chairman of the Council of the

Irish Medical Schools' and Graduates' Association. In 1920 he was invited to become the first president of the newly formed Section of Urology at the Royal Society of Medicine. He died at his home in Harley Street in 1921 and was buried in the west of Ireland.

TERENCE MILLIN

Terence Millin, the son of a lawyer, was born in St Helen's Bay, County Down, in 1903. He was educated at St Andrew's College in Dublin and in 1921 he won an entrance exhibition to Trinity College. The following year he became a foundation scholar in mathematics, a remarkable achievement for someone so young. He could not see any future in mathematics, so he transferred to the School of Physic in 1923, where he won almost every undergraduate distinction, including the Cunningham Medal in anatomy, before qualifying in 1927. Millin played rugby for Ireland against Wales in 1925.

Having won a surgical travelling prize Millin studied at the Middlesex Hospital and Guy's Hospital in London. He became a fellow of the Royal College of Surgeons in Ireland in 1928 and of the English College in 1930. He subsequently worked as senior house officer at the General Hospital, Northampton, and as assistant surgeon at Sir Patrick Dun's Hospital in Dublin. He then took up a post at All Saints' Hospital in London, as house surgeon and clinical assistant to Edward Canny Ryall, a specialist in genito-urinary surgery. He obtained this post through the influence of the Dublin surgeon Sir Thomas Myles, Ryall's cousin. Millin's talent for urology was soon recognised. He was appointed honorary assistant surgeon to All Saints' and he set up rooms in Harley Street. Later he became urologist to Southall Hospital, The Royal Masonic Hospital, The Chelsea Hospital for Women, and St Helier Hospital, Carshalton. During this period of development he maintained his interest in rugby and he was elected a vice-president of the London-Irish Rugby Football Club.

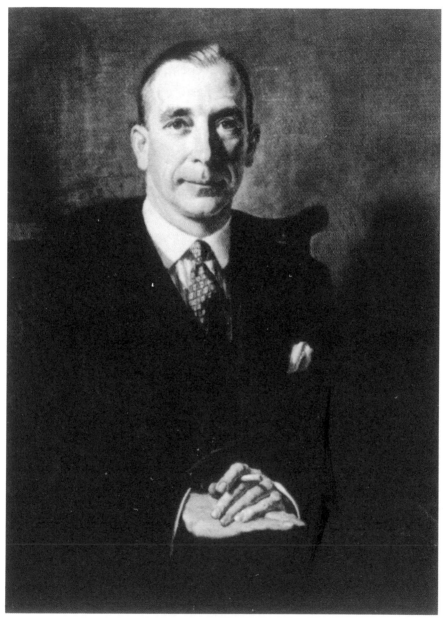

36.3   Terence Millin 1903–1980 (Courtesy of RCSI)

NEW APPROACH TO PROSTATECTOMY

Millin became an expert at transurethral resection of the prostate. The first highlight of his career was when he demonstrated the technique to Lord Moynihan in the early thirties. In 1945 he published a paper in *The Lancet* in which he introduced a new method of prostatectomy. It was entitled 'Retropubic prostatectomy. A new extravesical technique', and it began confidently:

> The operation which I am presenting in this paper is, I believe, original. Although this report is based on a relatively small series of 20 cases, the procedure represents, in my view, a great advance in the treatment of prostatic obstruction.[3]

The paper made an extraordinary impact. A leading article in the same issue of *The Lancet* compared the innovation with Archimedes' discovery of his Principle, and the explorations of Stanley and Livingstone. It continued:

> Yet in this year of 1945, eighty years after the birth of surgical craftsmanship, and in the surgery of the prostate, a branch of operative technique commoner, more important, more closely studied, and more widely pursued than most, T J Millin has discovered a method that is not only quite new, but also simpler, safer, and better than those now in use....[4]

Not only did Millin describe a new operation, he also created many new instruments with which to perform it efficiently. It was in 1944 that the idea of the retropubic approach first occurred to him:

> I was doing a total cystectomy and saw the anatomy of the prostate laid bare from the outside instead of the usual view one got from inside the bladder. It seemed to me then that the logical approach to the prostate was the direct one. After all it is a subvesical organ, even if it does encroach into the bladder when enlarged. Why on earth should we open first the top and then the bottom of the bladder to get at an organ that can be approached without opening the bladder at all?[5]

He performed the first retropubic operation in August 1945, and two months later he described twenty cases at the French Urological Congress in Paris. He subsequently introduced the technique to an audience of British surgeons:

> Later, I presented a case at the Royal Society of Medicine, having filled the patient up with beer beforehand. I introduced him as a man who had had a prostatectomy eight days before and showed them the scar on his tummy which still had the stitches in. I then asked him to pass water and, because of the beer, I thought he'd never stop. Everyone wanted to know what I'd done, but I told them to wait until the following morning when they could read it in the Lancet.[5]

INTERNATIONAL ACCLAIM

The paper in *The Lancet* brought Millin international acclaim and he travelled the world demonstrating his technique and operating on influential people. Although interesting, these journeys were very demanding. He also had a number of bizarre experiences, such as the occasion when he recalled 'being driven to examine the President of Turkey in a bullet-proof car and operating on him in the presence of the entire Turkish Cabinet — suitably gowned up. It was rather like the birth of a royal baby, except I was delivering a Presidential prostate'.[5]

As might be expected of a mathematical scholar, he had a very lucid mind, and this was reflected in the clarity of his clinical presentations and lectures. In 1947 he published a book entitled *Retropubic Surgery*. His operation became the standard approach to prostatectomy until the more recent technical advances in transurethral surgery made the latter the norm.

Apart from his work on prostate surgery Millin made significant contributions to the urological aspects of gynaecology and to the treatment of bladder cancer.

PRIVATE LIFE

Millin retired early from the British National Health Service but continued to operate at a private clinic in Queen's Gate, London, which he had established with Charles Reed. At the peak of his success he bought a farm in Doneraile, County Cork:

> I was overwhelmed with work, and because of taxation, was working for a small proportion of my income. My elder daughter was congenitally deaf and we heard of opportunities in Ireland for special tuition. And, after all, I am an Irishman. I graduated at Trinity and, though city bred, I'd always hankered after the country life. I'd established a team at the Queen's Gate Clinic in London and, in 1950, I set up a routine where I worked for a month over there, living over the shop, and then spent a month farming in County Cork.... It was a great period of my life. I drove my own tractors and spent one month dressed like a surgeon and the other month dressed like a farm labourer.[5]

CONTRIBUTIONS TO SURGERY IN IRELAND

Millin went out of his way to encourage young Irish surgeons who were training in England. He also used his talent and influence to promote the interests of the Royal College of Surgeons in Ireland. He became its president in 1963 and, as an international figure, did a great deal for the image of the institution. Working closely with Dr Harry O'Flanagan, the registrar of the college, he inaugurated a major fund-raising campaign which led to a substantial phase of building and expansion. In order to be near the college he sold his farm and moved to a house in the Dublin Mountains. When he had completed the customary two years in office, he was persuaded to stay on for another year. During his presidency he played a major role in developing postgraduate surgical training in Ireland. He was scrupulously careful not to become involved in urological practice in Ireland, although his advice was always available to Irish colleagues if they requested it. Victor Lane, a former president of the Royal College of Surgeons in Ireland and one of the country's leading urologists, recalled:

> On several occasions he was invited to the Meath Hospital, Dublin, to observe the senior registrars performing retropubic operations — an exercise that he did his best to make easy for the registrar concerned, who was unlikely, however, to forget the experience —much as he would treasure the memory in later years.[6]

In 1961 the College of Surgeons received a substantial anonymous donation through Millin from one of his patients. This was used to refurbish one of the houses purchased in York Street as a Students' Union. It was named Millin House and it contained a meeting hall in which concerts and various student events were held. When the college was extended subsequently the building was demolished, but the student accommodation in the new development in the former Mercer's Hospital has been named Millin House. In his book *An Assembly of Irish Surgeons* the college's distinguished historian Professor J B Lyons has said that 'Terence Millin's pre-eminence among the 20th Century presidents cannot be disputed. No other has been so acclaimed'.[7] In 1979 the College of Surgeons decided to hold an annual Millin Lecture, which would be delivered by a young surgeon on some aspect of research.

HIGHLY REGARDED

Millin is remembered by his friends as a great story-teller and an excellent after-dinner speaker. Robert Cox, who worked for a brief period as Millin's assistant and subsequently became a consultant urologist at Westminister Hospital, recalls that Millin was 'a *very* fine after-dinner speaker with an enormous fund of hilariously funny stories — some said that he made them up as he went along!'[8]

He received many honours, including the honorary fellowships of the American and Royal Australasian Colleges of Surgeons. He was made an honorary member of the Urological Section of the Royal Society of Medicine in 1978, and as he was unable to travel to London, he was presented with the honour at a special function in Trinity College.

He died from carcinoma of the larynx in July 1980, following a long and painful illness. After his death Dr Anthony Walsh, the pioneer of renal transplantation in Ireland, wrote in *The Lancet*:

> He was certainly one of the giants of surgery in the past half-century and it can be said of him, as of few doctors, that everything he wrote in his prime is still well worth reading.[9]

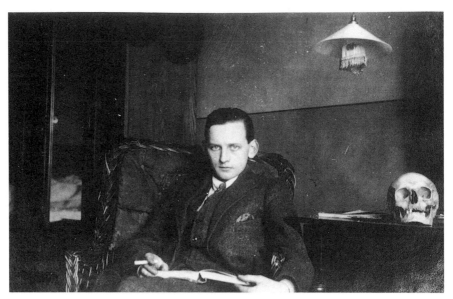

37.1   Peter Kerley in 1922, when he was a student in Dublin.

37 *The radiology of heart failure*

Medical students and doctors all over the world are taught how to identify Kerley lines on the chest X-ray films of patients suffering from various degrees of cardiac failure. The man who first described them was Peter James Kerley, a pioneer in the development of radiology and one of the authors of a famous textbook on the subject. He was born on 27 October 1900 in Dundalk, County Louth, the fourth son and thirteenth child of Michael and Matilda Kerley. His father, who owned an egg-exporting business, was one of thirteen sons of a farmer from County Louth. His mother was a daughter of Bernard Henry of Draperstown, County Antrim, a middle man in the flax business. His mother's brother, Augustine Henry, studied medicine and natural history in Galway, and he had a very distinguished career. He spent twenty years in China as a doctor with the Imperial Maritime Customs Service, during which time he studied the flora of China. On his return to Ireland he was appointed professor of forestry at the Royal College of Science (later University College) Dublin.

EARLY EDUCATION

When Peter Kerley was quite young his father died and his mother and eldest brother Austin took over the management of the family's egg-exporting business. Kerley went to school at St Mary's College in Dundalk, which was run by the Christian Brothers. His uncle, Augustine Henry, was impressed by the boy's intellectual ability and he decided to encourage and assist with his further education at University College Dublin. Kerley graduated MB in 1923 and he proceeded to MD in 1932.

His early ambition was to be an ear, nose and throat surgeon. He went to Vienna to study this subject, but there he was so impressed by the Holzknecht School of Radiology, at that time a centre of the new science, that he decided to pursue a career in radiology instead. In 1925 he went to Cambridge to take the Diploma in Medical Radiology and Electrology. Soon afterwards he was appointed to the Royal Chest Hospital in London, and in 1929 he joined the consultant staff of Westminster Hospital. In the same year he married Olivia MacNamee from Enniskillen, County Fermanagh, and they were to have two daughters.

CONTRIBUTIONS TO RADIOLOGY

Kerley's *Recent Advances in Radiology* was published in 1931. This was the first English language textbook of radiology to be directed at general physicians and general practitioners. In the preface he drew attention to the high mortality rate among the pioneers of radiology:

> The amazing progress of radiology during the last ten years is entirely due to the heroic efforts of the early workers, many of whom sacrificed health and life to increase our knowledge of X-rays. By 1921 the mortality among X-ray workers was so high that it occasioned grave public concern — some openly stated that the cost in human life did not warrant further research. This attitude did not deter radiologists from continuing their work....[1]

Kerley's own exposure to radiation in the early days caused him some concern all his life.

Kerley was elected a fellow of the Royal College of Physicians in 1943, and the following year he received the Röntgen Award of the

British Institute of Radiology. The experiences of his friends in Vienna and a visit there in 1938 left him with an abiding hatred of Nazism. It was for this reason that he joined the war effort, although he was not eligible for call-up. He enlisted with the Royal Army Medical Corps and rose to the rank of major. He served in Singapore, and after being invalided home from there he was posted to York.

In 1944 he was demobilised at the request of the Ministry of Health and invited to set up a programme of screening for tuberculosis by mass miniature radiography. This was a major challenge. He toured the country, ensuring that there were enough radiographers to take films and doctors to interpret them. He played a key role in launching a service which was one of the greatest contributions to public health in England in the post-war years. He was awarded the CBE for this work.

Kerley also gave very valuable advice when the mass radiography service was being established in Ireland. During this time he worked closely with James Deeny, formerly chief medical officer in the Department of Health. Deeny recalled one occasion at a meeting in the Custom House when Kerley turned very pale shortly after arriving from London. 'I have done it again', he said, as Deeny rose to call for an ambulance.[2] However, Kerley would not have an ambulance and asked to be driven instead to the rooms of his former classmate Bob Davitt in Fitzwilliam Square, where he recovered after an injection of adrenalin. Kerley calmly told Deeny that he developed an anaphylactic reaction when he ate lobster, and that there must have been some in the pâté that he had eaten on the plane during his flight from London.

In 1947 Kerley was appointed consultant radiologist to the International Refugee Organisation. This entailed visiting concentration camps and displaced persons' camps all over Western Europe to advise on the medical aspects of repatriation, with particular reference to the control of tuberculosis.

INTERNATIONAL REPUTATION

Because of his reputation, Kerley was called to consult in the treatment of many famous people, including King George VI. It was Kerley who diagnosed the bronchial neoplasm which claimed the king's life. Kerley's daughter Barbara recalls that her father:

....formed a sadly brief friendship with the King through their shared love of fishing. For the rest of his active life he always sent the first salmon he caught each season to the Queen Mother. Shortly before he died the King invested him with the CVO for his services. The King gave him his CVO at a private audience, because typically my father said he could not attend the regular investiture because he was going fishing![3]

During the 1950s and 60s, in addition to his hospital appointments, Kerley had a flourishing private practice, numbering Winston Churchill among his patients. He also continued to act as radiologist to the British Royal Family.

In 1939 Kerley was one of the founder members of the Faculty of Radiology in London, and he was elected president in 1952, serving in the post for three years. In 1955 he undertook an arduous lecture tour of India, the Far East and Australia, during which he made many life-long friends. He followed this with lecture tours to the USA and Canada. The Americans respected him for his fearless acceptance of their diagnostic challenges and for his obviously unparalleled skill in X-ray interpretation of chest and heart disease. He was the author of many original papers and editor of the *Journal of the Faculty of Radiologists*, later renamed *Clinical Radiology*. He was very influential in the development of radiology as a specialty and he was adviser on the subject to the Ministry of Health in the United Kingdom.

During his time as consultant at the Westminster Hospital, thoracic surgery developed into a major sub-specialty and he became one of the world's leading cardio-thoracic radiologists. His experience in this field was enhanced by his association with the National Heart Hospital. He gained eponymous fame for his description of the lines which can be observed on the chest X-ray films of patients suffering from various degrees of heart failure and raised venous pressure. These lines are now known as Kerley lines.

A severe attack of passive hyperaemia always leaves permanent radiological evidence behind it. The interlobar pleura remains thickened, and the shadows of the perivasular lymphatics persist as fine, sharp lines, most marked at the bases and near the hila. This appearance simulates fibrosis and bronchiectasis. The differential diagnoses is made on the screen by noting the normal expansion in the apparently fibrotic area.[4]

Kerley was co-editor with Cochrane Shanks of the world-famous, six-volume *Textbook of X-Ray Diagnoses*, which became the definitive text on radiology and which was known among radiologists as 'The Bible'. The first edition was published in 1938, with E W Twining of Manchester as co-editor. Subsequent editions were updated by Kerley and Shanks, and they then dedicated the rights of future editions to the Royal College of Radiologists, under whose auspices the book continues to be published.

Kerley enjoyed teaching and his reporting sessions at the National Heart Hospital were said to have been particularly stimulating. They were widely attended 'not only for the opportunity they offered of seeing and listening to a great teacher but for the chance to hear his comments on the people and places he had met and visited over the years'.[5] At the Westminster, with Sir Ivan Magill, Sir Stanford Cade and Sir Clement Price-Thomas, he formed a quartet of medical skill which was unique in London. In 1976 he was awarded the gold medal of the Royal College of Radiologists and two years later he was present at the first Pergamon-Kerley Lecture at the college. He was honoured by several radiological bodies around the world, and in 1962 he became one of the first honorary fellows of the Faculty of Radiologists of Ireland. His daughter recalls that this honour gave him particular pleasure. He was knighted in 1972.

Kerley was a keen sportsman with an interest in golf, shooting and fishing. He went on regular fishing excursions to rivers in Ireland, England, Scotland and Norway:

> What he really enjoyed was to collect half a dozen of his medical friends and have a fortnight's fishing for salmon and trout, with a comfortable inn (with good food) as a base. I can't think anyone said no to that invitation if they could help it.... His great invention in fishing was the 'Kerley special', a dry fly which could catch sea trout, grilse, even salmon.[6]

Kerley had a quick wit and an infectious sense of humour. In his early days he was a famous practical joker; once he succeeded in slipping a pike into the goldfish pool outside the Dorchester Hotel! He was celebrated among his friends at his London clubs for his ability as a raconteur. It has been said that only a Boswell could do him justice, and that whatever he did, whether work or play, he did it with style.

At a memorial service in the Chapel of the Royal Victorian Order, following Kerley's death in 1979, Sir Thomas Lodge outlined his achievements, and concluded by observing:

> There is a passage in Virgil which begins: Felix qui potuit rerum cognoscere causas. Happy is he who can discern the causes of things — a most appropriate motto for the arms of Peter Kerley.[7]

ROBERT COLLIS
1900–1975

38 A champion of child health

Robert Collis was a man of many talents. A paediatrician who made contributions to medical science, he also wrote plays and several books. He was a champion of the poor and campaigned for the eradication of the Dublin slums. After the Second World War he faced the daunting challenge of helping the children of the infamous Belsen death camp in Germany. He made significant contributions to paediatrics, particularly to neo-natal care in Ireland, before setting out to help to establish paediatric services in Nigeria.

Collis was a member of a family whose connections with medicine stretch back to the early years of the last century. His grandfather Maurice Collis, a surgeon in the Meath Hospital, described an operation for vesicovaginal fistula, and his father, a lawyer, was chairman of the Board of the Meath Hospital. Collis spent his early childhood playing with his brothers and sisters in the large gardens of their home at Killiney. His twin brother John Stewart and his other brother Maurice were both to become well-known writers.

EASTER REBELLION

Collis' first school was at Bray, where he developed what was to become a life-long passion for rugby football, and when he was fourteen his father sent him to Rugby School in England. He was at home on holidays in 1916 when the Easter rebellion started. Each day of the rebellion Robert Collis cycled to the Meath Hospital from Killiney, wearing Red Cross armlets which got him through both sides safely. He helped at the hospital, which was near Jacob's Biscuit Factory, the site of some of the fiercest fighting. Collis found that his sympathies gradually changed in favour of the insurgents. A few days after the rebellion, he read that the leaders of the uprising had been court martialled and shot. He was shocked by this, and he later recalled:

> As I walked up Grafton Street I suddenly realised that I was an Irishman. I knew that I was on the side of the people of Ireland. I did not realise much more then. I did not feel any violent nationalistic surge of feelings. It was a deep compassion for the people, particularly the poor of Ireland. Class and religion had no part in it.[1]

Collis returned to Rugby after the holidays and, continuing to excel in sport, he became captain of the school rugger 15. He was not very gifted academically, but the headmaster told him that he might be able to realise his ambition of becoming a doctor 'as that did not require any great intelligence'.[2]

MEDICAL STUDIES

In the spring of 1918 Collis joined a cadet battalion outside London to train for the Irish Guards, but the war ended and he was demobilised before seeing any action. He had planned to return to Dublin to study medicine at Trinity College, but the university had not yet resumed normal operations after the war. His English friends urged him to go to Trinity College in Cambridge, and this was supported by his father, who was somewhat suspicious of his Irish nationalist sympathies. During his time at Cambridge he developed an interest in research and he helped Sir Joseph Barcroft at night with his physiological experiments.

   Collis had to stop all his study when he developed an acute illness during which he noticed red, raised eruptions like blotches on the front of his shins. His doctor identified these blotches as erythema nodosum and he concluded that Collis was suffering from rheumatic fever. He treated him with large doses of salicylate, and his mother took him to the south of France.

On recovering, Collis spent a year at Yale on an exchange scholarship. There he continued his study of anatomy and physiology, but he also attended a course on English poetry and modern drama. This brief introduction to literature would have a significant impact on him later. Whilst at Yale he became very ill again and this time he developed a pleural effusion. His doctors suspected that he had tuberculosis, but Collis refused to accept this and he clung to the earlier diagnosis of rheumatic fever. He returned to Cambridge where he finished his pre-clinical courses before going on to King's College Hospital in London for clinical teaching.

PAEDIATRIC TRAINING

As a student at King's, Collis came under the influence of the great paediatrician, Sir Frederick Still, and he was determined that he too would become a paediatrician. While at King's he began to play rugby again, and he came to the attention of Bethel Solomons, the famous master of the Rotunda Hospital who had once been an international rugby player himself. Solomons arranged a trial for Collis and he was selected to play against France. Solomons also arranged for Collis to do his practical midwifery course at the Rotunda Hospital. During this course all the young doctors spent time visiting women in labour in their homes in the Dublin slums. Collis was horrified by the poverty he witnessed and he resolved that he would eventually come back to Dublin and help rid the city of these shameful slums. He returned to King's College Hospital where he became house physician, working for a time under Kinnear Wilson, the famous neurologist. When he was finished his residency at King's, Still invited him to become his last house physician at the Hospital for Sick Children in Great Ormond Street.

JOHNS HOPKINS HOSPITAL

Whilst working at Great Ormond Street Collis continued to play rugby for Ireland, and he also managed to become a member of the Royal College of Physicians. He then won a Rockefeller Research Fellowship which allowed him to work in the Children's Department of the Johns Hopkins Hospital in Baltimore. Here he worked closely with Professor Ned Park, who had just been appointed to the chair of paediatrics and who subsequently became one of the leading figures in American paediatrics. Collis took over the children's allergy clinic and he began to write a thesis on allergies. Park had decided to set up a children's heart clinic and he asked Collis to visit a number of cardiac clinics and then to set one up at Johns Hopkins. Collis complied with his wishes and he established the first children's cardiac clinic at the hospital. This clinic would later become one of the most celebrated in the world, as it was here that Helen Taussig and Alfred Blalock introduced modern cardiac surgery for congenital heart conditions.

IMPORTANT DISCOVERY

When his American scholarship came to an end, Collis was appointed as a research fellow at the Hospital for Sick Children at Great Ormond Street. His research was primarily on the aetiology of rheumatic fever, and he also kept up clinical contact by doing a clinic once a week. It was at this clinic that he came up against the problem of erythema nodosum again. There were two predominant views at that time on the aetiology of erythema nodosum. The British believed that it was of rheumatic origin, whilst on the Continent it was thought to be related to tuberculosis. Collis heard of a child who had developed recurrent erythema nodosum and he went to see her at home. The child was unwell with a sore throat and her mother told Collis that the erythema nodosum usually followed such infections. Collis admitted the child to hospital and, as predicted, she had an attack of erythema nodosum a few days later. He proceeded to do some tests and found that she was insensitive to tuberculin inoculation. He then prepared an extract of streptococcus and injected some of it into her skin. The injection produced generalised erythema nodosum all over the body. He described this case and two other similar cases in a paper entitled 'A new conception of the aetiology of erythema nodosum' which was published in the *Quarterly Journal of Medicine* in 1932. He concluded the paper by stating that 'the above facts suggest that erythema nodosum is a type of hypersensitive tissue response to different bacterial allergens and that the allergens responsible for erythema nodosum in London are commonly tuberculin and haemolytic streptococcal endotoxin'.[3]

NEO-NATAL WORK IN DUBLIN

His father was anxious that Collis should return to Dublin and he suggested that he should join the staff of the Meath Hospital. The hospital had one ward of ten cots, but many children attended the out-patients, so Collis was appointed as assistant physician to Sir John Moore. Moore was the oldest member on the staff and had been one of the last students to work under William Stokes.

Bethel Solomons was Master of the Rotunda at this time and he invited Collis to develop a neo-natal department in the hospital. Not much was known about neo-natal paediatrics and Collis and the staff nurse who was appointed to work with him had to learn as they went along. They developed a special incubator which could be made cheaply and which was later used widely in the Third World. They also developed the nasogastric technique as a safe way of feeding the infants:

> The nurse, now Sister Moran, found that it was much easier and safer to feed these premature babies by stomach tube than by any other way before they had learned to suck. She introduced a simple method which could be taught in a few minutes to young nurses. It saved time, the whole procedure taking less than three minutes. It was much safer than the risk of drowning the baby when fed by spoon, and was altogether satisfactory.[4]

At first the unit concentrated on babies born within the hospital, but later a new neo-natal hospital was built in the grounds of the Rotunda, and this allowed Collis to take in critically ill new-born babies from outside.

THE FOUNDING OF THE IRISH PAEDIATRIC CLUB

Collis was the moving spirit behind the foundation in 1933 of the Irish

Paediatric Club, which was later to develop into the Irish Paediatric Association. A number of doctors who have made significant contributions to the development of paediatrics in Ireland were present at the first meeting, including Ella Webb, Dorothy Price, Kathleen Lynn, Coleman Saunders, John Shanley and Robert Steen. This first meeting was held in Dorothy Price's home at 10 Fitzwilliam Place. She was a great-granddaughter of the obstetrician Evory Kennedy and she was largely responsible for the elimination of childhood tuberculosis in Ireland. Coleman Saunders was very actively involved in the planning of Our Lady's Hospital for Sick Children in Crumlin; John Shanley was a pioneer in paediatric surgery, and Robert Steen was a pathfinder in paediatric cardiology. Collis was elected honorary secretary of the new society at its first meeting.

LITERARY WORK AND OTHER INTERESTS

Collis lived at 26 Fitzwilliam Square with his wife Phyllis and two young sons, Dermot and Robert. Paediatrics was not a lucrative specialty and during the first ten years of his practice Collis seldom earned more than £350 a year, and during the first years he made less than £200. The house in Fitzwilliam Square, although chosen by Collis, was actually acquired by his father, and subsequently leased from him. Collis published his first autobiographical book *The Silver Fleece* in 1936, when he was thirty-six years old. This was well received and it brought him to the attention of literary circles in Dublin. He used the resultant fame and prestige to begin a campaign on behalf of the unfortunate people living in the city's slums.

Collis was one of the founder members of the Citizens Housing Council, which campaigned for better housing for the poor. The writer Frank O'Connor was one of the directors of the Abbey Theatre at the time and he suggested to Collis that he should write a play about the Dublin slums. Collis agreed and he wrote *Marrowbone Lane*, with some advice from his friends Lennox Robinson and Seán O'Faoláin. As it turned out, the play was not performed at the Abbey but it was accepted by Micheál MacLiammóir and Hilton Edwards for the Gate Theatre. The well-known actress Shelagh Richards played the leading role and the play was a considerable success.

Until his old age Collis was quite at odds with any form of organised religion, but this did not prevent him from developing a close working relationship with clergymen of different denominations in his efforts to improve the conditions of the poor. He was a particularly close friend of Father John Hayes, founder of Muintir na Tíre, the Irish farming cooperative movement. During his middle years he became interested in philosophy:

> Being very much a man of social action he yet strove to link head, heart and soul through theosophy in his middle years. He read a lot of philosophy, was particularly fond of Donne, Locke and Hume and became interested in the Golden Dawn theosophical movement of which Yeats was a member.[5]

THE BELSEN CONCENTRATION CAMP

Towards the end of the Second World War Collis joined the Red Cross, as did a number of other Irish doctors, including the vascular surgeon Nigel Kinnear. Collis was asked to go to Belsen concentration camp which had just been uncovered by the advancing British Army. He was horrified when he arrived there and witnessed for himself the piles of dead which were in some places ten feet high and the emaciated conditions of the inmates who were still alive. There were many children in the camp so Collis immediately set up a children's hospital. He had the enthusiastic support of a brilliant young Dutch woman named Han Hogerzeil, a lawyer who spoke five languages. The work was very tiring and demanding and they carried it out with great enthusiasm under difficult conditions. Eventually, as the children began to make progress, plans were made to repatriate them to their own countries. Collis travelled with one group of frail Jewish children to Prague. He arranged to take some of the children who had not been claimed by relatives, back to Dublin with him, and he set up a hospital at Fairy Hill in Howth for this purpose. He also took two of the children into his own home. In 1947 he published a book with Han Hogerzeil entitled *Straight On*. It gives a harrowing account of their experiences in Belsen.

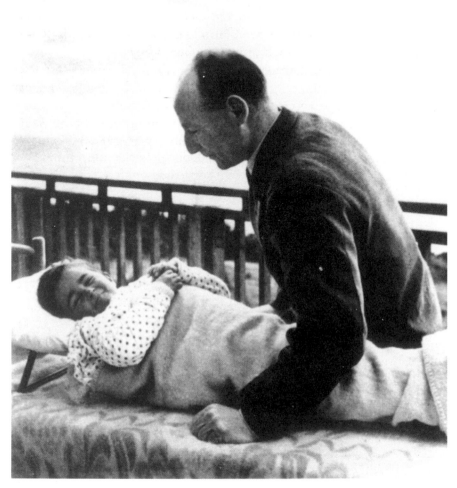

38.1   Robert Collis at Fairy Hill Hospital, Howth, County Dublin, with one of the children from Belsen Concentration Camp.

THE NATIONAL CEREBRAL PALSY CLINIC

After the war, when Collis returned to Dublin, he threw his energies into starting a clinic for children with cerebral palsy, and this became the National Cerebral Palsy Clinic. Soon after he had started the clinic he remembered a child he had seen at a children's Christmas party in one of the Dublin theatres; the child was very badly handicapped but he had a remarkable face. When Collis made enquiries he was told that the child was Christy Brown. He now set out to locate the boy and he eventually traced him to 54 Stanaway Road. Collis went to considerable trouble to arrange transport for Christy so that he could attend the clinic. Christy could not use his upper limbs but he had learned to write with his left foot. He made progress at the clinic and some years later Collis received a telegram from him which read 'Am writing my autobiography, please come and help'.[6] Collis went at once to encourage the young author. He also arranged for the publication of the book, entitled *My Left Foot*, which became an immediate success and launched Christy Brown upon his writing career.

PAEDIATRICS IN NIGERIA

Collis' personal life had become very complicated after the war. He had fallen in love with Han Hogerzeil and he kept in contact with her when he returned from Germany. He parted on an amicable basis from his first wife, but he felt that it would be difficult to continue his practice in Dublin as he and Han had decided to marry. He looked around for suitable opportunities abroad and one came when he was offered the post of director of the paediatric department at the new Nigerian Medical School at Ibadan.

Collis became head of the Department of Paediatrics at the University of Ibadan in 1957. At Ibadan he was faced with the grim realities of life in Nigeria, where the child death-rate among the uneducated was 50 per cent in many places. On his second day there he saw 92 children at the general out-patient clinic of the hospital. He soon realised that malnutrition was a major cause of ill health and death in the country, and he began to address the whole issue of prevention. He obtained support from the Rockefeller Foundation and he went on to develop Institutes of Child Health at Ibadan and Lagos.

His son Robert, who had studied medicine, joined his father's unit as a houseman in 1959:

I joined my father's unit after six months of paediatrics in Singapore under Elaine Field, a prominent tropical paediatrician. Though I was familiar with many of the syndromes I was not prepared for the magnitude of the problems, the hordes of infants and children that arrived at the hospitals *in extremis* every day. By the time I arrived it was apparent to my father that a specialist unit in a London-style teaching hospital was not even a good place for teaching Nigerian medical personnel basic preventive paediatrics which was singularly lacking throughout the nation. As a consequence he was in the process of setting up an Institute of Child Health which would research the needs of a rural community and run community clinics where preventive paediatrics could be taught. He was also frustrated that a full department of Paediatrics with a Chair had not been created.

It was however delightful to see him in action again. His obvious love for his patients and his outgoing fun-loving demeanour endeared him to the Nigerians and helped him to be an effective agent of change. Comic relief from the daily tragedy of very sick children was obtained on the polo field where he taught me to play the game on small stallions who came from the race track and could not be stopped or turned once they got into full stride.[7]

In 1962 Collis moved to Lagos to become professor of paediatrics and director of the Institute of Child Health there. Subsequently he went to Zaria in northern Nigeria to establish the Department of Paediatrics in the new Ahmadu Bello University, where he was also appointed dean. He was in Nigeria during a very unsettled political period. He developed close friendships with many of the political leaders of the country and he used his influence to advance the cause of child health. He was subsequently very distressed when many of these friends, who had promoted his work in Nigeria, were assassinated during the political upheaval. He wrote two books about this period, the first *A Doctor's Nigeria* and the second *Nigeria in Conflict.*

PILGRIM'S END

Collis resigned from his academic commitments in Nigeria in 1970 and he returned to Ireland. He was seventy, but he was still full of energy and ideas and he had no intention of retiring. He became consultant to the National Association of Cerebral Palsy and examiner in Final Medicine at both Trinity College and University College Dublin. Between 1973 and 1975 he spent periods of up to three months working in a leper colony in the village of Dichpalli, near Hyderabad in southern India, where he took part in trials of a new drug treatment for leprosy in children. He also organised a cricket tournament among the lepers, and he was himself an active participant in the games. He celebrated his seventy-fifth birthday at Dichpalli: his team-mates presented him with batting gloves and a cap in recognition of his services as a player! Shortly after this, in May 1975, he was fatally injured in a riding accident in County Wicklow. In the same year his autobiography *To Be A Pilgrim* was published posthumously. In a foreword Christy Brown wrote:

Robert Collis has led a many-rainbowed life in so many spheres: physician, paediatrician, child psychologist, writer, playwright — a life so varied and diffuse as to be almost impossible to pin down between the covers of any book, and, like many another rare thing, the things that go unsaid are as valid and meaningful as those that are said so beautifully.[8]

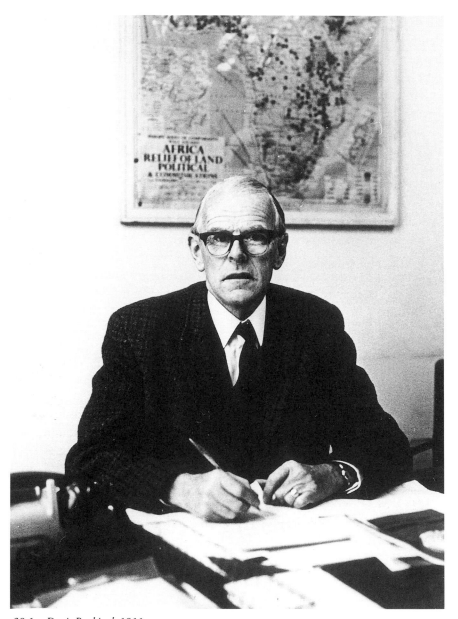

39.1   *Denis Burkitt b 1911*

DENIS BURKITT
b 1911

Denis Burkitt will occupy a unique place in the history of medical achievement. The first to describe a common and lethal form of childhood cancer in Africa, he was also the first to discover the cure for the condition. Following these achievements he embarked on a series of studies which helped to establish the link between many diseases of Western civilisation and the lack of dietary fibre. Burkitt, more than any other person, is responsible for the remarkable revolution which has taken place in Western diet over the last twenty years.

He was born in 1911, the son of James Burkitt, a county surveyor, and the family lived at Lawnakilla near Enniskillen, County Fermanagh. James Burkitt was a very practical man and he was also an able naturalist. He was the first to identify individual birds by ringing their legs with metal bands of different patterns. This system allowed him to plot their territories and their distribution. His biography, together with those of several very eminent Irish scientists, such as Robert Boyle, Lord Kelvin and Ernest Walton, appeared in a book entitled *Ten famous Irish scientists* which was published in 1984. The approach adopted by James Burkitt to identify the territorial distribution of birds around his house in Fermanagh bore similarities to the approach which would be adopted years later by his son Denis when identifying tumour distribution in Africa.

Denis, together with his younger brother Robin, was sent to preparatory school at Portora Royal School in Enniskillen, which Oscar Wilde and Samuel Beckett also attended. The Burkitts spent only two years at the school. In a row between two groups of boys, Denis had his glasses broken and his eye was injured. All efforts to save the eye failed and eventually it was removed. Denis was only eleven at the time. After being discharged from hospital he was sent with his brother to preparatory school at Tre-Arddur Bay near Holyhead in north Wales. He subsequently went to secondary school at Dean Close in Cheltenham.

A STUDENT AT TRINITY COLLEGE

In 1929 Denis Burkitt returned to Dublin to enrol at the School of Engineering at Trinity College. During his first year at college he became an active member of a Bible Study group which met in rooms at 'No 40' and this experience was to have a major influence on his career. At the end of his first year he changed his subject to medicine.

> I think the thing that strikes me looking back is the total absence of any medical research being done to my knowledge when I was at Trinity. Teaching was poor and almost totally lacking with visual aids. I remember Professors writing up long screeds on the blackboard before the lecture and we students going in early to copy them all down.[1]

Norman Moore, consultant psychiatrist and former director of St Patrick's Hospital in Dublin, was Burkitt's classmate at Trinity. They both lived in residential accommodation at number 19 Botany Bay, where Burkitt shared rooms with his brother Robin. Moore remembers Burkitt as 'an unassuming, industrious and much respected member of our year'.[2] Moore and Burkitt pursued their clinical studies at the Adelaide Hospital. At the end-of-term examinations before graduation, Burkitt won the Hudson prize and silver medal. Moore recalls: 'This was generally thought to have entitled him to one of the two coveted posts of successive house physician and surgeon at his teaching hospital. The job was given to a more lowly placed and popular student, a rugby international who helped the hospital to win the rugby cup. The disappointment seemed a big one at that stage in his career, but he accepted it with characteristic dignity and indeed had the magnanimity to go back and fill the post at a later stage.'[2]

POSTGRADUATE EXPERIENCE

For three and a half years after graduating, Burkitt worked in hospitals in Chester, Dublin, Preston and Poole. In 1936 he attended a course in Edinburgh to prepare for the fellowship of the Royal College of Surgeons. He obtained the fellowship in 1938 and then signed on as a ship's surgeon on a voyage to Manchuria. As he travelled, Burkitt thought about his future and he resolved that he would work as a surgeon somewhere in the Third World. On his return to England in 1939 he decided to seek further surgical experience. He obtained a position as resident surgical officer at the Prince of Wales Hospital in Plymouth. There he met a nurse named Olive Rogers who shared his religious convictions and who would later become his wife.

WAR SERVICE

Burkitt left Plymouth and worked in Barnsley for a short period before applying to the Colonial Office early in 1941 for a position in the medical service in Africa. He was dismayed when his application was rejected because he had lost an eye. The Second World War was then at its height so Burkitt decided to join the Royal Army Medical Corps and he began training in Hampshire. He was then posted as an army surgeon to the 219 Field Ambulance Unit at Witton, near Norwich. He married in July 1943 and a few months later he had to leave his wife to embark on a troopship bound for Mombasa. At a railway station in the south of England, on his way to the boat, he came upon Norman Moore, his old classmate from Trinity College. Moore recalls:

> It was wartime and we were both in uniform. Denis was *en route* to embark that night on a transport ship for an unknown destination, leaving behind his newly married wife. To add to the disappointment of

these personal affairs, the war seemed to be going badly then and it was
the only time I have known Denis to appear sad and pessimistic.[2]

Burkitt worked as an army surgeon in East Africa and Ceylon. Aware
that the war was coming to an end, he sent a second application to the
Colonial Office asking them to reconsider their decision and requesting
a posting in Uganda.

WORK IN UGANDA

After the war Burkitt received an MD from Trinity College for a thesis
on 'Spontaneous rupture of abdominal viscera'. He had worked on this
thesis while he was in Ceylon. Before leaving for Uganda, where he had
succeeded in obtaining an appointment as medical officer with the
Colonial Office, he acted as locum for a general practitioner in the
village of Fivemiletown, fifteen miles from Laragh, County Fermanagh,
where his parents lived. In Uganda the Burkitts lived in a colonial-style
bungalow with a red corrugated roof and a veranda. Burkitt worked at a
hospital in Lira, where the facilities were very limited. He had to sterilise
surgical instruments over a primus stove and he sometimes had to ask a
local man who had no nursing experience to administer the anaesthetic
using ether. The alternative was a spinal block administered by himself.

During his work in the hospital Burkitt found that one of the most
common problems was a scrotal swelling due to hydrocele. Most of the
patients came from one particular area and the hydroceles were very
large. This prompted him to embark on his first study of the
geographical distribution of a disease. He found that 30 per cent of the
male population of the eastern section of the district suffered from
hydrocele, whereas only 1 per cent from the western section were
affected. This study, which was published in *The Lancet*, formed the first
of over three hundred scientific papers which would be published by
Burkitt. The cause of the hydrocele was subsequently found to be due to
a tiny filaria worm which was transmitted by a mosquito.

After eighteen months at Lira, Burkitt was transferred to Mulago
Hospital in Kampala, the capital of Uganda, where he had to cope with
a very busy surgical practice. He was rather distressed by the frequency
with which he had to perform amputations, particularly as there were

no artificial limbs available in Uganda. As a consequence, many patients had to beg or were dependent on relatives. During his first term on leave, Burkitt attended a five-month postgraduate course in orthopaedic surgery at the National Orthopaedic Hospital in London. Here he learned that inexpensive artificial limbs could be formed using plastic materials which had recently been developed for the aircraft industry. When Burkitt returned to Kampala he set up a small workshop to make plastic limbs, which revolutionised the quality of life for many disabled people. The centre developed and was eventually taken over by a full-time orthopaedic surgeon, becoming a training centre which attracted doctors from all over Africa.

BEGINNINGS OF TUMOUR RESEARCH

In 1957, when Burkitt had been in Kampala for ten years, he was asked by Hugh Trowell, a physician at the hospital, to see a five-year-old boy whose face was deformed by swellings on both sides of his upper and lower jaws. Burkitt had seen children with similar tumours in one jaw, and he knew that they had to be removed as they grew very rapidly and resulted in death in a couple of months if left untreated. However, he had never before seen swellings so symmetrically placed. He made careful notes of the child's condition and he took some photographs. Unfortunately the disease was too extensive to benefit from surgery. A few weeks later, when Burkitt was teaching some fifty miles east of Kampala, at Jinja at the head of the river Nile, he saw a girl with identical swellings to the five-year-old boy. He brought her and her mother back to Mulago Hospital where he examined the child carefully and photographed the lesions. As the disease progressed, swellings also became apparent in other parts of the girl's body. These two children died, but Burkitt was determined to try and elucidate the cause of their deaths.

He searched through the autopsy records of the hospital and found that when children died of jaw tumours, swellings were also found in other parts of the body. Careful examination of the records showed that tumours were almost unknown in children under two, the incidence peaked between the ages of six and eight, and then fell away during adolescence. He stimulated interest amongst the two pathologists in the medical school, and to their surprise they found that the histology of the tumours removed from the jaw was similar to the swellings found in other parts of the body and consisted of lymphatic tissue. Going back over old records, Burkitt discovered that the disease had been prevalent in the area for many years. He also discovered that patients with these tumours came more frequently from the north and east of Uganda than from the west and south. He immediately saw a parallel with his work on hydrocele and he resolved to work on the geographical distribution of the lymphoma which he had identified.

BURKITT'S LYMPHOMA

Burkitt decided to send a questionnaire to the many government and mission hospitals throughout Africa, seeking further information on the distribution of the tumour. He received two government grants, worth £10 and £15, to cover the cost of printing and posting the leaflets. He had a thousand leaflets printed with pictures of various forms of the tumour and a brief description of the clinical presentation. Based on the answers to the questionnaires, he plotted the distribution of the tumour on a large map of the African continent. He found a definite pattern in the distribution, as most of the tumours were contained in a band which stretched across Africa, running between 10 degrees north and 10 degrees south of the Equator. The five million square miles within this band became known as the Lymphoma Belt. Burkitt was very excited by his discovery and he published his results in the *British Journal of Surgery* in 1958. He reported his findings on thirty-eight cases with lymphoma, and his presentation of the typical findings is a masterpiece of clinical description. The prognosis was very grim, as Burkitt observed: 'Within two or three months of onset of symptoms their relatives removed the majority of the children from hospital in a moribund condition.'[3]

He was rather disappointed when this initial paper aroused little interest. However, in 1961 he published a more detailed version of the paper in *Cancer*. It was written in collaboration with a pathology colleague named Greg O'Conor, and this paper aroused great interest. Burkitt's epidemiological observations revealed that his lymphoma was a form of cancer which had environmental rather than genetic or racial origins. The cancer could affect African, Asian and European children if they lived within the Lymphoma Belt. Burkitt was invited to lecture on his lymphoma at the Middlesex Hospital in March, 1961. The title of his lecture was 'The commonest children's cancer in tropical Africa, a hitherto unrecognised syndrome'. A virologist named Tony Epstein from the Bland Sutton Institute was in the audience. He was researching possible links between viruses and tumour formation at the time and he was very excited by the lecture. Later he asked Burkitt if he would send him frozen specimens of tumours from Kampala. Burkitt agreed.

MEDICAL SAFARI

Burkitt now resolved to probe more deeply into the aetiology of the tumour and he planned a ten-thousand-mile medical safari across the Lymphoma Belt which would take ten weeks to accomplish. Two medical colleagues, Ted Wilson and Cliff Nelson, accompanied him on this journey. When they returned to Kampala they carefully analysed the distribution of the lymphoma. Altitude seemed to be important, but it appeared that climate might be the controlling influence. Burkitt embarked on further journeys across Africa, this time by aeroplane, and he found that the tumour was the commonest childhood cancer in the hot southern region of Nigeria, where rainfall averaged more than twenty inches per year. In contrast, it was unknown in the dry northern part of the country. There were marked similarities between the tumour distribution and an insect map of Africa, suggesting that a virus borne by insects might be the causative agent.

EPSTEIN-BARR VIRUS

In 1964 Tony Epstein, with the help of his assistants Bert Achong and Yvonne Barr, isolated a virus from tumour cells which had been sent to him from Kampala. The virus was a hitherto unknown member of the Herpes group. Achong was a graduate of University College Dublin and Yvonne Barr was a graduate of Trinity College Dublin. In 1966 a hypothesis was developed which could explain the distribution of the tumour. A link was discovered between the distribution of the lymphoma and the depressant effect of malaria on the immune system. It was argued that the Epstein-Barr virus could cause a proliferation of lymphoid cells which could then become malignant in individuals who had their defences weakened by severe malaria. This would explain why the distribution of the lymphoma matched the distribution of intense malaria in Africa.

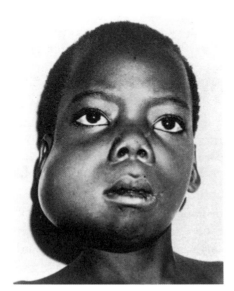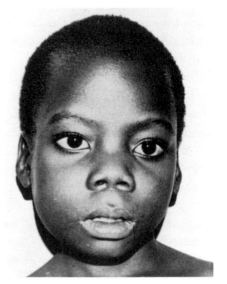

39.2   A boy aged seven with Burkitt's lymphoma involving his right mandible, (left) before treatment, (right) after treatment by Denis Burkitt

A CURE

Burkitt now set out to find a cure to help the unfortunate children under his care. Surgery was not the answer, as the tumours were often enormous and the disease frequently occurred in more than one part of the body. He could not try radiation as this form of therapy was unavailable anywhere in tropical Africa at that time. This left chemotherapy as the only option. He persuaded a major pharmaceutical company to give him a supply of methotrexate free on a trial basis. He did not use the high toxic levels normally administered as he did not have adequate monitoring facilities. However he soon began to obtain remarkable results. Many of his young patients achieved complete remission, without subsequent relapse, on the methotrexate therapy. He then began to achieve similar results with cyclophosphamide and vincristine. He had made a major breakthrough in cancer treatment. Burkitt's lymphoma was the only form of cancer at that time, apart from the very rare choriocarcinoma, which could be cured by chemotherapy alone. Burkitt was now internationally famous. Not only had he described a completely new form of tumour in children, but he had also found the treatment for the condition.

In 1967 two Americans working in Philadelphia, Werner and Gertrude Henle, discovered that infectious mononucleosis was caused by the Epstein-Barr virus. They also found that antibodies to the virus were very common in the blood of children from all over the world. Burkitt put a new hypothesis together to explain the aetiology of the lymphoma, accepting that the Epstein-Barr virus causes a common childhood infection. 'In normal lymphoid tissue this virus is usually harmless, but occasionally it causes a non-malignant proliferation that leads to infectious mononucleosis. In the presence of severe immunodepression, as results from very intense malaria, it can cause a malignant transformation and gives rise to Burkitt's lymphoma.'[1] Research still continues and more facts are emerging which throw new light on the condition. The lymphoma is endemic in the wet tropical zones of Africa, but with increasing awareness over the years sporadic cases have been reported in many other parts of the world, including Ireland.

DIET AND DISEASE

In April 1964 Burkitt began a new appointment with the Medical Research Council. He remained in Kampala but he had resigned his surgical post in favour of an African surgeon. Now he was free to concentrate on his geographical medical research. He had just returned from leave in Ireland, where he had worked out an ambitious programme for the following two years. This again involved travelling all over Africa and mapping out the incidence of various cancers in different parts of the continent. In the course of this work he discovered remarkable differences in the distribution of a number of different cancers. In 1966, after twenty years in Africa, Burkitt moved his base to the Medical Research Council offices in London. He continued to travel widely around the world, gathering information about environmental factors which might cause cancer. Early in 1967 Sir Richard Doll, the director of the Medical Research Council's statistics unit, introduced Burkitt to a retired naval physician named Peter Cleave. This meeting was to open up a whole new area of research and endeavour for Burkitt, which would become for him even more important than the discovery of the lymphoma. Cleave believed that diet was responsible for many of the common Western illnesses. Burkitt was readily convinced by the logic of his ideas as he already had a deep knowledge of the geographical distribution of disease. Cleave argued that many of the chronic diseases of Western people, such as coronary heart disease, gallstones, haemorrhoids, diverticular disease and others, were caused by over-refined food and a lack of fibre in the diet. Cleave's views had been ridiculed by the establishment and he was often dismissed as a food crank. As a consequence he had failed to make any significant progress in getting his ideas accepted widely. Burkitt by this time was an acknowledged expert on cancer research and he was invited to lecture all over the world. He decided to use the prestige which this gave him to advance Cleave's theories. He began collecting masses of information about the distribution of disease in the Third World which would help substantiate Cleave's claims.

During his travels in 1969, he met Alec Walker in Johannesburg. Walker had studied several very different ethnic groups and had found that they all had different disease patterns and that they consumed different foods. Walker had accumulated a mass of information on bowel transit times and stool weights of individuals on different diets. Burkitt began his own studies on bowel behaviour and his observations were eventually published together with those of Walker and other colleagues in *The Lancet* in 1972 and in the *Journal of the American Medical Association* in 1973. On the basis of his research Burkitt believed that he had substantiated Walker's claim that fibre could provide protection against bowel cancer. He published a paper on this subject in *Cancer* in 1971, entitled 'Epidemiology of cancer of the colon and rectum'. Though it was received somewhat sceptically by the medical profession of the time, it became a 'citation classic' in 1980, just ten years after its publication. Burkitt's first paper on his lymphoma also subsequently became a 'citation classic', making him one of the few men with two 'citation classics' in unrelated fields of medical endeavour.

One of his old colleagues from Kampala, Hugh Trowell, who had first drawn Burkitt's attention to children with lymphoma, now joined in the research in London. Trowell had already carried out some work in the area and had published *Non-infective Diseases in Africa* in 1960. As the work progressed both men became more and more aware of the relationship between fibre-deficient diets and the diseases of the Western World. They published the results of their research in a number of journals, and in 1975 they were co-authors of a book entitled *Refined Carbohydrate Foods and Disease; Some Implications of Dietary Fibre* which was published by Academic Press.

In 1976, at the age of sixty-five, Burkitt retired from the Medical Research Council and accepted an honorary appointment at St Thomas's Hospital. This position gave him an office in London where he could continue his work. In 1979 he published a book entitled *Don't Forget Fibre in Your Diet*, which was directed at the layperson. It was an immediate success and by the time the first few editions had appeared, over two hundred thousand copies had been sold around the world.

INTERNATIONAL RECOGNITION

Burkitt received many honours in recognition of his work. He was elected a fellow of the Royal Society in 1972. In 1974 he was made a Companion of the Order of St Michael and St George, and in 1978 he received the Gold Medal of the British Medical Association, the highest honour of that organisation. During these years he also received several top scientific awards in Europe and North America. In 1990 he was made a member of the prestigious 'Academie de Sciences' in Paris. He also received Irish honours, including an honorary fellowship of the Royal College of Surgeons in Ireland in 1973 and an honorary fellowship of the Royal College of Physicians of Ireland in 1976. In 1979 he was made an honorary fellow of Trinity College Dublin, the highest honour of the college.

A PERSONAL PHILOSOPHY

Burkitt still follows a busy schedule of lecturing to both undergraduates and graduates at different meetings around the world. He reminds the students and young doctors 'that life is not a sprint but a marathon', and that if they are to achieve anything of significance in medicine, they must be prepared to work hard for long periods. At the end of his lectures he is often approached by members of his audience who ask him to autograph their books. He frequently writes the following:

Attitudes are more important than abilities,
Motives are more important than methods,
Character is more important than cleverness,
And the heart takes precedence over the head.[1]

40 *A pathfinder in genetic research*

The major advances in genetic research that have taken place this century have been described as amounting to a 'revolution' in biology. These advances have also radically changed the practice of medicine. William Hayes was one of the key figures whose work played a central role in these dramatic developments. He was born on 18 January 1913 in Rathfarnham, County Dublin. His father, also named William, was a pharmacist and founder of William Hayes and Company, later Hayes Conyngham & Robinson, of 12 Grafton Street, Dublin. William Hayes senior was a very able man who built up a successful business and became president of the Pharmaceutical Society of Ireland. When he was seventy-one he married for a second time, to Miriam Harris, the daughter of a Church of England clergyman. Their only son, William, was brought up in a substantial Georgian house surrounded by fifty hectares of grazing land, which his father farmed as a hobby. William's father died when he was five years old, and he lived alone with his mother and grandmother during his early childhood.

SCHOOLDAYS

Hayes was educated at home by a governess until the age of ten, and

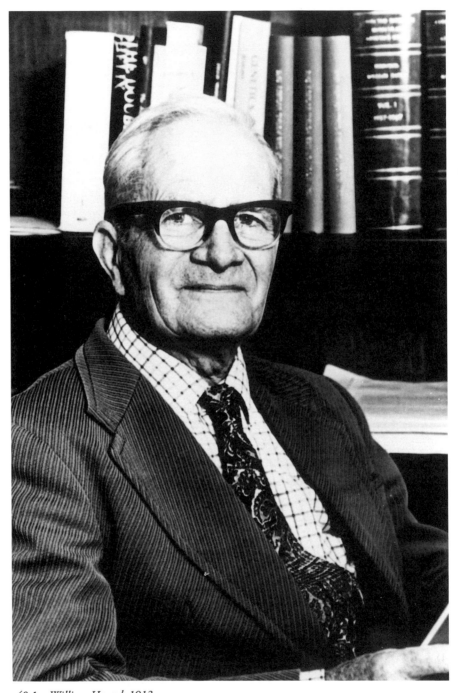

40.1   *William Hayes b 1913*

then he went to Castle Park, a preparatory school in Dalkey, County Dublin, where he was a classmate of the writer Patrick Campbell. From there he went to St Columba's College in Rathfarnham. During his early years at this school he began to develop an interest in science, especially in radio and electronics. He read a weekly technical radio journal and eventually he constructed his own crystal set. He was delighted to find that it worked, but unfortunately the set soon landed him in trouble:

> I had rigged an outdoor aerial of bare copper wire and earthed the instrument to a water pipe in the school dormitory where I and about twenty other boys slept. One stormy night the aerial collapsed on to uninsulated DC electric light cables supplying the building. My set blew up and started a fire which I extinguished with a device which covered my belongings and those of my neighbours with a thin layer of congealed white foam. A memorable night![1]

However, this did not dampen his enthusiasm for science, and he went on to construct more complex radios for friends who were prepared to pay for the components. Surprisingly, in view of his interests, he did not study science at school. He was encouraged to study literature and the classics by the headmaster who was a classical scholar. The mathematics teacher, Sandham Willis, was a remarkable man who encouraged his students to read far beyond the normal school curriculum. He would then discuss with his students the philosophical, social and political import of what they had read. Hayes was to benefit greatly from this.

During his penultimate year at school he wrote an essay on 'The Irish Free State', as a result of which he was selected to represent Ireland at an oratorical contest sponsored by an American newspaper, the *Washington Star*. He was flown to the United States where he had to deliver an address before an audience of some five thousand, which included the president of the United States and the ambassadors of the competing countries. Before leaving Ireland he had been given elocution lessons by the Irish actor Frank Fay at the Abbey School of Acting. He did not win the competition but he performed very well and he received an invitation to travel to Hollywood for a screen test. Fortunately for medical science he did not accept the offer! The high point of this remarkable experience was a visit to the White House where he was photographed with President Hoover.

MEDICAL STUDENT

During his last year at school some of his friends opted to study medicine at Trinity College and he decided to do the same. He found the study of physiology particularly exciting during his second year at the college and he began to perform some experiments of his own. He also enjoyed biochemistry and he set up his own small laboratory at home where he practised qualitative tests and did experiments on the effects of thyroxine on tadpole development. During his third year in university he decided to follow a career in bacteriology, when he came under the influence of the distinguished bacteriologist, Professor J W Bigger. His interest was stimulated further when he read two books, the novel *Martin Arrowsmith* by Sinclair Lewis and a history of *The Microbe Hunters* by Paul de Kruif, both of which as Hayes recalled 'rather glamourized the subject and certainly made me excited about it'.[1]

Towards the end of his time in Trinity College he read three papers to the Dublin University Biological Association, he won the Haughton Prize for medicine, and he was awarded the Adrian Stokes Memorial Travelling Fellowship for postgraduate study abroad. However he was unable to take advantage of the latter because of the outbreak of World War II. In 1936 he obtained a first class honours BA in natural science and in 1937 he qualified in medicine. He interned at the Victoria Hospital, Blackpool, Lancashire, where he fell in love with a young nurse named Nora Lee.

ASSISTANT TO J W BIGGER

Hayes returned to Ireland after six months to complete his internship at Sir Patrick Dun's Hospital. He then joined the Department of Bacteriology at Trinity College as an assistant lecturer to Professor Bigger, who had identified Hayes as a 'promising' student. The main duties of his new post involved routine diagnostic bacteriology and serology for a number of Dublin hospitals. He also assisted Bigger with the revision of his textbook *Handbook of Bacteriology*, the fifth edition of which was published in 1939. Shortly after Hayes joined the department a distinguished refugee from Nazi Germany, Professor Hans Sachs, came to work in the laboratory. Sachs had been professor of bacteriology at Heidelberg University and was well known for the Sachs-Gyorgy precipitation test for syphilis. It was Sachs who initiated Hayes into 'the mysteries of serology'. Hayes also met the noted theoretical physicist Edwin Schrödinger who was working at the Institute for Advanced Studies in Dublin at this time.

THE WAR YEARS

In July 1941 Hayes married Nora Lee at St Stephen's Church, Dublin. This was the beginning of a remarkable partnership and throughout his career Hayes received considerable support from his wife. In the same year Hayes joined the Royal Army Medical Corps. He served in India and rose to the rank of major. During the war his wife served in Britain with a plastic surgery unit. Hayes was based initially at Kasauli, a small station in the Himalayan foothills, but was later moved to the Central Laboratory at Poona. Because of the demands of wartime and the associated deprivations, Hayes had to improvise and use his ingenuity in the laboratory. He began work on penicillin, which was being imported into India for army use. This work led to an unexpected journey to the United Kingdom before the end of the war to meet Alexander Fleming and Howard Florey. Hayes wrote a book on the laboratory control of penicillin therapy when he returned to India.

Despite the practical difficulties associated with his laboratory work in India, Hayes managed to publish a number of research papers. It was during these years that he first developed his interest in bacterial genetics through his studies of phase variation in Salmonella enteritidis, which he noticed when typing the bacteria for diagnostic purposes.

LECTURER AT TRINITY COLLEGE

Hayes retired from the army in 1946 and the following year he was appointed lecturer in bacteriology at Trinity College Dublin. Around this time he also competed unsuccessfully for a fellowship of the college, which was regarded as a prestigious distinction and a sinecure for life:

My main competitors were the zoologist Dr J D Smythe and the botanist

Dr D A Webb. The principal formality of the competition was a public lecture to be delivered before the Board of the College while attired in full evening dress but with a black tie instead of a white one. We did not have the opportunity to listen to one another's performance but I was told that Smythe spoke most entertainingly about the habits of tapeworms which the Board seemed to find amusing and enjoyable. For my part I gave a straightforward account of my analysis of the plate method for penicillin assay which, however logical, must have seemed prosaic and unglamorous in comparison. I cannot remember the topic of Webb's dissertation. In the event, Smythe was awarded the Fellowship while I, as runner-up, won the Madden Prize of £150 which then seemed a princely sum.[1]

In 1949 his early research endeavours, including some on bacterial genetics, were rewarded when he received the degree ScD from Trinity College. In the same year he was elected president of the pathology section of the Royal Academy of Medicine in Ireland. In his presidential address he emphasised the recent developments in bacterial genetics and their significance for medicine. He worked at Trinity College for three years and during this period he lived at the family home at Edmonstown Park in Rathfarnham. These years in Dublin were clouded by the distress of his mother's last illness and her death in 1948.

RESEARCH ON BACTERIAL GENETICS

In 1950 Hayes was appointed senior lecturer in bacteriology at the Postgraduate Medical School at the Hammersmith Hospital in London. There he began to develop an interest in research on bacterial genetics, and he decided to attend a summer school on bacterial chemistry at Cambridge University. Here he met the Italian scientist Luca Cavalli-Sforza, who was then one of the leaders in bacterial genetics. It was a time of momentous developments in genetics.

In 1944, working with pneumococci at the Rockefeller Institute, Oswald Avery had identified DNA as the genetic blueprint that determines the way in which every organism develops. Two years later, A D Hershey, of the Cold Spring Harbor Laboratory in New York, demonstrated that when a bacterial virus (phage) attacks a bacterium it does so by squirting its DNA into the cell. Hershey was awarded a Nobel Prize in 1970 with Max Delbruck and Salvador Luria. Together these three men laid the basis for the understanding of the genetics of viruses and thus contributed critically to the development of molecular biology. In 1946 Joshua Lederberg, one of the youngest biologists ever to receive the Nobel Prize, working with Edward Tatum, demonstrated that colonic bacteria sometimes underwent a form of genetic exchange called conjugation. By mixing two strains of bacteria and finding that the offspring possessed characteristics of both, he proved that a mixing of genetic material or 'genetic recombination' had occurred.

The exact nature of the bacterial mating system was unknown when Hayes met Cavalli-Sforza at the Cambridge Summer School, but it was generally assumed that both parental types of bacteria were partners in contributing equal amounts of genetic material to their offspring. However, this model did not explain the results obtained in experiments.

In his research over the following two years, using a strain K^{12} of Escherichia coli, Hayes began to develop the hypothesis of one-way, partial transfer of genetic material during mating between two bacteria. He reported his hypothesis at the second European Symposium on Microbial Genetics held at Pallanza, Italy, in September 1952. It was here that Hayes first spoke to James Watson, who was then working with Francis Crick on the structure of DNA.

Watson was fascinated by Hayes' novel interpretation of the conjugation phenomena, which he unfolded at Pallanza. In his famous book *The Double Helix* Watson recalled:

> Cavalli-Sforza and Bill Hayes talked about the experiments by which they and Joshua Lederberg had just established the existence of two discrete bacterial sexes.
>
> Bill's appearance was the sleeper of the three-day gathering: before his talk no one except Cavalli-Sforza knew he existed. As soon as he had finished his unassuming report, however, everyone in the audience knew that a bombshell had exploded in the world of Joshua Lederberg....
>
> Bill's reasoning started from the seemingly arbitrary hypothesis that only a fraction of the male chromosomal material enters the female cell. Given this assumption, further reasoning was infinitely simpler.[2]

Watson kept in touch with Hayes after both men returned to England:

'as the fall progressed, I remained ensnared by bacterial matings, often going up to London to talk with Bill Hayes at his Hammersmith Hospital lab.'[3] Hayes was also visited for the first time by the French biologist Elie Wollman. It was an historic meeting. Wollman was very impressed with Hayes' work and he realised that a new era had dawned in genetic research. He also noted that Hayes had made his breakthrough in spite of working conditions which were so modest that they made his own musty attic in the Pasteur Institute look luxurious by comparison!

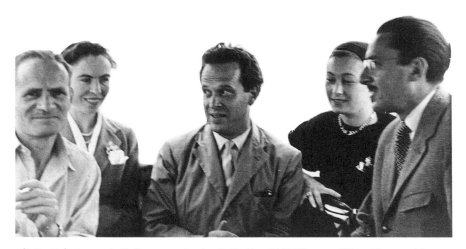

40.2   Relaxing at the Pallanza meeting in 1952: (L to R) William and Nora Hayes and Luca Cavalli-Sforza. The names of the other two people are not known. It was at this meeting that Hayes made a major impression on the scientists present, as James Watson has recorded in his book The Double Helix.

HFR HAYES

On both Wollman's and Watson's recommendation, Hayes was invited to participate in the 1953 Cold Spring Harbor Symposium on 'Viruses', which was organised by Max Delbruck. At the same symposium, James Watson presented the Watson-Crick structure for DNA, the biggest breakthrough in biology since the discoveries of Mendel. Hayes read a paper on 'Sexual differentiation in E. coli' and he mentioned that he had isolated a new sub-strain of E. coli, K^{12}, that produced recombinants a thousand to ten thousand times more frequently than normal. Until then genetic recombination in bacteria had been a rare event, and as a consequence was very difficult to study. The new Hfr (high frequency of recombinants) strain was named Hfr Hayes to distinguish it from a similar strain discovered by Cavalli-Sforza two years previously. These strains permitted the genetic analysis or gene mapping of E. coli, and subsequently it led to the genetic analysis of other bacteria. The strain HfrH would become famous through the definitive work on bacterial sexuality of Elie Wollman and François Jacob at the Pasteur Institute in Paris. Jacob later shared a Nobel Prize with Jacques Monod and Andre Lwoff. Hayes, together with Jacob and Wollman, showed that in bacterial matings the chromosome is transferred from the male (Hfr) strain to the female strain from a fixed point known as the origin, in a fixed direction linearly as a function of time. Many years later, at a dinner party, Hayes was sitting next to an American biochemist who, on hearing Hayes' name, asked, 'Are you, by any chance, Hfr HAYES?' Hfr strains became an essential tool in bacterial and molecular genetics for many years, and are still in use today in strain construction. It is only since the introduction in recent years of recombinant DNA techniques in the field of genetic engineering that their use has declined.

FURTHER DISCOVERIES

Delbruck was impressed by Hayes and he invited him to work for six months in his laboratory at the California Institute of Technology, Pasadena. Hayes remembers that he accepted this offer with alacrity. He published a paper with Watson in 1953 entitled 'Proposing a model of genetic transfer during bacterial mating'. They planned to work together at Caltech, but after Watson's success with the structure of DNA, he became engrossed in the problem of the structure of RNA. However, Watson and Hayes got to know each other better, as Hayes recalls: 'At that time he had recently learnt to drive and had bought a car jointly with de Mars, but no one would go on trips with him except my wife and I! So we had several expeditions together up the San Gabriel Mountains where Jim took me for strenuous walks on which I found it hard work to keep pace with him.'[1]

Hayes now began to concentrate his research on the kinetics of conjugation, and he continued his work when he returned to London. Apart from his discovery of the one-way transfer of only part of the donor chromosome to recipient cells, Hayes proposed that fertility in bacteria was controlled by a genetic factor which was not part of the chromosome. This is the sex factor F (also identified by Lederberg and Cavalli-Sforza) and he correctly interpreted its role:

> Oddly, the ability to be a donor was something a male bacterium could pass to a female: bacterial masculinity was itself a genetic element that could be transmitted by conjugation. Hayes discovered not just bacterial sex but bacterial sex change. He called the genetic element the sex factor, often written F for short. The bacterium that had got it was F^+.[4]

This sex factor turned out to be the prototype of a totally new group of extra-chromosomal elements called plasmids, which determine important bacterial functions. The significance of these factors is appreciated increasingly in genetic research today, and they already have an established place in the concept of the bacterial cell. T D Brock in his book *The Emergence of Bacterial Genetics* accords Hayes a central position in the development of modern genetic research, and he divides research on bacterial genetics into two phases: pre-Hayes and post-Hayes.[5]

THE MOLECULAR GENETICS UNIT

In 1957 Hayes founded the British Medical Research Council's Microbial Genetics Unit at the Hammersmith Hospital in London. This was later renamed the Molecular Genetics Unit and it has contributed many original discoveries to microbial and molecular genetics. Hayes held the post of director of the new institute for over ten years. Stuart Glover was one of the first to join Hayes in the new unit in Hammersmith. Although he was also a graduate of Trinity College, he did not know Hayes before coming to London, but he did remember seeing his name on a door in Trinity. Glover was elated by their first meeting and he stayed to work with Hayes for sixteen years, first in

London and later in Edinburgh.

> As Director he did not interfere with the work of his staff but was
> invariably available for help, advice and encouragement.... He created an
> environment in which good research could be done with a minimum of
> hassle.
>   Bill Hayes was above all a social man. Seldom was he happier than
> when hosting a party for his staff so that we would meet the good and
> the great who frequently beat a track to his Unit. Delbruck, Luria, Jacob,
> Wollman, were the first among many names famous to me from the
> literature that became flesh and blood in Bill Hayes' hospitable home.[6]

Hayes acquired a second home on the Mediterranean island of Gozo,
long before the island appeared in package travel brochures. It was a
converted farmhouse and it provided a wonderful retreat for Hayes, his
wife Nora and his son Michael. He enjoyed the annual holidays he spent
on the island with the mixture of outdoor life, the sun and the sea. He
used these vacations to recharge his batteries and he liked to relax by
reading and painting. He also took a keen interest in the Gozo people.

FAMOUS TEXTBOOK

Hayes was elected a fellow of the Royal Society in 1964, and in the same
year he published his classic work *The Genetics of Bacteria and their
Viruses*. He wrote, edited and typed the book, working day and night.
He was so absorbed by the project that his wife Nora said that for two
years she had a silent house. She also protected him from telephone
conversations during this creative period. The book was very successful
and it was republished in 1968 with extensive revisions. It was widely
adopted as a standard textbook in the field of bacterial genetics and for
several years was the only advanced general textbook available. It was
translated into several languages and was very influential in channelling
the attention of a whole generation of leading biologists into the field of
bacterial genetics. There are very few instances in the history of
biological science when a single textbook has had such influence in its
field and has been such a successful teaching instrument.

The international success of the book enabled Hayes and his wife to visit the USSR on the proceeds from the Russian translation of the work. They were treated very well by Soviet geneticists, some of whom accompanied them on their expeditions: 'in the hierarchical mode of the times in the USSR, Bill and Nora were embarrassed by always being hustled by their hosts to the head of any queue in railway station, airport or hotel.'[7]

Hayes had visited universities in Czechoslovakia in the early sixties, and he was very shocked when the USSR sent tanks into Prague in 1968. He protested officially and wrote several letters, including one to the president of the USSR. He also cancelled arranged visits to two or three universities whose governments had dispatched tanks to Czechoslovakia. He took an equally strong stand when the Americans were bombing Vietnam, refusing all official invitations to the USA.

Hayes was regularly asked to lecture at major scientific meetings. He was Mendel Lecturer of the Genetical Society in 1965. He was invited to contribute to the famous Festshrift *Phage and the Origins of Molecular Biology*, published in honour of Max Delbruck in 1966. He published *Experiments in Microbial Genetics* with Royston Clowes in 1968, and this proved to be another very influential book.

FROM EDINBURGH TO AUSTRALIA

In 1968 Hayes moved with his team to Edinburgh University where he was appointed professor of molecular genetics and honorary director of the Molecular Genetics Research Unit. The research unit in Edinburgh became pre-eminent in a much-vaunted field of science, and several members of its staff went on to hold chairs in genetics in both British and North American universities. In 1971 Hayes was elected president of the Genetical Society. However, he found that the demands made on him because of his international fame, together with the administrative burdens associated with his new post, left him little time for personal research. He was also on constant call to serve on university and Royal Society committees, but he saw himself as a bench-working scientist rather than a committee man. It was because of these considerations that in 1974 he accepted the post of professor of genetics at the Centre for Advanced Studies in Canberra, as he thought it would allow him time to pursue more basic research.

As might have been expected, given his senior position in the world of genetic research, there continued to be international demands on his time and expertise. He also made frequent professional visits to Europe and America, and personal visits to friends and family in Ireland and Scotland.

After his retirement in 1978 he spent a year as Sherman Fairchild distinguished scholar at the California Institute of Technology, where he worked with his old friend Max Delbruck. Following this, Hayes became visiting fellow to the Department of Botany at the Australian National University from 1980 to 1986.

During his life he received several honorary degrees, including the degree of D Sc from the universities of Leicester, Kent and the National University of Ireland, and LL D from the University of Dublin. The Nobel prize-winner James Watson has written the following about his association with Hayes forty years ago, when Watson himself was in the process of unravelling the structure of DNA:

> I first met Bill Hayes in Italy at the meeting in Pallanza in September, 1952. His talk came out of the dark since no one there knew he was doing such experiments. His discovery of the donor F$^+$ strains revolutionized K^{12} genetics which Lederberg until then had so dominated. Upon my return to Cambridge, I went in several times to the Hammersmith Hospital and at least once visited Bill and Nora's house in Richmond.... Working with Bill was a pleasure since underneath his modesty was a deep intelligence coupled to a real desire to do first class science. Later we so admired his massive book on the Genetics of Bacteria and their Viruses.[8]

REFERENCES

Introduction
1. W Wilde. 1841. Molyneux correspondence in *Dublin University Magazine*, xviii: 485
2. G Cleghorn. 1758. 'A proposal for furthering the intentions of this society by Mr Cleghorn' in *Medical and Philosophical Memoirs* (The Repository), 1: 308–12, in the library of the Royal College of Physicians of Ireland.

Chapter 1 Allen Mullen
1. J T Gilbert. 1859. *A History of the City of Dublin*. McGlashan and Gill, Dublin, II: 147–9.
2. K T Hoppen. 1970. *The Common Scientist in the 17th Century*. Routledge and Keegan Paul, London, pp 37–8.
3. Marquis of Lansdowne. 1927. *The Petty Papers*. Constable, London, pp 90–92.
4. J Ware. 1739. *The Whole Works of Sir James Ware Concerning Ireland*, revised and improved, by Walter Harris. Dublin, I, II: 206.

Chapter 2 Bernard Connor
1. B Connor. 1698. *History of Poland, its Ancient and Present State*. London, I: 200.
2. *Ibid*, I: 183–4.
3. *Ibid*, II: 292.
4. R H Dalitz and G C Stone. 1981. 'Doctor Bernard Connor: Physician to Jan III Sobieski and author of The History of Poland 1698' in *Oxford Slavonic Papers*, XIV: 14–35.
5. B Connor. 1698. *History of Poland, its Ancient and Present State*. London, II: 307.
6. *Ibid*, II: 310.
7. S Szpilczynski. 1974. 'Bernard O'Connor from Ireland: aulic physician to the Polish King Jan III Sobieski. A contribution to the development of medical thinking at the turn of the century' in *Proceedings of the XXIII International Congress of the History of Medicine*. Wellcome Institute of the History of Medicine, London, 1: 762–71.
8. B Connor. 1694. 'An extract of a letter from Bernard Connor, M.D. to Sir Charles Walgrave, published in French at Paris: giving an account of an extraordinary humane skeleton, whose vertebrae of the back, the ribs, and several bones down to the Os Sacrum, were all firmly united into one solid bone, without joynting or cartilage' in *Philosophical Transactions*, 215: 21–7.
19. B Connor. 1698. *History of Poland, its Ancient and Present State*. London, II: 316–22.
10. *Ibid*, I. Preface.
11. W Hayley. 1699. *A Sermon Preached in the Parish Church of St Giles in the Fields at the Funeral of Bernard Connor who Departed This Life October 30, 1698*. London, p 32.

Chapter 3 Fielding Ould
1. F Ould. 1742. *A Treatise of Midwifry*. Nelson and Connor, Dublin, p 4.
2. *Ibid*, p XVI.
3. *Ibid*, p 71.
4. A H McClintock. 1858. 'On the rise of the Dublin School of Midwifery' in *The Dublin Quarterly Journal of Medical Science*, XXV, 49: 1–20.
5. J D H Widdess. 1963. *A History of the Royal College of Physicians of Ireland*. Livingstone, Edinburgh, p 65.

Chapter 4 George Cleghorn
1. J C Lettsom. 1783. *The Works of John Fothergill. Charles Dilly in the Poultry*. London, p XCIX.
2. G Cleghorn. 1751. *Observations on the Epidemical Diseases in Minorca from the Year 1744 to 1749*. Wilson at Plato's Head in the Strand. London, p 175.
3. *Ibid*, p 176.
4. R Collins. 1849. *A Short Sketch of the Life and Writings of Joseph Clarke*. Longman, London, p 107.
5. G Cleghorn. 1758. 'A proposal for furthering the intentions of this Society by Mr. Cleghorn. Medical and Philosophical Memoirs (RCPI)' in *Repository*, 1: 308–12.
6. T J Pettigrew. 1817. *Memoirs of the Life and Writings of the late John Coakley Lettsom*. Nichols, Son and Bently. London, II: 364.
7. R Collins. 1849. *A Short Sketch of the Life and Writings of Joseph Clarke*. Longman, London, p 14.
8. *Ibid*, p 23.
9. *Ibid*, p 16.

Chapter 5 Samuel Clossy
1. T P C Kirkpatrick. 1924. *The History of Doctor Steevens' Hospital.* University Press, Dublin, p 118.
2. M H Saffron. 1967. *Samuel Clossy M.D.* Haffner Publishing Company, New York, p LXXXI.
3. *Ibid,* p LXXXII.
4. S Clossy. 1764. 'Letter to George Cleghorn' in *Repository of the Medico-Philosophical Society* (No. 85). Royal Irish Academy, Dublin.
5. M H Saffron. 1974. 'The Influence of Dublin on American Medicine' in *Proceedings of the XXIII International Congress of the History of Medicine.* Welcome Institute, London, 1: 841–5.
6. M H Saffron. 1967. *Samuel Clossy,* p LIII.
7. *Ibid,* p LXX.
8. *Ibid,* p LXXII.

Chapter 6 John Crawford
1. J E Wilson. 1942. 'An early Baltimore physician and his medical library' in *Annals of Medical History,* pp 63–80.
2. E F Cordell. 1899. 'Sketch of John Crawford' in *Johns Hopkins Hospital Bulletin,* 102: 158–62.
3. R W Doetsch. 1964. 'John Crawford and his contribution to the doctrine of contagium vivum' in *Bacteriological Reviews,* 28, 1: 87–96.

Chapter 7 Abraham Colles
1. R McDonnell. Ed. 1881. *The Works of Abraham Colles.* New Sydenham Society, London, p 5.
2. *Ibid,* p 10.
3. Sir W Stokes. 1902. *Operative and Clinical Surgery.* Ed W Taylor. Bailliere Tindall & Cox, London, p 398.
4. A Colles. 1814. 'On the fracture of the carpal extremity of the radius' in *The Edinburgh Medical and Surgical Journal,* 10: 182–6.
5. R W Smith. 1847. *Treatise on Fractures in the Vicinity of the Joints.* Dublin, p 129
6. A Colles. 1837. *Practical Observations on the Venereal Disease, and on the Use of Mercury.* Sherwood, Gilbert and Piper, London, p 304.
7. M Fallon. 1972. *Abraham Colles.* Heinemann, London, p 210.

Chapter 8 John Cheyne
1. T J Pettigrew. 1886. *Medical Portraits — John Cheyne.* London, p 1.
2. J Cheyne. 1843. *Essays on Partial Derangement of the Mind.* Curry, Dublin, p 3.
3. *Ibid,* p 16.
4. W Wilde. 1846. The editor's preface, *Dublin Quarterly Journal of Medical Science,* 1: i–xviii.
5. J Cheyne. 1818. 'A case of apoplexy, in which the fleshy part of the heart was converted into fat' in *Dublin Hospital Reports,* 2: 216–23.
6. W Stokes. 1846. 'Observations on some cases of permanently slow pulse' in *Dublin Quarterly Journal of Medical Science,* 11, III: 73–85.
7. J Cheyne. 1843. *Essays on Partial Derangement of the Mind.* Curry, Dublin, p 28.
8. *Ibid,* p 30.
9. *Ibid,* p 38.

Chapter 9 Arthur Jacob
1. A Jacob. 1819. 'An account of a membrane in the eye, now first described', communicated by James Macartney MD, FRS in *Philosophical Transactions,* pp 300–7.
2. A Jacob. 1827. 'Observations respecting an ulcer of peculiar character, which attacks the eyelids and other parts of the face' in *Dublin Hospital Reports,* 4: 232–9.
3. L B Sommerville-Large. 'Arthur Jacob' in *What's Past is Prologue — A Retrospect of Irish Medicine.* Eds W Doolin and O Fitzgerald. Dublin, 1952.
4. M Fallon. 1979. *The Sketches of Erinensis.* Skilton and Shaw, Dublin, p 75.
5. *Ibid,* p 77.
6. S L L Bigger. 1837. 'An inquiry into the possibility of transplanting the cornea, with the view of relieving blindness (hitherto deemed incurable) caused by several diseases of that structure' in *Dublin Journal of Medical Science,* II: 408–17.

Chapter 10 Robert Adams
1. M Fallon. 1979. *The Sketches of Erinensis.* Skilton and Shaw, Dublin, p 203.

2. R Adams. 1827. 'Cases of diseases of the heart accompanied with pathological observations' in *Dublin Hospital Reports*, IV: 353–453.
3. W Stokes. 1854. *Diseases of the Heart and Aorta.* Hodges and Smith, Dublin, p 191.
4. R Adams. 1840. 'Chronic rheumatic arthritis of the knee joint' in *Dublin Journal of Medical Science,* 17: 520–22.
5. R Adams. 1860. 'Richmond, Whitworth and Hardwicke Hospitals' in *Dublin Hospital Gazette,* 7: 321–4.
6. British Medical Association. 1867. Thirty-fifth Annual Meeting. *British Medical Journal,* 2: 159–65.
7. J Herrick. 1942. *A Short History of Cardiology.* C C Thomas, Springfield, Illinois.

Chapter 11 Robert Graves
1. W Stokes. 1868. 'The life and labours of Graves' in R J Graves *Studies in Physiology and Medicine.* London, p XXII.
2. L H Ormsby. 1892. *Medical History of the Meath Hospital and County Dublin Infirmary.* Fannin, Dublin, p 46.
3. W Stokes. 1868. 'The life and labours of Graves' in R J Graves *Studies in Physiology and Medicine.* London, p LIX.
4. 'Newly observed affection of the thyroid gland in females' in *London Medical and Surgical Journal* (1835), VII, 2: 516.
5. D Reisman. 1922. 'The Dublin Medical School and its influence upon medicine in America' in *Annals of Medical History,* 4: 86–96.
6. S Taylor. 1989. *Robert Graves.* Royal Society of Medicine, London, p 75.
7. W. Gibson. 1841. *Rambles in Europe.* Lea and Blanchard, Philadelphia, p 214.
8. H Cushing. 1940. *The Life of Sir William Osler,* Oxford University Press, London, p 1008.
9. W Stokes. 1868. 'The life and labours of Graves' in R J Graves *Studies in Physiology and Medicine.* London, p LXII.
10. *Ibid,* p LXVII.
11. *Ibid,* p LXXXII.

Chapter 12 Francis Rynd
1. L H Ormsby. 1883. *Medical History of the Meath Hospital and County Dublin Infirmary.* Dublin, p 206.
2. F Rynd. 1845. 'Neuralgia — Introduction of fluid to the nerve' in *Dublin Medical Press,* 13: 167–8.
3. F Rynd. 1861. 'Description of an instrument for the subcutaneous introduction of fluids in affections of the nerves' in *Dublin Quarterly Journal of Medical Science,* 32: 13.
4. Obituary. 1861. *Dublin Quarterly Journal of Medical Science,* 32: 64, 248.
5. L H Ormsby. 1883. *Medical History of the Meath Hospital and County Dublin Infirmary.* Dublin, p 209.

Chapter 13 Dominic Corrigan
1. J L Thornton. 1968. 'A diary of James Macartney 1770–1843, with notes on his writings' in *Medical History,* XII: 164–73.
2. D J Corrigan. 1832. 'On permanent patency of the mouth of the aorta or inadequacy of the aortic valves' in *Edinburgh Medical and Surgical Journal,* 37: 225–245.
3. T Cuming. 1822. 'A case of diseased heart, with observations' in *Dublin Hospital Reports,* 3: 319–34.
4. R T H Laënnec. 1827. *A Treatise on the Diseases of the Chest and Mediate Auscultation.* Translated by J Forbes. Underwood, London, p 554.
5. D J Corrigan. 1838. 'On cirrhosis of the lung' in *Dublin Journal of Medical Science,* 13: 266–86.
6. W Stokes. 1902. *Operative and Clinical Surgery.* Ed. W. Taylor. Bailliere, Tindall and Cox, London, p 432.
7. R H Mayor. 1945. *Classic Descriptions of Disease.* Charles Thomas, Illinois, p 354.
8. J Dowling. 1952. 'A country doctor looks back' in *Journal of the Irish Medical Association,* XXXI, 184: 277–84.
9. D Corrigan. 1862. *Ten Days in Athens, with Notes by the Way.* Longman, London, p 112.
10. *Ibid,* p 197.
11. D Corrigan. 1867. 'Address in Medicine. Annual Meeting of the BMA at Dublin' in *British Medical Journal,* 2: 103–107.
12. W Stokes. 1902. *Operative and Clinical Surgery.* Ed. W. Taylor. Bailliere, Tindall and Cox, London, p 430.

Chapter 14 John Houston
1. R G Butcher. 1846. 'Memoir of the life and writings of the late John Houston, MD' in *Dublin Quarterly Journal of Medical Science,* II, 294–302.

2. W Gibson. 1841. *Rambles in Europe*. Lea and Blanchard, Philadelphia, p 217.

3. J Houston. 1844. 'On the microscopic pathology of cancer' in *Dublin Medical Press*, 12: 5–8.

4. J D H Widdess. 1948. 'The beginnings of medical microscopy in Ireland' in *Irish Journal of Medical Science*, 668–78.

5. J Houston. 1830. 'Observations on the mucous membrane of the rectum' in *Dublin Hospital Reports*, 5: 158–65.

Chapter 15 William Stokes

1. W Stokes. 1902. *Operative and Clinical Surgery*. Ed. W Taylor. Bailliere, Tindall and Cox, London, p 400.

2. J B Herrick. 1942. *A Short History of Cardiology*. Thomas, Springfield, p 122.

3. W Stokes. 1846. 'Observations on some cases of permanently slow pulse' in *Dublin Quarterly Journal of Medical Science*, 11, 3: 73–85.

4. R Mulcahy. 1955. 'Diseases of the heart and aorta. A Modern Clinical Review' in *Irish Journal of Medical Science*, 350: 53–66.

5. W Stokes. 1854. *Diseases of the Heart and the Aorta*. Hodges and Smith, Dublin, p 139.

6. H A Snellen. 1984. *History of Cardiology*. Donker Academic Publications, Rotterdam, p 163.

7. Lady Ferguson. 1896. *Sir Samuel Ferguson in the Ireland of his Day*. Blackwood, Edinburgh, II: 109.

8. B O'Brien. 1978. 'William Stokes' in *Journal of the Irish Medical Association*, 71: 18, 598–601.

9. J Dowling. 1952. 'A country doctor looks back' in *Journal of the Irish Medical Association*, XXXI: 184, 277–84.

10. W M Dickson. 1902. *Trinity College Dublin*. Robinson, London, p 259.

11. Obituary. 1900. 'Sir William Stokes' in *Dublin Quarterly Journal of Medical Science*, LX: 240.

Chapter 16 Robert Collins

1. R Collins. 1835. *A Practical Treatise on Midwifery*. Longman, London, p 388.

2. *Ibid*, p 389.

3. *Ibid*, p 390.

4. *Ibid*, preface.

5. J C Ferguson. 1830. 'Auscultation, the only unequivocal evidence of pregnancy' in *Dublin Medical Transactions*, 1: 64.

6. D C Nagle. 1830. 'On the use of the stethoscope for the detection of twins in utero' in *The Lancet*, I: 232–4.

7. T D O'Donel Browne. 1947. *The Rotunda Hospital*. Livingstone, Edinburgh, p 176.

Chapter 17 Robert William Smith

1. W R Wilde. 1846. The editor's preface, *Dublin Quarterly Journal of Medical Science*, 1, 1: i–xlviii.

2. W Stokes. 1898. *William Stokes*. T Fisher Unwin, London, p 126.

3. R W Smith. 1847. *A Treatise on Fractures in the Vicinity of the Joints*. Hodges and Smith, Dublin, p 164.

4. C Cameron. 1886. *History of the Royal College of Surgeons in Ireland*. Fannin, Dublin.

5. W Stokes. 1854. *Diseases of the Heart and the Aorta*. Hodges and Smith, Dublin.

6. W Stokes. 1867. 'President's Address' in *British Medical Journal*, 2, 101–2.

7. 'Dr Robert W Smith of Dublin' in *British Medical Journal* (1873), 2: 358.

8. Editorial note on Smith's death, in *Dublin Journal of Medical Science* (1873), LVI: 429.

Chaper 18 William Brooke O'Shaughnessy

1. R Lewins. 1832. Letter in *The Lancet*, I: 244.

2. W B O'Shaughnessy. 1831. Letter in *The Lancet*, I: 401–4.

3. W B O'Shaughnessy. 1831. 'Experiments on the blood in cholera' (Letter) in *The Lancet*, I: 490.

4. T Latta. 1832. Letter in *The Lancet*, II: 275.

5. W B O'Shaughnessy. 1832. Letter in *The Lancet*, II: 281.

6. Editorial. 1932. *The Lancet*, 284–6.

7. P Astrup. 1985. *The Early Development of Blood Gas and Blood Acid-Base Measurements in Anaesthesia. Essays on Its History*. Eds J Rupreht, M J Van Lieburg, J A Lee and W Erdmann. Springer-Verlag, Berlin, p 181.

8. M Donovan. 1845. 'On the physical and medicinal qualities of India kemp (Cannabis Indica), with observations on the best mode of administration, and cases illustrative of its powers' in *Dublin Journal of Medical Science*, XXVI: 368–402.

9. B McNicholl. 1973. 'Irish Blood — and Electrolytes' in *Journal of the Irish Medical Association*, 66, 14: 388–90.

Chapter 19 Robert Bentley Todd
1. R B Todd. 1853. *Farewell Address at King's College.* W Tyler, London, p 6.
2. L S Beale. 1870. 'Lecture on medical progress: in memoriam R B Todd' in *British Medical Journal,* 1: 485.
3. J Collier. 1934. 'Inventions and outlook in neurology' in *The Lancet,* II: 855.
4. R B Todd. 1849. 'On the pathology and treatment of convulsive diseases' in *London Medical Gazette,* 8: 661–71.
5. R B Todd. 1845. *Anatomy of the Brain, Spinal Cord and Ganglions.* Sherwood, Gilbert and Piper, London, p X.

Chapter 20 Thomas Andrews
1. P G Tait and A Crum Brown. 1889. *The Scientific Papers of Thomas Andrews with a Memoir.* Macmillan, London, p XII.
2. *Ibid,* p 19.
3. *Ibid,* p 17.
4. *Ibid,* p XIV.
5. *Ibid,* p XVII.
6. T W Moody and J C Beckett. *Queen's, Belfast.* Faber and Faber, London, p 162.
7. P G Tait and A Crum Brown. 1889. *The Scientific Papers of Thomas Andrews with a Memoir.* Macmillan, London, p XXIV.
8. *Ibid,* p XLIX.
9. *Ibid,* p 316.
10. C S Breathnach. 1985. 'Andrews' in *Irish Medical Journal,* 78, 11: 338.
11. P G Tait and A Crum Brown. 1889. p LIII.

Chapter 21 William Wilde
1. T G Wilson. 1942. *Victorian Doctor.* Methuen, London.
2. L B Sommerville-Large. 1944. 'Dublin's Eye Hospitals' in *The Irish Journal of Medical Science,* XV: 534–7.
3. W R W Wilde. 1853. *Practical Observations on Aural Surgery and the Nature and Treatment of Diseases of the Ear.* Churchill, London. Preface.
4. P Froggatt. 1965. 'Sir William Wilde and the 1851 Census of Ireland' in *Medical History,* 9: 302–27.
5. W R W Wilde. 1841. 'Sir Thomas Molyneux Bart MD, FRS' in *Dublin University Magazine,* 18: 305–27, 470–90, 604–19, 744–64.
6. C A Cameron. 1913. *Reminiscences of Sir Charles A Cameron.* Hodges Figgis, Dublin.
7. T de Vere White. 1967. *The Parents of Oscar Wilde.* Hodder and Stoughton, London, p 228.
8. P Harbison. 1991. *Beranger's Views of Ireland.* Royal Irish Academy, Dublin, p 6.

Chapter 22 Samuel Haughton
1. S Haughton. 1873. *Principles of Animal Mechanics.* Longmans, Green, London. Preface.
2. N D McMillan. 1988. 'Rev. Samuel Haughton and the age of the earth controversy' in *Science of Ireland.* Eds J Nudds, N D McMillan, D Weaire and S McKenna Lawlor. Trinity College Dublin, pp 151–61.
3. S Haughton. 1873. *Principles of Animal Mechanics.* Longmans, Green, London, pp 139–40
4. S Haughton. 1866. 'On Hanging' in *Philosophical Magazine* (July), p 8.
5. J J Abraham. 1958. *Surgeon's Journey.* Heinemann, London, p 46.
6. 'Proceedings of the Dublin Pathological Society (1878)' in *Dublin Quarterly Journal of Medical Science,* 66, 172–4.

Chapter 23 Arthur Leared
1. Obituary. 1879. *Medical Times and Gazette,* 25 Oct, p 488.
2. C D T James. 1972. 'Medicine and the 1851 exhibition' in *Proceedings of the Royal Society of Medicine,* 65, 693–6.
3. A Leared. 1856. 'On the self-adjusting double stethoscope' in *The Lancet,* II: 138.
4. A Leared. 1854. 'On the pancreatic juice in relation to the digestion of fat' in *Medical Times and Gazette,* 8: 568–70.
5. A Leared. 1891. *Marocco and the Moors.* Ed. Sir R Burton. 2nd Edition. Sampson Low, London. Preface, III.
6. *Ibid,* introduction, V.
7. *Ibid,* p 132.
8. *Ibid,* p 141.
9. A Leared. 1879. *A Visit to the Court of Morocco.* Sampson Low, London, p 19.

Chapter 24 Francis Cruise
1. F R Cruise. 1912. *Sir Dominic Corrigan*. Catholic Truth Society, London, p 8.
2. F R Cruise. 1865. 'The utility of the endoscope as an aid in the diagnosis and treatment of disease' in *Dublin Quarterly Journal of Medical Science*, 39: 329–63.
3. *The Lancet*. 1865. I: 327–8.
4. W Stokes. 1866. 'An address delivered before the medical society of the King and Queen's College of Physicians in Ireland' in *The Medical Press and Circular*, II: 609–11.
5. J Dowling. 1952. 'A country doctor looks back' in *Journal of the Irish Medical Association*, XXXI, 184: 277–84.
6. F R Cruise. 1887. *Thomas à Kempis*. Kegan Paul and Trench, London, p 31.
7. *Ibid*, p VIII.
8. C A Cameron. 1886. *History of the Royal College of Surgeons in Ireland*. Fannin, Dublin, p 571.
9. J H Pollock. 1959. 'Colleagues and chariots: A reverie' in *Journal of the Irish Medical Association*, XLV: 143–4.

Chapter 25 Edward Hallaran Bennett
1. F J O'Rourke. 1970. *The Fauna of Ireland*. Mercier Press, Cork, p 43.
2. E H Bennett. 1866. 'On the possibility of naturalizing the ringed snake in Ireland' in *Proceedings of the Natural History Society of Dublin*, V: 27–30.
3. E H Bennett. 1864–71. Private diary.
4. T G Moorehead. 1942. *A Short History of Sir Patrick Dun's Hospital*. Hodges Figgis, Dublin, pp 127–8.
5. E H Bennett. 1882. 'Fractures of the metacarpal bones' in *Dublin Journal of Medical Science*, LXXIII: 72–5.

Chapter 26 Henry Newell Martin/Harold J C Swan
1. M Foster. 1897. Obituary. 'Henry Newell Martin' in *Proceedings of the Royal Society of London*, LX: XX–XXIII.
2. H Sewall. 1911. 'Henry Newell Martin, professor of biology in Johns Hopkins University 1876–1893' in *Johns Hopkins Bulletin*, 22: 327–33.
3. H N Martin. 1895. *Physiological Papers*. Johns Hopkins Press, Baltimore, p 1.
4. L T Morton. 1983. *A Medical Bibliography*. Gower, London.
5. W B Fye. 1985. 'H Newell Martin — A remarkable career destroyed by neurasthemia and alcoholism' in *Journal of the History of Medicine*, 40: 133–66.
6. J Swan. 1991. Personal communication.
7. J B Lyons. 1991. Personal communication.
8. J Swan. 1991. 'Development of the pulmonary artery catheter' in *Disease-a-Month*, XXXVII, 8: 485–508.
9. J W Hurst. 1988. 'H J C Swan' in *Clinical Cardiology*, 11: 727–728.

Chapter 27 Charles MacMunn
1. D Keilin. 1966. *The History of Cell Respiration and Cytochrome*. Cambridge University Press, Cambridge, pp 335–57.
2. C A MacMunn. 1887. 'Further observations on myohaematin and the histohaematins' in *Journal of Physiology*, 8: 51–65.
3. W Stokes. 1871. 'On some requirements of clinical teaching in Dublin' in *Dublin Quarterly Journal of Medical Science*, 51: 38–52.

Chapter 28 Charles Donovan
1. P Krishnaswami. 1955. 'Col. C Donovan. Physician, physiologist and discoverer' in *Indian Journal of History of Medicine*, 1, 2: 33–8.
2. C Donovan. 1903. 'On the possibility of the occurrence of tryansomiasis in India' in *British Medical Journal*, 2: 79.
3. R Ross. 1903. 'Note on the bodies recently described by Leishman and Donovan' in *British Medical Journal*, 2: 1261–2.
4. J A Weaver and P Froggat. 1987. 'The Wild Geese' in *The Ulster Medical Journal*, 56; suppl., S31–S56.
5. Obituary. 1951. 'Charles Donovan' in *British Medical Journal*, 2: 1158.
6. Obituary. 1952. 'Lieut-Colonel Charles Donovan' in *The Irish Naturalists' Journal*, X: 258–9.

Chapter 29 Almroth Wright
1. L Colebrook. 1954. *Almroth Wright*. William Heinemann, London, p 11.

2. *Ibid*, p 12.
3. W Bulloch. 1938. *The History of Bacteriology*. Oxford University Press, London, p 117.
4. Zachari Cope. 1966. *Almroth Wright*. Nelson, London, p 165.
5. L Colebrook. 1954. *Almroth Wright*. William Heinemann, London, p 194.
6. M Holroyd. 1989. *Bernard Shaw. The Pursuit of Power*. Chatto and Windus, London, p 161.
7. L Colebrook. 1954. *Almroth Wright*. William Heinemann, London, p 195.
8. H Cushing. 1940. *The Life of Sir William Osler*. Oxford University Press, London, p 789.

Chapter 30 Gordon Holmes
1. J F Fulton. 1946. *Harvey Cushing*. Blackwell, Oxford, p 399.
2. Wilder Penfield. 1971. 'Lights in the great darkness' in *Journal of Neurosurgery*, 35: 377–83.
3. B D Parsons Smith. 1982. 'Sir Gordon Holmes' in *Historical Aspects of the Neurosciences*. Eds F Clifford Rose and W F Bynum. Raven Press, New York.
4. C S Breathnach. 1975. 'Sir Gordon Holmes' in *Medical History*, 19: 194–200.

Chapter 31 Walter Clegg Stevenson
1. J Joly. 1931. 'In Memoriam. Walter Clegg Stevenson' in *Irish Journal of Medical Science*, 6th series, 134–5.
2. W C Stevenson. 1914. 'An economical method of using radium for therapeutic purposes' in *The Medical Press*, 97, NS: 251–2.
3. W C Stevenson. 1929. 'The uses of radium in medicine' in *The Medical Press*, 128 NS: 409–12.
4. J Stevenson. 1991. Personal communication.

Chapter 32 Robert Foster Kennedy
1. I K Butterfield. 1981. *The Making of a Neurologist*. Stellar Press, London, p 1.
2. *Ibid*, p 30.
3. *Ibid*, p 34.
4. *Ibid*, p 40.
5. *Ibid*, p 51.
6. F Kennedy. 1918. 'The nature of nervousness in soldiers' in *War Medicine*, pp 1–10
7. I K Butterfield. 1981. *The Making of a Neurologist*. Stellar Press, London, p 78.
8. 1991. Personal communication.

Chapter 33 Adrian Stokes
1. Obituary. 1928. 'Adrian Stokes' in *Guy's Hospital Reports*, 78: 1–17.
2. Obituary. 1927. 'Adrian Stokes' in *British Medical Journal*, II: 615–18.
3. B Stokes. 1991. Private collection of material relating to Adrian Stokes.
4. N P Hudson. 1966. 'Adrian Stokes and yellow fever research: a tribute' in *Transactions of the Royal Society of Tropical Medicine and Hygiene*, 60, 2: 170–74.

Chapter 34 Ivan Whiteside Magill
1. Obituary. 1987. 'Sir Ivan Magill' in *British Medical Journal*, 1: 62–3.
2. A W Edridge. 1987. Editorial 'Sir Ivan Whiteside Magill' in *Anaesthesia*, 42: 231–3.
3. V McCormick. 1967. *The Kirkpatrick Lecture*.
4. J W Dundee. 1987. 'Anaesthetics' in *The Ulster Medical Journal*, 56, (Suppl. 87–90).
5. H A Condon. 1987. 'Sir Ivan Magill. A supplementary bibliography' in *Anaesthesia*, 42: 1096–7.
6. A W Edridge. 1987. Obituary 'Ivan Whiteside Magill' in *The Lancet*, I: 55.

Chapter 35 Edward Joseph Conway
1. M Maizels. 1969. 'Edward Joseph Conway' in *Biographical Memoirs of Fellows of the Royal Society*, 15: 69–82.
2. Conway correspondence. Courtesy of Dr Kevin McGeeney, University College Dublin.
3. E J Conway. 1951. 'Science and the physician' in *Irish Journal of Medical Science*, 310: 441–52.
4. *The Irish Times*. 1953. Portrait Gallery — 'E J Conway FRS'. Saturday, 3 January.

Chapter 36 Peter Freyer and Terence Millin
1. P J Freyer. 1901. 'A clinical lecture on total extirpation of the organ' in *British Medical Journal*, 2: 125–9.
2. J B Lyons. 1984. *Brief Lives of Irish Doctors*. Blackwater Press, Dublin, p 122.
3. T J Millin. 1945. 'Retropubic prostatectomy. A new extravesical technique' in *The Lancet*, II: 693–6.

4. Editorial. 1945. 'Eureka' in *The Lancet*, II: 711.
5. M O'Donnell. 1967. 'Surgeon extraordinary' in *World Medicine*, 3 Oct, pp 22–4.
6. V Lane. 1980. 'T J Millin' in *British Medical Journal*, 2: 234.
7. J B Lyons. 1984. *An Assembly of Irish Surgeons*, pp 152–6.
8. R Cox. 1991. Personal communication.
9. A Walsh. 1980. 'Terence John Millin' in *The Lancet*, II: 270–1.

Chapter 37 Peter Kerley
1. P Kerley. 1931. *Recent Advances in Radiology*. Churchill, London, p V.
2. J Deeny. 1991. Personal communication.
3. B Phillips. 1991. Personal communication.
4. P Kerley. 1933. 'Radiology in heart disease' in *British Medical Journal*, II: 594–7.
5. Obituary. 1979. *The Lancet*, I: 735.
6. Obituary. 1979. *British Medical Journal*, 1, 1095.
7. Sir T Lodge. 1979. 'Sir Peter Kerley — A man of many talents.' Funeral oration.

Chapter 38 Robert Collis
1. R Collis. 1975. *To Be a Pilgrim*. Secker & Warburg, London, p 18.
2. *Ibid*, p 19.
3. W R F Collis. 1932. 'A new conception of the aetiology of erythema nodosum' in *Quarterly Journal of Medicine*, 1 (N.S.), 141–56.
4. R Collis. 1975. *To Be a Pilgrim*. Secker & Warburg, London, p 77.
5. D Collis. 1991. Personal communication.
6. R Collis. 1975. *To Be a Pilgrim*. Secker & Warburg, London, p 135.
7. R Collis. 1991. Personal communication.
8. R Collis. 1975. *To Be a Pilgrim*. Secker & Warburg, London, p IX.

Chapter 39 Denis Burkitt
1. D Burkitt. 1991. Personal communication.
2. N Moore. 1991. Personal communication.
3. D Burkitt. 1958. 'A sarcoma involving the jaws in African children' in *British Journal of Surgery*, 46: 218–23.

Chapter 40 William Hayes
1. W Hayes. Personal communication from unpublished autobiographical details prepared for the Royal Society.
2. J D Watson. 1968. *The Double Helix*. Wiedenfeld and Nicolson, London, pp 141–3.
3. *Ibid*, p 147.
4. H F Judson. 1979. *The Eighth Day of Creation, Makers of the Revolution in Biology*. Simon and Schuster, New York, p 386.
5. T D Brock. 1990. *The Emergence of Bacterial Genetics*. Cold Spring Harbour Laboratory Press, New York, p 87.
6. S Glover. 1991. Personal communication.
7. J Crofton. 1991. Personal communication.
8. J D Watson. 1991. Personal communication.

SELECT BIBLIOGRAPHY

1977. 'Old masters' in *Irish Journal of Medical Science*, 146, 7: 185–9.

Allison, R S. 1972. *The Seeds of Time*. Belfast General and Royal Hospital, Belfast.

Bailey, H and W J Bishop. 1959. *Notable Names in Medicine and Surgery*. H K Lewis, London.

Browne, O'Donel, T D. 1947. *The Rotunda Hospital*. Livingstone and Edinburgh.

Cameron, C A. 1886. *History of the Royal College of Surgeons*. Fannin, Dublin.

Coakley, D. 1988. *The Irish School of Medicine*. Town House, Dublin.

Doolin, W. 1987. *Dublin's Surgeon-Anatomist*. Ed. J B Lyons. Royal College of Surgeons in Ireland, Dublin.

Doolin, W and O Fitzgerald. Eds. 1952. *What's Past Is Prologue*. Dublin.

Fleetwood, J F. 1983. *The History of Medicine in Ireland*. 2nd ed. Skellig Press, Dublin.

Kirkpatrick, T P C. 1912. *History of the Medical Teaching in Trinity College*. Hanna and Neale, Dublin.

Kirkpatrick, T P C and Jellet, H. 1913. *The Book of the Rotunda Hospital*. Adlard, London.

Lyons, A S and R J Petrucelli. 1978. *Medicine. An Illustrated History*. Abrams, New York.

Lyons, J B. 1978. *Brief Lives of Irish Doctors*. Blackwater, Dublin.

Lyons, J B. 1984. *An Assembly of Irish Surgeons*. Glendale, Dublin

Major, R H. 1945. *Classic Descriptions of Disease*. 3rd ed. Thomas, Illinois.

Mollan, C, W Davis and B Finucane. Eds. 1985. *Some People and Places in Irish Science and Technology*. Royal Irish Academy, Dublin.

Morton, L T. 1983. *A Medical Bibliography* (Garrison and Morton). Gower, Hampshire.

O'Brien, E, A Crookshank, G Wolstenholme. 1984. *A Portrait of Irish Medicine*. Ward River Press, Dublin.

O'Rahilly, R. 1949. *A History of the Cork Medical School*. Cork University Press, Cork.

Packard, F. 1932. *History of Medicine in the United States*. Paul B Hoeber, New York.

Taylor, W B. 1845. *History of the University of Dublin*. London.

Widdess, J D H. 1963. *A History of the Royal College of Physicians of Ireland*. Livingstone, Edinburgh.

Widdess, J D H. 1984. *The Royal College of Surgeons in Ireland*. Dublin.

Wilde, W. 1846. The editor's preface in *Dublin Quarterly Journal of Medical Science*, 1: I-XLVIII.

INDEX